Advances in the Development of New Drugs and Treatment Targets for Brain Cancers

Advances in the Development of New Drugs and Treatment Targets for Brain Cancers

Editors

Luis Exequiel Ibarra
Laura Natalia Milla Sanabria
Nuria Arias Ramos

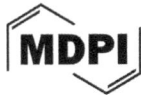

Basel • Beijing • Wuhan • Barcelona • Belgrade • Novi Sad • Cluj • Manchester

Editors

Luis Exequiel Ibarra
Institute of Environmental
Biotechnology and Health
(INBIAS)
National Council for Scientific
and Technical Research
(CONICET) and National
University of Río Cuarto
(UNRC)
Río Cuarto
Argentina

Laura Natalia Milla Sanabria
Institute of Environmental
Biotechnology and Health
(INBIAS)
National Council for Scientific
and Technical Research
(CONICET) and National
University of Río Cuarto
(UNRC)
Río Cuarto
Argentina

Nuria Arias Ramos
Department of Endocrine and
Nervous System
Pathophysiology
Instituto de Investigaciones
Biomedicas Alberto Sols
(IIBM)
Madrid
Spain

Editorial Office
MDPI
St. Alban-Anlage 66
4052 Basel, Switzerland

This is a reprint of articles from the Special Issue published online in the open access journal *Brain Sciences* (ISSN 2076-3425) (available at: https://www.mdpi.com/journal/brainsci/special_issues/1T19O4Z206).

For citation purposes, cite each article independently as indicated on the article page online and as indicated below:

Lastname, A.A.; Lastname, B.B. Article Title. *Journal Name* **Year**, *Volume Number*, Page Range.

ISBN 978-3-7258-1403-9 (Hbk)
ISBN 978-3-7258-1404-6 (PDF)
doi.org/10.3390/books978-3-7258-1404-6

© 2024 by the authors. Articles in this book are Open Access and distributed under the Creative Commons Attribution (CC BY) license. The book as a whole is distributed by MDPI under the terms and conditions of the Creative Commons Attribution-NonCommercial-NoDerivs (CC BY-NC-ND) license.

Contents

Luis Exequiel Ibarra, Laura Natalia Milla Sanabria and Nuria Arias-Ramos
Advances in the Development of New Drugs and Treatment Targets for Brain Cancers
Reprinted from: *Brain Sci.* 2024, 14, 526, doi:10.3390/brainsci14060526 1

**Corneliu Toader, Lucian Eva, Daniel Costea, Antonio Daniel Corlatescu,
Razvan-Adrian Covache-Busuioc, Bogdan-Gabriel Bratu, et al.**
Low-Grade Gliomas: Histological Subtypes, Molecular Mechanisms, and Treatment Strategies
Reprinted from: *Brain Sci.* 2023, 13, 1700, doi:10.3390/brainsci13121700 5

**Matías Daniel Caverzán, Lucía Beaugé, Paula Martina Oliveda, Bruno Cesca González,
Eugenia Micaela Bühler and Luis Exequiel Ibarra**
Exploring Monocytes-Macrophages in Immune Microenvironment of Glioblastoma for the
Design of Novel Therapeutic Strategies
Reprinted from: *Brain Sci.* 2023, 13, 542, doi:10.3390/brainsci13040542 24

**Ammu V. V. V. Ravi Kiran, G. Kusuma Kumari, Praveen T. Krishnamurthy, Asha P. Johnson,
Madhuchandra Kenchegowda, Riyaz Ali M. Osmani, et al.**
An Update on Emergent Nano-Therapeutic Strategies against Pediatric Brain Tumors
Reprinted from: *Brain Sci.* 2024, 14, 185, doi:10.3390/brainsci14020185 48

Nuria Arias-Ramos, Cecilia Vieira, Rocío Pérez-Carro and Pilar López-Larrubia
Integrative Magnetic Resonance Imaging and Metabolomic Characterization of a Glioblastoma
Rat Model
Reprinted from: *Brain Sci.* 2024, 14, 409, doi:10.3390/brainsci14050409 70

**Irlã Santos Lima, Érica Novaes Soares, Carolina Kymie Vasques Nonaka,
Bruno Solano de Freitas Souza, Balbino Lino dos Santos and Silvia Lima Costa**
Flavonoid Rutin Presented Anti-Glioblastoma Activity Related to the Modulation of Onco
miRNA-125b Expression and STAT3 Signaling and Impact on Microglia Inflammatory Profile
Reprinted from: *Brain Sci.* 2024, 14, 90, doi:10.3390/brainsci14010090 87

Ana Alves, Ana M. Silva, Joana Moreira, Claúdia Nunes, Salette Reis, Madalena Pinto, et al.
Polymersomes for Sustained Delivery of a Chalcone Derivative Targeting Glioblastoma Cells
Reprinted from: *Brain Sci.* 2024, 14, 82, doi:10.3390/brainsci14010082 101

**Takumi Hoshimaru, Naosuke Nonoguchi, Takuya Kosaka, Motomasa Furuse,
Shinji Kawabata, Ryokichi Yagi, et al.**
Actin Alpha 2, Smooth Muscle (ACTA2) Is Involved in the Migratory Potential of Malignant
Gliomas, and Its Increased Expression at Recurrence Is a Significant Adverse Prognostic Factor
Reprinted from: *Brain Sci.* 2023, 13, 1477, doi:10.3390/brainsci13101477 115

**Corina Tamas, Flaviu Tamas, Attila Kovecsi, Georgiana Serban, Cristian Boeriu and
Adrian Balasa**
The Role of Ketone Bodies in Treatment Individualization of Glioblastoma Patients
Reprinted from: *Brain Sci.* 2023, 13, 1307, doi:10.3390/brainsci13091307 127

**Miguel Hernández-Cerón, Víctor Chavarria, Camilo Ríos, Benjamin Pineda,
Francisca Palomares-Alonso, Irma Susana Rojas-Tomé, et al.**
Melatonin in Combination with Albendazole or Albendazole Sulfoxide Produces a Synergistic
Cytotoxicity against Malignant Glioma Cells through Autophagy and Apoptosis
Reprinted from: *Brain Sci.* 2023, 13, 869, doi:10.3390/brainsci13060869 140

Irene Guadalupe Aguilar-García, Ismael Jiménez-Estrada, Rolando Castañeda-Arellano, Jonatan Alpirez, Gerardo Mendizabal-Ruiz, Judith Marcela Dueñas-Jiménez, et al.
Locomotion Outcome Improvement in Mice with Glioblastoma Multiforme after Treatment with Anastrozole
Reprinted from: *Brain Sci.* **2023**, *13*, 496, doi:10.3390/brainsci13030496 . . . . **154**

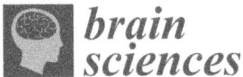

Editorial

Advances in the Development of New Drugs and Treatment Targets for Brain Cancers

Luis Exequiel Ibarra [1,2,*], Laura Natalia Milla Sanabria [1,2] and Nuria Arias-Ramos [3]

1 Instituto de Biotecnología Ambiental y Salud (INBIAS), Universidad Nacional de Rio Cuarto (UNRC) y Consejo Nacional de Investigaciones Científicas y Técnicas (CONICET), Rio Cuarto X5800BIA, Argentina; lmilla@exa.unrc.edu.ar
2 Departamento de Biología Molecular, Facultad de Ciencias Exactas, Fisicoquímicas y Naturales, Universidad Nacional de Rio Cuarto, Rio Cuarto X5800BIA, Argentina
3 Instituto de Investigaciones Biomédicas Sols-Morreale, Consejo Superior de Investigaciones Científicas-Universidad Autónoma de Madrid (CSIC-UAM), 28029 Madrid, Spain; narias@iib.uam.es
* Correspondence: libarra@exa.unrc.edu.ar

Brain tumors are a significant concern for the global medical community, with over 300,000 cases reported annually worldwide [1]. While some tumors are benign, many can become malignant and invade healthy brain tissue. Advances in diagnosis and treatment, such as improved imaging, targeted therapies, and minimally invasive surgeries, have improved outcomes and quality of life for patients. Despite these advancements, brain and other central nervous system (CNS) tumors are the fifth most common type of cancer and the most common among children [2].

Various criteria such as the location, type, grade, invasiveness, and potential spread of a brain tumor can restrict the success of its treatment. The blood–brain barrier (BBB) can hinder the efficacy of some medications, and tumors can become resistant to treatments with prolonged exposure [3]. Neurological impairment resulting from therapies such as surgery and radiation therapy can also affect a patient's quality of life [4]. The problems highlight the intricate nature of handling brain tumors and the necessity for continuous research to enhance results. Ongoing research is focused on comprehending the biology of brain tumors, discovering new treatment targets, and creating breakthrough medicines like immunotherapy and tailored drug delivery systems. These endeavors show potential for enhancing results and increasing survival rates in the future.

This Editorial refers to the Special Issue "Advances in the Development of New Drugs and Treatment Targets for Brain Cancers". The Special Issue features original research articles and review articles that discuss new therapy tactics and target medications, emphasizing the significance of brain tumors at cellular and molecular levels.

Nineteen manuscripts were submitted for consideration for the Special Issue, and all of them were subject to a rigorous review process. In total, ten papers were finally accepted for publication and inclusion in this Special Issue (seven articles and three reviews). The contributions are listed below:

1. Aguilar-García, I.G.; Jiménez-Estrada, I.; Castañeda-Arellano, R.; Alpirez, J.; Mendizabal-Ruiz, G.; Dueñas-Jiménez, J.M.; Gutiérrez-Almeida, C.E.; Osuna-Carrasco, L.P.; Ramírez-Abundis, V.; Dueñas-Jiménez, S.H. Locomotion Outcome Improvement in Mice with Glioblastoma Multiforme after Treatment with Anastrozole. Brain Sci. 2023, 13, 496. https://doi.org/10.3390/brainsci13030496
2. Caverzán, M.D.; Beaugé, L.; Oliveda, P.M.; Cesca González, B.; Bühler, E.M.; Ibarra, L.E. Exploring Monocytes-Macrophages in Immune Microenvironment of Glioblastoma for the Design of Novel Therapeutic Strategies. Brain Sci. 2023, 13, 542. https://doi.org/10.3390/brainsci13040542
3. Hernández-Cerón, M.; Chavarria, V.; Ríos, C.; Pineda, B.; Palomares-Alonso, F.; Rojas-Tomé, I.S.; Jung-Cook, H. Melatonin in Combination with Albendazole or Albendazole

Citation: Ibarra, L.E.; Milla Sanabria, L.N.; Arias-Ramos, N. Advances in the Development of New Drugs and Treatment Targets for Brain Cancers. Brain Sci. 2024, 14, 526. https://doi.org/10.3390/brainsci14060526

Received: 2 May 2024
Accepted: 14 May 2024
Published: 22 May 2024

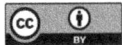

Copyright: © 2024 by the authors. Licensee MDPI, Basel, Switzerland. This article is an open access article distributed under the terms and conditions of the Creative Commons Attribution (CC BY) license (https://creativecommons.org/licenses/by/4.0/).

Sulfoxide Produces a Synergistic Cytotoxicity against Malignant Glioma Cells through Autophagy and Apoptosis. *Brain Sci.* **2023**, *13*, 869. https://doi.org/10.3390/brainsci13060869

4. Tamas, C.; Tamas, F.; Kovecsi, A.; Serban, G.; Boeriu, C.; Balasa, A. The Role of Ketone Bodies in Treatment Individualization of Glioblastoma Patients. *Brain Sci.* **2023**, *13*, 1307. https://doi.org/10.3390/brainsci13091307
5. Hoshimaru, T.; Nonoguchi, N.; Kosaka, T.; Furuse, M.; Kawabata, S.; Yagi, R.; Kurisu, Y.; Kashiwagi, H.; Kameda, M.; Takami, T.; et al. Actin Alpha 2, Smooth Muscle (ACTA2) Is Involved in the Migratory Potential of Malignant Gliomas, and Its Increased Expression at Recurrence Is a Significant Adverse Prognostic Factor. *Brain Sci.* **2023**, *13*, 1477. https://doi.org/10.3390/brainsci13101477
6. Toader, C.; Eva, L.; Costea, D.; Corlatescu, A.D.; Covache-Busuioc, R.-A.; Bratu, B.-G.; Glavan, L.A.; Costin, H.P.; Popa, A.A.; Ciurea, A.V. Low-Grade Gliomas: Histological Subtypes, Molecular Mechanisms, and Treatment Strategies. *Brain Sci.* **2023**, *13*, 1700. https://doi.org/10.3390/brainsci13121700
7. Alves, A.; Silva, A.M.; Moreira, J.; Nunes, C.; Reis, S.; Pinto, M.; Cidade, H.; Rodrigues, F.; Ferreira, D.; Costa, P.C.; et al. Polymersomes for Sustained Delivery of a Chalcone Derivative Targeting Glioblastoma Cells. *Brain Sci.* **2024**, *14*, 82. https://doi.org/10.3390/brainsci14010082
8. Ravi Kiran, A.V.V.V.; Kumari, G.K.; Krishnamurthy, P.T.; Johnson, A.P.; Kenchegowda, M.; Osmani, R.A.M.; Abu Lila, A.S.; Moin, A.; Gangadharappa, H.V.; Rizvi, S.M.D. An Update on Emergent Nano-Therapeutic Strategies against Pediatric Brain Tumors. *Brain Sci.* **2024**, *14*, 185. https://doi.org/10.3390/brainsci14020185
9. Lima, I.S.; Soares, É.N.; Nonaka, C.K.V.; Souza, B.S.d.F.; dos Santos, B.L.; Costa, S.L. Flavonoid Rutin Presented Anti-Glioblastoma Activity Related to the Modulation of Onco miRNA-125b Expression and STAT3 Signaling and Impact on Microglia Inflammatory Profile. *Brain Sci.* **2024**, *14*, 90. https://doi.org/10.3390/brainsci14010090
10. Arias-Ramos, N.; Vieira, C.; Pérez-Carro, R.; López-Larrubia, P. Integrative Magnetic Resonance Imaging and Metabolomic Characterization of a Glioblastoma Rat Model. *Brain Sci.* **2024**, *14*, 409. https://doi.org/10.3390/brainsci14050409

Glioblastoma (GBM) is the most aggressive type of glioma in adult patients and has the highest occurrence among malignant tumors. Patients typically have a limited survival span with conventional treatments, largely due to factors such as incomplete surgical resection and glioma cell infiltration, which contribute to a poor prognosis. Contribution 5 delved into the exploration of actin family genes as potential biomarkers for assessing brain invasion and distant recurrence in gliomas. The study uncovered the significant role of ACTA2 as a migratory factor in malignant gliomas, correlating with recurrence. Understanding the migratory mechanisms in malignant gliomas holds paramount importance for the development of forthcoming therapeutic strategies, with ACTA2 emerging as a promising candidate for targeted therapeutic interventions.

Various endeavors are currently being made in preclinical models of GBM to discover new molecular or cellular targets for treating malignant glioma. Estrogen receptors have been found in GBM tumor cells, suggesting a potential application of hormone-based therapies. While not a typical treatment for GBM, various studies suggest it may have a role in combination therapy. Contribution 1 evaluated the functional significance of anastrozole treatment's anticancer effect by altering ERα and GPR30 expression in GBM xenografts. As a result, there was an improvement in walking movement, perhaps due to a decrease in the size of the brain tumor in the right motor region.

Contribution 10 aimed to discover new MRI and metabolomic indicators of GBM and their effects on healthy tissue utilizing a C6 glioma rat model. The authors studied an advanced-stage GBM tumor model by using in vivo multiparametric MRI evaluations and ex vivo metabolomic HRMAS MRS studies, due to the challenges posed by GBM and the growing recognition of the importance of multiparametric MRI in understanding its pathophysiology.

Recent studies have emphasized the cellular metabolism reprogramming process, which plays a crucial role in establishing the cellular microenvironment for tumor development and the invasion of GBM cells in normal brain tissue. Contribution 4 examined the potential use of ketones (KBs) and the glucose–ketone index (GKI) in predicting tumor aggressiveness in patients with GBM in a prospective clinical investigation, emphasizing novel biomarkers like KBs or GKI that are easier to measure.

Considering the composition of the GBM tumor microenvironment (TME), recent efforts have been placed on understanding the microenvironment surrounding tumor cells and the interaction between these cellular and acellular components in different preformed tumor niches to design new treatment options. Contribution 2 offers a comprehensive review of the pivotal role played by a primary cellular immune component in GBM, namely monocytes/macrophages. It elucidates how, over the past decade, this population has increasingly been recognized as a cell target in the formulation of novel therapeutic approaches. Within this field of study, Contribution 9 described a new intervention involving rutin on the viability and regulation of miRNA-125b and STAT3 expression in GBM cells. It also examined the impact on the inflammatory profile and STAT3 expression in microglia during indirect interactions with GBM cells. Its findings confirm the anti-glioma properties of the flavonoid, which can also influence microglia to adopt a more effective anti-tumor behavior, making it a potential candidate for supplemental treatment for GBM.

Drug repositioning is a successful strategy used to explore existing drugs for new clinical uses. Evidence suggests that it can enhance therapeutic effects by utilizing alternative cell death mechanisms like autophagy or ferroptosis, leading to improved anticancer effects and the activation of the immune system. Contribution 3 investigated the combined effects of melatonin with albendazole or albendazole sulfoxide on GBM cells to determine whether they have an additive or synergistic lethal effect. The authors discovered that the combination therapies resulted in a much higher rate of apoptotic and autophagic cell death in GBM. Albendazole and albendazole sulfoxide suppressed proliferation regardless of melatonin. The data support the further assessment of these various medication combinations as a viable method to assist in the treatment of GBM.

The scientific community has directed a considerable amount of attention towards both natural and synthetic chalcones, owing to their diverse range of reported biological activities, notably their demonstrated antitumor effects mediated through the inhibition of various molecular targets. In Contribution 7, novel nanoparticles (polymersomes) were developed as alternative drug delivery systems to facilitate the encapsulation and sustained release of these promising anti-GBM chalcone compounds, exhibiting notable selectivity against GBM cells.

This Special Issue also discusses various types of brain tumors in addition to GBM. Low-Grade Gliomas (LGGs) are a diverse group of brain tumors that develop from glial cells and are identified by their unique histopathological and molecular features. Contribution 6 thoroughly analyzes LGGs, detailing their subtypes, histological characteristics, and molecular components. By studying the World Health Organization's grading system, 5th edition, more details were included due to a thorough understanding of new laboratory techniques, especially genetic analysis. Finally, Contribution 8 analyzed nanotechnology-based treatment options for childhood brain tumors in the revision. Pediatric brain tumors are the most common type of pediatric cancer and present a significant barrier for treatment due to their ability to spread to nearby tissues, limiting the effectiveness of surgery as the only treatment option. Nanotechnology delivery systems may efficiently penetrate the BBB. By including receptors that are highly expressed in both blood–brain barrier cells and cancer cells, these systems can differentiate cancer cells from healthy ones and target therapeutic drugs specifically to malignant cells.

This Special Issue requested manuscripts on novel therapeutic approaches and target medications as well as the significance of brain tumors at the cellular and molecular levels. We wanted to gather relevant expertise from experienced authors on the issue. Both the scholarly community and the general public can freely access the content upon publication.

Conflicts of Interest: The author declares no conflicts of interest.

References

1. Miller, K.D.; Ostrom, Q.T.; Kruchko, C.; Patil, N.; Tihan, T.; Cioffi, G.; Fuchs, H.E.; Waite, K.A.; Jemal, A.; Siegel, R.L.; et al. Brain and other central nervous system tumor statistics. *CA Cancer J. Clin.* **2021**, *71*, 381–406. [CrossRef] [PubMed]
2. Ostrom, Q.T.; Francis, S.S.; Barnholtz-Sloan, J.S. Epidemiology of Brain and Other CNS Tumors. *Curr. Neurol. Neurosci. Rep.* **2021**, *21*, 68. [CrossRef] [PubMed]
3. McFaline-Figueroa, J.R.; Lee, E.Q. Brain Tumors. *Am. J. Med.* **2018**, *131*, 874–882. [CrossRef] [PubMed]
4. Roth, P.; Pace, A.; Le Rhun, E.; Weller, M.; Cohen-Jonathan Moyal, E.; Coomans, M.; Giusti, R.; Jordan, K.; Nishikawa, R.; Winkler, F.; et al. Neurological and vascular complications of primary and secondary brain tumours: EANO-ESMO Clinical Practice Guidelines for prophylaxis, diagnosis, treatment and follow-up. *Ann. Oncol.* **2021**, *32*, 171–182. [CrossRef] [PubMed]

Disclaimer/Publisher's Note: The statements, opinions and data contained in all publications are solely those of the individual author(s) and contributor(s) and not of MDPI and/or the editor(s). MDPI and/or the editor(s) disclaim responsibility for any injury to people or property resulting from any ideas, methods, instructions or products referred to in the content.

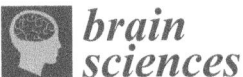

Review

Low-Grade Gliomas: Histological Subtypes, Molecular Mechanisms, and Treatment Strategies

Corneliu Toader [1,2], Lucian Eva [3,4,*], Daniel Costea [5,*], Antonio Daniel Corlatescu [1], Razvan-Adrian Covache-Busuioc [1], Bogdan-Gabriel Bratu [1], Luca Andrei Glavan [1], Horia Petre Costin [1], Andrei Adrian Popa [1] and Alexandru Vlad Ciurea [1,6]

1. Department of Neurosurgery, "Carol Davila" University of Medicine and Pharmacy, 020021 Bucharest, Romania; corneliu.toader@umfcd.ro (C.T.); antonio.corlatescu0920@stud.umfcd.ro (A.D.C.); razvan-adrian.covache-busuioc0720@stud.umfcd.ro (R.-A.C.-B.); bogdan.bratu@stud.umfcd.ro (B.-G.B.); luca-andrei.glavan0720@stud.umfcd.ro (L.A.G.); horia-petre.costin0720@stud.umfcd.ro (H.P.C.); andreiadrianpopa@stud.umfcd.ro (A.A.P.); prof.avciurea@gmail.com (A.V.C.)
2. Department of Vascular Neurosurgery, National Institute of Neurology and Neurovascular Diseases, 077160 Bucharest, Romania
3. Department of Neurosurgery, Dunarea de Jos University, 800010 Galati, Romania
4. Department of Neurosurgery, Clinical Emergency Hospital "Prof. Dr. Nicolae Oblu", 700309 Iasi, Romania
5. Department of Neurosurgery, "Victor Babes" University of Medicine and Pharmacy, 300041 Timisoara, Romania
6. Neurosurgery Department, Sanador Clinical Hospital, 010991 Bucharest, Romania
* Correspondence: elucian73@yahoo.com (L.E.); costea.daniel@umft.ro (D.C.)

Abstract: Low-Grade Gliomas (LGGs) represent a diverse group of brain tumors originating from glial cells, characterized by their unique histopathological and molecular features. This article offers a comprehensive exploration of LGGs, shedding light on their subtypes, histological and molecular aspects. By delving into the World Health Organization's grading system, 5th edition, various specificities were added due to an in-depth understanding of emerging laboratory techniques, especially genomic analysis. Moreover, treatment modalities are extensively discussed. The degree of surgical resection should always be considered according to postoperative quality of life and cognitive status. Adjuvant therapies focused on chemotherapy and radiotherapy depend on tumor grading and invasiveness. In the current literature, emerging targeted molecular therapies are well discussed due to their succinctly therapeutic effect; in our article, those therapies are summarized based on posttreatment results and possible adverse effects. This review serves as a valuable resource for clinicians, researchers, and medical professionals aiming to deepen their knowledge on LGGs and enhance patient care.

Keywords: low-grade gliomas; astrocytoma; oligodendroglioma; ependymoma; rare low-grade gliomas; pediatric low-grade gliomas; neuropathology and classification; molecular pathways; outcome; treatment strategies; surgery; radiation therapy; targeted therapies; immune therapies

1. Introduction

The prognosis for patients with lower-grade diffuse gliomas (LrGGs), classified as grades II and III, is showing signs of improvement, though it varies based on the molecular subtype of the tumor. Despite these advancements in survival, both the tumors themselves and the treatments employed to combat them frequently result in considerable cognitive impairments. These impairments can be both objective (measurable through cognitive testing) and subjective (as they are perceived by the patients themselves). Neoplasms of the central nervous system (CNS) are categorized according to their cellular origin and distinct histological characteristics, which are indicative of their probable clinical course. Among these neoplasms, gliomas, which arise from CNS glial cells, constitute a significant subgroup. These glial neoplasms are further divided into astrocytomas, oligodendrogliomas, mixed oligo-astrocytic, and mixed glioneuronal tumors, with each originating from different glial cell types, such as astrocytes or oligodendrocytes. The World Health Organization (WHO) employs a grading system for gliomas that spans from grade 1 (least aggressive) to grade 4 (most aggressive) and is based on a range of histological characteristics, including cellular atypia, proliferative patterns, and necrosis presence. Specifically, low-grade gliomas (LGGs) are classified as grade 1 gliomas, which are devoid of these histological markers, or grade 2 gliomas, which exhibit only cellular atypia [1].

Low-grade astrocytic tumors include diffuse astrocytomas, pilomyxoid astrocytomas, and pleomorphic xanthoastrocytomas (WHO grade 2), as well as SEGA and pilocytic astrocytomas (WHO grade 1). Oligodendrogliomas and oligoastrocytomas (WHO grade 2) represent low-grade oligodendroglial tumors. Additionally, specific low-grade glioneuronal tumors such as gangliogliomas and dysembryoplastic neuroepithelial tumors are categorized under WHO grade 1 [2]. In the revised taxonomy of diffuse gliomas, a substantial proportion have been reclassified based on IDH 1/2 mutation status and the 1p/19q codeletion, leading to the anticipated redundancy of the oligoastrocytoma category and the redefinition of gliomatosis cerebri as a growth pattern [3].

Assessing the incidence of low-grade gliomas poses a challenge due to the recent transition to a molecular-based classification. Cancer registries are gradually integrating changes from the 2016 WHO neuropathological categorization. Based on previous classifications, the estimated yearly incidence rates in the U.S. for grade 2 astrocytomas, oligodendrogliomas, and mixed gliomas are 0.51, 0.25, and 0.20 per 100,000 individuals, amounting to 1180, 690, and 610 cases, respectively. There is a higher prevalence of low-grade gliomas among white people compared to people, with lower rates in American Indians/Alaska Natives and Asian/Pacific Islanders. Astrocytomas commonly peak between ages 30 and 40 years old, whereas oligodendrogliomas peak at ages 40–45. Males are slightly more affected by low-grade gliomas [4,5].

The precise etiological factors for low-grade gliomas are not fully understood. Exposure to ionizing radiation, particularly among childhood leukemia survivors, is a recognized environmental risk factor. Intriguingly, a history of allergies or asthma seems to confer some protective effect against gliomas, suggesting the potential involvement of the immune system. Although rare inherited tumor syndromes contribute to a minority of cases, familial glioma occurrences and research pointing to increased glioma risk in close relatives imply more complex genetic factors. Recent genome-wide associations have identified gene variants correlated with a heightened risk of gliomas, including low-grade types. Notably, the g allele of CCDC26 on chromosome 8 elevates the risk of specific gliomas sixfold. This allele is present in about 40% of patients with certain glioma types compared to 8% in the general population. The mechanism of this variant is yet to be elucidated, and due to the overall low incidence of glioma, screening for this allele is not currently recommended [6].

2. Historical Overview of the 2021 WHO Classification: Molecular Intricacies and the Pathway to Targeted Therapies

Molecular advancements have substantially addressed the complexities in brain tumor classification. As a result, many brain tumors are now characterized by distinct molecular alterations. The 2021 5th Edition of the WHO Classification of Tumors of the Central Nervous System enhances the fundamental shifts introduced in the 2016 4th Edition, recognizing several new tumor entities, each assigned an official WHO grade. This edition notably incorporates methylome profiling, particularly pertinent for low-grade gliomas and glioneuronal tumors. The 2021 classification is significant for several reasons, such as its integration of molecular markers, improved diagnostic accuracy, the potential for personalized treatment, advancements in research, and potential better patient outcomes. These neoplasms are frequently categorized based on specific genetic changes such as FGFR1, MYB/MYBL1, BRAF, or IDH1/2, identified through DNA methylation profiles [7]. For pediatric-type low-grade gliomas and glioneuronal tumors (pLGG/GNTs), evidence suggests that MAP kinase pathway alterations are prevalent, albeit with variable manifestations and not always definitively. The 2021 WHO classification reflects the advancing comprehension of these tumors, where a specific genetic alteration can define a tumor, aid in its diagnosis, be common across different tumors, or be one of several alterations within a tumor type. Some diagnoses may not necessitate any demonstrated alteration, while others are yet to be discovered. The 2021 WHO's "hybrid taxonomy" encapsulates the current understanding of CNS tumors' clinical, histological, and molecular aspects, paving the way for more precise tumor classification and targeted therapies. The classification organizes gliomas, glioneuronal tumors, and neuronal tumors into six families. Three of these families correspond with pLGG/LGNT: pediatric-type diffuse low-grade gliomas [5], circumscribed astrocytic gliomas [8], and glioneuronal and neuronal tumors [9]. Moreover, six of the fourteen newly recognized tumor types in the 2021 WHO classification are categorized as pLGG/GNTs. Under "pediatric type diffuse low-grade gliomas," three new tumor types are introduced: "diffuse astrocytoma, MYB or MYBL1-altered"; "polymorphous low-grade neuroepithelial tumor of the young (PLNTY)"; and "diffuse low-grade glioma-MAPK altered". The category of glioneuronal and neuronal tumors includes three new additions: "Diffuse glioneuronal tumor with oligodendroglioma-like features and nuclear clusters (DGONC)"; "myxoid glioneuronal tumor (MGT)"; and "multinodular and vacuolating tumor (MVNT)" [10].

Patients with low-grade gliomas typically present at a younger median age compared to those with anaplastic gliomas or glioblastomas, usually diagnosed in their late twenties to mid-forties, although diagnosis over the age of 60 is possible. Seizures, ranging from generalized tonic–clonic to subtle partial seizures, are a frequent symptom, particularly in cases with oligodendroglial histology, likely due to their frequent cortical involvement. The widespread availability of CT and MRI scans has led to the incidental diagnosis of many patients while seeking care for unrelated conditions like migraines or head injuries [11,12]. Low-grade gliomas rarely present with specific focal deficits such as speech difficulties or unilateral weakness, as these tumors tend to infiltrate rather than disrupt critical brain structures. Neuroimaging is typically indicative of a low-grade glioma. Over 95% of these tumors are located in the cerebral hemispheres, with a near-even distribution across the frontal and temporal lobes and fewer in the occipital lobe. In CT scans, these tumors often appear as hypodense areas. Approximately 20% of low-grade gliomas, especially oligodendrogliomas, demonstrate calcification on CT. Additionally, around a quarter of these tumors show some contrast enhancement on CT, usually presenting as patchy rather than ring-like enhancement. Originating primarily in the white matter, those with an oligodendroglial component may extend into the cortex. MRI is more effective than CT in delineating these tumors, typically appearing as T1-hypointense and T2/FLAIR-hyperintense. MRI's susceptibility-weighted imaging can detect calcifications or occasional hemorrhages which are more common in oligodendrogliomas than astrocytomas. Advanced imaging techniques like PET scanning and magnetic resonance spectroscopy can aid in differentiating tumor types, though they are not always necessary. A key subject of ongoing research is utilizing magnetic resonance spectroscopy to monitor low-grade glioma progression and response to treatment by identifying elevated levels of 2-hydroxyglutarate in IDH mutant gliomas [13].

Traditionally, diffuse infiltrating gliomas were identified and classified based on their morphological characteristics, which can be observed under light microscopy following hematoxylin and eosin (H&E) staining. Tumors characterized by elevated cellular density and nuclear atypia but with sparse mitotic figures were classified as low-grade gliomas. However, the subjective assessment of "rare" mitotic activity led to inconsistencies in grading by neuropathologists. To mitigate this, the Ki-67 stain, which marks proliferating cells, is utilized, with low-grade gliomas typically exhibiting less than 10% labeling. Further classification into subtypes like low-grade astrocytoma, oligodendroglioma, or oligoastrocytoma is achieved through the tumor's cellular architecture and immunohistochemical staining [14]. Astrocytomas are noted for their pronounced fibrillary structures and strong reactivity to specific protein markers, whereas oligodendrogliomas possess scant cytoplasm and characteristic "fried egg" nuclei [15].

The advent of molecular neuropathology has profoundly augmented the understanding and categorization of low-grade gliomas. TP53 mutations, frequently observed in astrocytomas but uncommon in oligodendrogliomas, were among the early molecular distinctions recognized. The 1990s uncovered that most oligodendrogliomas exhibit distinct chromosomal losses, findings generally exclusive to TP53 mutations [16]. This led some experts to advocate for a molecular-based classification, positing it to be more objective and reflective of tumor behavior. A pivotal discovery was the prevalence of mutations in the IDH gene, involved in the Krebs cycle, in a majority of low-grade gliomas. The frequent IDH1 R132H mutation, in particular, can be readily detected, offering significant insights into glioma pathogenesis [17–19].

Within the WHO 2021 framework, histopathological grading adheres to the principles set by the WHO 2016 criteria, with the presence of necrosis and/or microvascular proliferation indicative of a grade 4 tumor, specifically classified as astrocytoma IDH mutant CNS WHO grade 4. Despite this continuity, a definitive criterion for differentiating grades 2 and 3 based on mitotic count remains unestablished [20]. Furthermore, while the Ki-67/MIB-1 proliferative index correlates with tumor grade, it lacks a universally accepted threshold for predicting increased recurrence risk [21]. In this context, the category of diffuse astrocytoma, IDH-wild-type, corresponding to CNS WHO grades II or III but lacking glioblastoma molecular characteristics, is now considered rare and has been removed from the CNS WHO5 classification [22]. Recent studies have led to the reclassification of IDH mutant grade 2 and 3 astrocytomas as "diffuse low-grade astrocytomas," owing to their prognostic similarities. This reclassification questions the previous grouping of grade 3 and 4 astrocytomas as "high-grade," given the distinct differences in molecular profiles and clinical outcomes between IDH mutant grade 3 astrocytomas and IDH-wild-type grade 4 glioblastomas [4].

Genomic analyses have shown that the majority of grade II and III diffuse astrocytomas, IDH-wild-type, harbor genomic alterations and clinical outcomes akin to primary glioblastoma, grade IV [23]. One particular study indicated that histopathologic grade II or III IDH-wild-type diffuse astrocytic gliomas, characterized by chromosomal anomalies such as +7/−10, EGFR amplification or TERT promoter mutations, are prognostically equivalent to histologically confirmed glioblastoma [24]. Moreover, the diagnosis of IDH mutant diffuse astrocytoma grade 2 is now strictly limited to cases without anaplastic histopathological features, significant mitotic activity, and the homozygous deletion of CDNK2A/B [25].

In-depth genomic investigations regarding various cancers have revealed a previously underappreciated prevalence of molecular alterations affecting the cellular epigenome [26]. This epigenome comprises DNA modifications, histones, their associated marks, and other chromatin-binding factors, all of which collectively orchestrate gene expression. The critical role of epigenomic dysfunction has been identified in several primary brain tumors, including gliomas [27]. Among these, mutations in isocitrate dehydrogenase 1 and 2 (IDH1 and IDH2) and the H3.3 histone-encoding genes H3F3A and HIST1H3B are particularly notable. IDH mutations result in a widespread pattern of DNA and histone hypermethylation, owing to the generation of the oncometabolite 2-hydroxyglutarate [28,29], while H3.3 mutations directly impact histone marks, chromatin accessibility, and gene expression [30]. These disruptions, complex and cell-specific, appear to fundamentally deviate from normal developmental pathways, contributing to the pathogenesis of glioma. Although pivotal in adult and/or high-grade glioma variants, IDH and H3.3 mutations are infrequently associated with pediatric low-grade gliomas (pLGG). Some studies have detected H3.3 K27M mutations in subgroups of pilocytic astrocytomas and glioneuronal tumors, which are typically more aggressive than their H3.3-mutant counterparts. Yet, these pLGG variants often have longer patient survival compared to high-grade gliomas with H3.3 mutations [31].

Epigenomic profiles have become indispensable markers in pLGG and other primary CNS tumors. Specifically, global DNA methylation profiling has enabled the identification of distinct "signatures" that often define brain tumor subtypes, laying the groundwork for systematic pLGG classification. Recent research employing global methylation profiling has been instrumental in characterizing various gliomas, and similar methodologies are expected to further refine pLGG classification in the future [32].

The discovery of key genetic alterations in pLGG has opened avenues for targeted therapies, particularly those addressing the commonly altered MAPK pathway in these tumors (Figure 1).

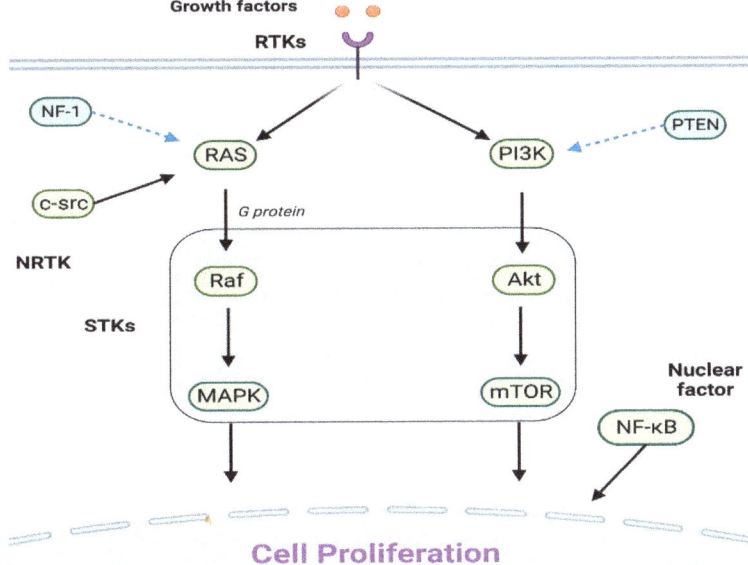

Figure 1. An explanation of the primary cell proliferation pathways: The PI3K/Akt/mTOR and Ras/Raf/MAPK routes are the main pathways. When growth factors attach to receptor tyrosine kinases (RTKs), they can trigger either the Ras/Raf/MAPK or PI3K/Akt/mTOR pathways. The key players in these pathways, Raf, MAPK, Akt, and mTOR, have been identified as serine/threonine-specific protein kinases (STKs). Additionally, the intracellular tyrosine kinase c-src can initiate the Ras/Raf/MAPK pathway. It is worht noting that the nuclear factor NF-κB also significantly contributes to cell proliferation.

Selumetinib (AZD6244), an oral MEK1/2 inhibitor, has undergone extensive testing in pLGG. Initial trials established its optimal dosage and demonstrated encouraging outcomes in terms of partial responses and progression-free survival [33,34]. These results have led to additional studies, with emerging evidence suggesting the potential efficacy of MEK inhibitors even in the absence of characteristic BRAF mutations. Consequently, two major studies are currently evaluating selumetinib as a primary treatment option for pLGG. Other MEK inhibitors, such as trametinib, binimetinib, and cobimetinib, are also being explored for their applicability in pLGG [35,36]. While their deployment in treating low-grade gliomas is still in preliminary stages, the initial findings are promising. These inhibitors typically exhibit similar side effects, including dermatological and gastrointestinal reactions. Some, particularly in adult populations, have been associated with cardiac and ocular adverse effects [33,37]. The determination of the most effective MEK inhibitor for pLGG is still underway.

Direct BRAF inhibitors such as dabrafenib and vemurafenib also show potential for pLGG treatment. They specifically target BRAF kinases and have shown significant responses in pLGG with BRAFV600 mutations [38,39]. Ongoing studies are exploring these inhibitors for BRAF mutant pLGG. However, it is crucial to note that first-generation BRAF inhibitors might not be suitable for tumors with BRAF fusion due to potential adverse effects [40]. Second-generation inhibitors, which do not have this limitation, are being tested in ongoing trials and may offer a promising avenue [41]. Trametinib effectively treated progressive pLGG, achieving disease control in all subjects. Nonetheless, treatment-related side effects posed challenges for some patients, and a subset experienced disease recurrence after discontinuing MEKi [42] (Figure 2).

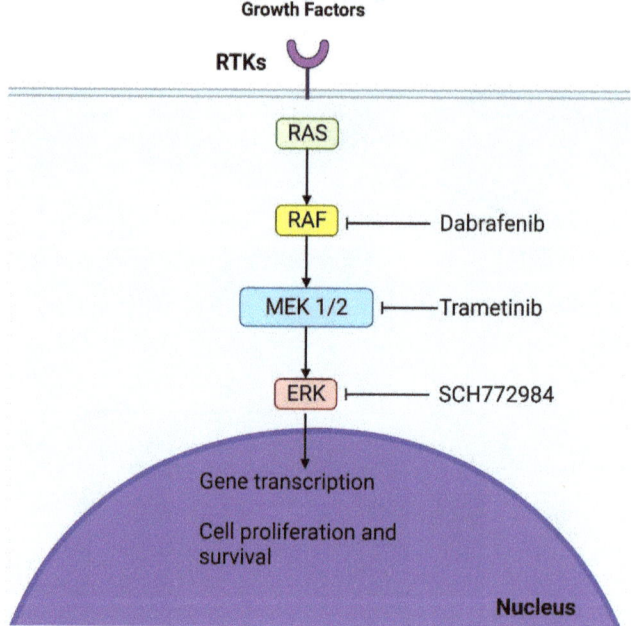

Figure 2. Mechanisms of action of dabrafenib and trametinib: These agents, which are BRAF and MEK inhibitors, respectively, act at two distinct sites within the MAPK (mitogen-activated protein kinase) pathway. By binding to their respective targets, they halt the oncogenic signaling cascade, culminating in cell cycle arrest.

3. Specificities of WHO 2021 Classification of Brain Tumors

In the WHO CNS5 guidelines, the grading of central nervous system (CNS) tumors has been substantially revised: the transition from Roman to Arabic numerals for grading supersedes previous practices, and grading is now consistently implemented within specific tumor types rather than comparatively across different types. The significance of this specific change involves more clarity and universality for the classification, more precision and adaptability, and greater alignment with other classifications leading to their easier use in the research field, which ultimately benefits patients. This entity-specific grading approach for CNS tumors differs from other organ systems where neoplasms are graded according to type-specific systems, such as those for breast or prostate cancers [43]. The rationale behind adopting intra-type grading within WHO CNS5 is multifaceted: first, to provide greater grading flexibility relative to each tumor type; second, to emphasize the biological consistency within tumor types over the prediction of clinical behavior; and third, to synchronize with WHO's grading protocols for non-CNS tumors [10]. In tandem with these grading modifications, nomenclature changes have been made to reflect molecular characteristics in accordance with cIMPACT-NOW Update 6 and to standardize terminology across all classifications within the WHO Blue Books, especially those pertaining to peripheral nerve and soft-tissue tumors [44].

The revised classification introduces fourteen new types within the categories of Gliomas, Glioneuronal Tumors, and Neuronal Tumors, along with updates to the nomenclature of existing entities. A key example is the reclassification of diffuse midline glioma, now termed "H3 K27-altered" instead of "H3 K27M-mutant," to recognize a range of pathogenic mechanisms influencing these tumors [45].

Significantly, WHO CNS5 differentiates diffuse gliomas based on the patient's age, distinguishing between "adult-type" and "pediatric-type". This distinction acknowledges the clinical and molecular differences between these groups and aims to guide more effective treatment strategies for CNS tumors in both demographics [10]. Additionally, the classification now recognizes infant-type hemispheric glioma as a separate high-grade glioma category characterized by a unique molecular profile, including fusion genes involving ALK, ROS1, NTRK1/2/3, or MET, predominantly seen in newborns and infants [46].

4. Rare Entities in Low-Grade Gliomas

4.1. MYB/MYBL1 Alterations

Pediatric-type diffuse low-grade gliomas (pLGG) with MYB/MYBL1 alterations constitute a distinct subset of IDH-wild-type and H3-wild-type tumors, notable for their benign clinical course and favorable prognosis [47]. In 2021, the World Health Organization updated their CNS tumor classification to include two categories of these pLGGs: angiocentric glioma with MYB-QKI fusions and diffuse astrocytoma with various MYB/MYBL1 alterations [4]. Most of the existing studies on these gliomas have focused on their clinicopathologic characteristics, with less emphasis on their radiologic features [48]. The primary treatment strategy for pLGGs with MYB/MYBL1 alterations is comprehensive surgical resection, as complete removal is often correlated with a positive outcome [49].

The 2016 WHO update on CNS tumors offered valuable insights but did not thoroughly delineate pediatric gliomas and their prognostic outcomes. Specifically, the IDH-wild-type/H3-wild-type low-grade tumors remained a heterogeneous group. Despite their typically benign nature and rare progression to anaplastic forms in children, there was a lack of distinction between pediatric and adult tumor types. Research showed different molecular markers in tumors between children and adults, with pediatric low-grade gliomas predominantly exhibiting alterations in the BRAF, FGFR, and MYB/MYBL1 genes, while IDH1/2 mutations were less common [50]. This distinction was further emphasized by cIMPACT-NOW in their fourth update [47].

In its 2021 revision, the WHO introduced a classification for pediatric-type diffuse low-grade gliomas, encompassing four subtypes: (1) diffuse astrocytoma, MYB- or MYBL1-altered; (2) angiocentric glioma; (3) polymorphous low-grade neuroepithelial tumor of the young; and (4) diffuse low-grade, MAPK pathway-altered glioma [8]. This discussion focuses on the first subtype. There are few studies on the radiologic characteristics of MYB/MYBL1-altered gliomas. In a study by Chiang et al., 46 such tumors were evaluated, with 23 pre-operative MR images being reviewed. The majority of patients presented with epilepsy, and the tumors were predominantly located in the cerebral hemispheres, although some were found in the diencephalon and brainstem. Upon T1 imaging, these tumors typically appeared iso- to hypointense, while T2/FLAIR imaging often revealed mixed signals or hyperintensity. Only one case showed faint and diffuse contrast enhancement, and no diffusion restriction was observed [51]. In cases where complete resection is not possible, additional chemotherapy and radiation are considered. MYB/MYBL1 alterations can be considered distinctive in the field of oncology due to their unique molecular characteristics and implications, giving them an important role in the context of personalized medicine and hinting toward their potential as therapeutic targets.

4.2. Angiocentric Glioma

Angiocentric glioma (AG) is a unique brain tumor often associated with treatment-resistant epilepsy in children and young adults which can be effectively managed through neurosurgical intervention. An analysis of case reports since its initial identification revealed several key findings: (1) seizures are the most common initial symptom; (2) magnetic resonance imaging (MRI) typically reveals a supratentorial, non-enhancing lesion that is T1-hypointense and/or T2-hyperintense; (3) these tumors display specific histopathological features; and (4) outcomes following complete tumor resection are generally positive [52]. First identified in 2005 [4,53] and recognized as a distinct entity by 2007 [4], AG was initially categorized under "other glioma" in the 2016 WHO edition. However, in the latest classification, it is included among "pediatric-type low-grade diffuse gliomas".

Due to the rarity of AG, gaining a comprehensive understanding has been challenging, but it is now graded as 1 in the 2021 WHO Classification. Commonly presenting with persistent, drug-resistant epilepsy in children, AG accounts for a small proportion of tumors in the German Neuropathology Reference Center [54]. A study by Kurokawa et al. reported a median patient age of 13. AGs are typically located in the supratentorial cortex, with a slight preference for the temporal lobe, although occurrences in the brainstem have been documented. MRI scans often reveal a single, T2-hyperintense lesion with no enhancement and a distinctive cortical rim on T1-weighted images [54,55].

Histologically, AG is characterized by an infiltrative growth pattern with uniform, bipolar spindle-shaped cells. Its hallmark features include perivascular cell arrangement around blood vessels and a horizontal cell stream beneath the pia-arachnoid structures. While some regions may resemble schwannomas, others can exhibit an epithelioid appearance. Key characteristics include the near absence of mitoses, microvascular proliferation, and necrosis. The tumor cells typically test positive for GFAP and negative for Olig2. EMA tests indicate ependymoma-like differentiation, corroborated by electron microscopy findings [53].

Some researchers postulate that AG originates from bipolar radial glia during embryogenesis, displaying ependymal features. Tests for IDH1-R132H, BRAF V600E, and neuronal antigens generally yield negative results, and the Ki-67 proliferation index is usually low. While rare anaplastic features have been noted, their clinical significance is not fully understood. Most AGs are associated with an MYB, QKI gene fusion, but the 2021 WHO Classification considers this only as a recommended, not mandatory, diagnostic criterion [4].

4.3. Diffuse Low-Grade MAPK Pathway-Altered Gliomas

The mitogen-activated protein kinase (MAPK) pathway is crucial in regulating a variety of cellular functions, including cell growth, differentiation, apoptosis, and more. This pathway is activated by signaling molecules such as FGF, EGF, IGF, and TGF binding to their respective cell surface receptors, initiating a cascade of cytoplasmic protein kinase activations. This series of activations leads to the phosphorylation of multiple proteins and nuclear transcription factors, ultimately affecting gene expression [56,57].

The dysregulation of the MAPK signaling pathway has been implicated in a range of diseases, including inflammatory, immunological, and degenerative disorders. Its aberration is also associated with the initiation and progression of various neoplasms due to factors such as abnormal receptor expression or genetic mutations activating receptors and downstream signaling molecules. This includes CNS tumors like pilocytic astrocytomas and gangliogliomas [58].

The recent WHO classification of CNS tumors has introduced a new category within pediatric-type diffuse low-grade gliomas: diffuse low-grade gliomas with MAPK pathway alterations. These tumors typically develop in childhood and can occur anywhere in the CNS, often presenting with epilepsy [59].

The exact prevalence of these tumors is somewhat uncertain, as specialized molecular testing is required for diagnosis, but they are considered relatively rare. Radiologically, they often appear as variably enhancing masses with cystic components. Histologically, these tumors exhibit diverse morphologies, usually displaying non-extensive infiltration patterns. On a molecular level, they are characterized by alterations in the genes associated with the MAPK pathway and are distinct in that they lack IDH1/2 and H3F3A mutations and CDKN2A deletion. Several subtypes of these tumors have been identified, with the most common alterations involving FGFR1 and BRAF mutations [9].

4.4. Polymorphous Low-Grade Neuroepithelial Tumor of the Young (PLNTY)

Polymorphous low-grade neuroepithelial tumor of the young (PLNTY) is an exceptionally rare, slowly progressing tumor that was recently incorporated into the World Health Organization classification of central nervous system tumors. Initially identified and characterized by Huse et al. in 2017, PLNTY was subsequently classified in the WHO Central Nervous System Tumors later that same year [60]. This tumor predominantly affects the temporal lobe (observed in approximately 80% of cases), although instances in other brain regions, like the parietal, frontal, and occipital lobes, have been documented. PLNTY typically presents in children and young adults, with an average age of onset around 20.6 years and a slight female predominance. It is categorized among long-term epilepsy-associated brain tumors (LEATs), which are commonly associated with seizures and often resistant to standard antiepileptic drugs [61]. However, symptoms of PLNTY may include headaches, dizziness, or visual disturbances.

Genetically, PLNTY is characterized by a unique DNA methylation profile and frequently involves alterations in the mitogen-activated protein kinase (MAPK) pathway, including the BRAF proto-oncogene and fibroblast growth factor receptors 2 and 3 (FGFR2 and FGFR3). These genetic alterations, such as BRAF-V600E mutations or FGFR2 and FGFR3 fusions, often coexist. BRAF-V600E mutations are more common in young adults, while FGFR2 fusions tend to be more prevalent in younger patients. The exact role of these genetic changes in the development of PLNTY is not fully understood [62,63].

The histology of PLNTY can vary, but it typically includes an oligodendroglioma-like component. This tumor type exhibits a range of cellular morphologies, from cells with uniformly small round nuclei to those with anisonucleosis or distinct nuclear features. Other features often observed include perivascular pseudorosetting and calcifications, while mitosis, necrosis, vascular proliferation, inflammation, and certain other cell features are typically absent. Immunostaining has shown positive staining for glial markers such as GFAP and Olig2, albeit with weak or focal expression, but CD34 expression was notably prominent and consistently observed across tumor cells and neuronal elements. Some tumor cells may exhibit antibodies for the BRAF p.V600E mutation, while the Ki-67 proliferation index is generally low, though higher values have been reported. Neuronal markers EMA and IDHp.R132H tend to be negative, and ATRX mutations and chromosome 1p/19q codeletion are absent as well [64].

5. Pediatric Low-Grade Gliomas: A Special Consideration

Tumors originating in the central nervous system (CNS) are the most commonly diagnosed solid tumors among children, with an estimated incidence rate of 5.4–5.6 cases per 100,000 individuals. These tumors can sometimes represent a cause of cancer-related mortality in this age group, with approximately 1 in every 100,000 diagnoses resulting in a fatal outcome. Among CNS tumors, pediatric-type low-grade gliomas (pLGGs) represent about 30% of brain tumor diagnoses in children. These tumors, classified as WHO grade 1 or 2 malignancies, encompass a variety of histological subtypes and can develop anywhere along the neural axis [65].

Children with low-grade gliomas typically present with both generalized and localized symptoms, often experiencing these symptoms for at least six months before diagnosis. General symptoms related to increased intracranial pressure due to ventricular obstruction include morning headaches, nausea, vomiting, and lethargy. Physical examination might reveal signs like impaired upward gaze, abnormalities of the sixth cranial nerve, or papilledema, often indicating tumor growth in regions such as the cerebellum, optic chiasm/hypothalamus, dorsally exophytic brainstem, or tectum. The manifestation of individual tumors varies depending on their location, frequently resulting in neurological deficits, seizures, and endocrinopathies in localized areas. For instance, cerebellar tumors often lead to ataxia and dysmetria, while cerebral hemisphere tumors may cause seizures, hemiparesis, or behavioral changes. Tumors affecting the hypothalamus and pituitary gland can lead to obesity, growth failure, diabetes insipidus, hormonal irregularities, and visual field impairment due to optic chiasm compression. Optic pathway gliomas, which can occur anywhere along the visual pathway, are more commonly bilateral or affect the chiasm and postchiasmatic regions in children with neurofibromatosis type 1. Symptoms of optic pathway gliomas include visual field impairments, reduced visual acuity, optic nerve atrophy, proptosis, or strabismus [66,67].

Brainstem low-grade gliomas typically progress slowly, often being detected after months to years. Although they do not extensively infiltrate the brainstem, dorsally exophytic and cervicomedullary tumors can cause lower cranial nerve deficits (e.g., dysphagia, dysarthria, abnormal breathing), as well as long tract signs such as hemiparesis, spasticity, hyperreflexia, and Babinski's sign. Cervicomedullary tumors may also present with torticollis, long tract signs, and sensory loss due to upper cervical cord involvement; hydrocephalus is a common manifestation of focal brainstem tumors [68].

Upon neuroimaging, pediatric low-grade gliomas typically exhibit certain characteristics. MRI usually reveals these tumors to be hypointense on T1-weighted and hyperintense on T2-weighted sequences, with varying degrees of enhancement post-gadolinium. Pilocytic astrocytomas often appear as well-circumscribed tumors with cystic components and an enhancing nodule, while diffuse fibrillary astrocytomas are less well-defined and show lesser enhancement post-gadolinium. Accurate histological verification usually requires a surgical biopsy or complete tumor resection. In cases like optic pathway or hypothalamic gliomas in children, diagnostic biopsies might be avoided if MRI characteristics are consistent with low-grade glioma, particularly in the presence of neurofibromatosis type 1. Deep midline and brainstem tumor biopsies should be approached cautiously as these tumors often show no progression upon serial MRI evaluations [69].

Postoperative staging can sometimes involve an MRI scan of the surgical site within 24–48 h after surgery to differentiate between residual tumor and postoperative changes. In cases where dissemination or leptomeningeal involvement is suspected, a comprehensive evaluation should include spinal imaging and cerebrospinal fluid cytology testing [68]. A key feature of pediatric low-grade glioma (pLGG) is the abnormal activation of the mitogen-activated protein kinase (MAPK) pathway, suggesting that targeting this pathway with small-molecule inhibitors like MEK inhibitors could be a promising treatment strategy [42].

6. Treatment Modalities, Approaches, Outcomes, and Prognosis in Low-Grade Glioma

Achieving an optimal integrated diagnosis in neuro-oncology involves harmonizing histological categorization with genomic characterization. This process draws upon both histologically and genetically defined compendia of neoplasms. Despite the extensive nature of these compendia, certain correlations are commonly observed, with frequent integrations appearing in a manageable number of routine diagnoses. This approach is exemplified by the classification of 'Diffuse low-grade glioma, MAPK pathway-altered' as a specific tumor subtype [47].

In recent years, methylome profiling has emerged as a key method in CNS tumor classification. This technique, which analyzes genome-wide DNA methylation patterns, has gained significant attention in the academic field and is increasingly fundamental in the molecular taxonomy of CNS neoplasms [70]. While methylome profiling can sometimes serve as an indicator of genetic aberrations—for instance, a methylation signature akin to an IDH-wild-type glioblastoma may be identified without direct IDH mutation assays—it cannot completely replace mutation detection, especially in situations where targeted treatments or clinical trials require precise molecular aberrations [71]. Consequently, the molecular analysis of WHO grade II or III diffuse astrocytic, IDH-wild-type gliomas in adult patients is highly recommended. The presence of chromosomal aberrations such as +7/−10, EGFR amplification, or TERT promoter mutation should lead to a reclassification to WHO grade IV, significantly impacting both treatment strategies and prognostic expectations [72].

In pediatric low-grade glioma (pLGG), negative prognostic indicators include older age, astrocytic histology, large tumor size (>4–6 cm), midline crossing tumors, neurological deficits, and poor performance status. Conversely, presenting with seizures, particularly in neurologically intact individuals, is often viewed as a favorable prognostic factor. Pignatti et al. developed a scoring system in 2002, assigning points to various risk factors, and this system was validated across multiple trials [73]. The University of California, San Francisco's (UCSF) more recent scoring system considers age, performance score, tumor size, and eloquent involvement in determining prognosis. Patients aged 55–60 years have a 5-year survival rate of 30% to 40%, with each additional year of age further diminishing their prognosis; however, those surviving beyond two years post-diagnosis may experience prolonged progression-free survival (PFS) despite challenging prognoses [74,75].

Tissue acquisition is crucial in accurately diagnosing, prognosing, and treating pLGG, as pathognomonic imaging is lacking. Needle biopsies can result in misdiagnosis rates of over 50%, making surgical resection the preferred method for tumor characterization. The support for extensive surgical resection is growing, as is evidence of its efficacy, although randomized controlled trials are still needed. This strategy was first proposed in 2001, and subsequent institutional studies, including one from the UCSF, have affirmed its effectiveness. Notably, the UCSF's study demonstrated that a extent of resection (EOR) greater than 90% significantly improves overall survival (OS), with a 5-year survival rate of 97% versus 76% for EORs less than 90% [76]. The Johns Hopkins Hospital reported similar findings, indicating that gross total resection (GTR) can enhance both overall survival and progression-free survival (PFS). However, factors such as the involvement of the corticospinal tract, tumor volume, and oligodendroglioma histology can impede complete resection [77].

In a cohort study examining low-grade gliomas (LGGs), a significant correlation was found between both the residual volume post-surgery ($p = 0.006$) and the extent of surgical resection ($p < 0.001$) with overall survival among various LGGs. However, this correlation varied across the three LGG molecular subtypes. In the IDHmut-Codel subgroup, overall survival was significantly associated with the extent of resection ($p = 0.01$), but neither pre- nor postoperative tumor volumes showed a significant relationship. In contrast, in the IDHmut-Noncodel subgroup, preoperative volume ($p = 0.018$), postoperative volume ($p = 0.004$), and the degree of resection ($p = 0.002$) each were associated with overall survival. For the IDHwt subtype, there was no significant association between tumor volumes or resection extent and overall survival [78].

The relationship between the extent of surgical resection and overall survival is particularly noted in molecularly characterized IDH mutant astrocytomas and oligodendrogliomas. This association appears more pronounced in astrocytomas, potentially because of the higher efficacy of non-surgical therapies in oligodendrogliomas or their generally longer survival periods, which could mask the survival benefits of surgical intervention [79,80]. Patel et al. reported in their 2018 study involving a cohort of 74 patients with WHO grade II diffuse gliomas that the extent of glioma resection correlated with overall survival in the IDH-wild-type subgroup but not in the IDH mutant subgroup. However, this study had limitations, such as an incomplete description of IDH mutation testing protocols and a lack of stratification by 1p/19q-codeletion status [81].

Prospective trials and retrospective studies have not consistently shown the significant prognostic effects of extent of resection (EOR) on overall survival (OS) and progression-free survival (PFS), but cognitive and quality of life outcomes post-surgery remain important considerations. The average preoperative cognitive function score in the LGG cohort, as measured by the EORTC score, was 80.9, compared to 70.9 in the high-grade glioma (HGG) group. Postoperatively, the LGG group's scores remained stable, while the HGG group showed significant improvement at 1- and 6-month follow-ups. In the LGG cohort, cognitive function changes varied, with 24% reporting improvement and 20% experiencing deterioration at 1 month postoperatively [82]. The rapid growth rate of IDH-wild-type gliomas may exert more pressure on adjacent brain structures than IDH mutant gliomas, suggesting that more aggressive surgical resection could improve cognitive outcomes by relieving mass effects and associated edema [83]. Postoperative experiences differ among patients, with some experiencing relief and others facing the stress of cancer diagnosis and ongoing surveillance or treatment. Notably, lower preoperative cognitive function scores have been observed in females compared to males [84].

Neuronavigation and brain mapping technologies, including functional MRI and cortical stimulation mapping, aid in precise resections while preserving quality of life. Neurosurgeons can customize procedures to individual brain structures, thereby minimizing permanent deficits. Brain mapping has shown efficacy in reducing permanent deficit rates, increasing gross total resection (GTR) rates, and providing survival benefits. Ideally, a prospective, multicenter trial would address this issue definitively, but challenges in recruitment, follow-up, and ethical considerations make organizing such a trial complex [85,86].

In neuro-oncology, temozolomide has gained attention as a chemotherapy drug, especially due to its ease of oral administration, lower toxicity compared to PCV (procarbazine, lomustine, and vincristine), effective penetration of the blood–brain barrier, and proven effectiveness against glioblastoma. Phase 2 studies have shown temozolomide to be effective against growing LGGs, whether previously exposed to radiation or not, on standard 5-day or alternate schedules like 3 weeks on followed by 1 week off, or 7 weeks on followed by 4 weeks off. Temozolomide has also been associated with improved quality of life outcomes [87].

In the realm of glioma treatment, there exist pivotal inquiries concerning the potential of temozolomide to either supplant radiotherapy or complement it in the management of low-grade gliomas (LGGs). Presently, ongoing clinical trials are diligently endeavoring to elucidate these quandaries. A phase 3 investigation spearheaded by a consortium of European and Canadian researchers is actively scrutinizing this matter by juxtaposing radiotherapy against temozolomide therapy for individuals afflicted with LGGs, with careful consideration being given to the chromosomal 1p status. This comprehensive study aims to assess a gamut of clinical outcomes, encompassing the likes of progression-free survival (PFS), neurocognitive functionality, and overall quality of life [88,89]. Furthermore, there are concerted endeavors to ascertain the advantages of amalgamating temozolomide with radiotherapy, particularly in the context of high-risk LGGs. The Radiation Therapy Oncology Group (RTOG) has successfully concluded its phase 2 inquiry (RTOG 0424), while the Eastern Cooperative Oncology Group (ECOG) has embarked upon a phase 3 exploration (ECOG E3F05). The overarching objective of these initiatives, in conjunction with similar studies unfolding in Europe, is to elucidate the role that temozolomide plays within the treatment paradigm for LGG [88,89].

In a separate investigation, a phase II trial delineated its primary objective as evaluating the response to temozolomide (TMZ) among pediatric patients grappling with recurrent or progressive LGG. The inception of this trial emanated from the Preston Robert Tisch Brain Tumor Center at Duke University Medical Center and subsequently expanded to encompass additional clinical sites. Notably, TMZ was administered orally under fasting conditions, with treatment cycles recurring at 28-day intervals. The observed outcomes encompassed partial response (PR) in three patients and minimal response (MR) in one patient, while 42% of patients exhibited stable disease (SD), and an equivalent percentage showed progressive disease (PD) after a minimum of two treatment cycles [90].

In a tangentially related vein, there exists substantiating evidence derived from the RTOG trial (RTOG 9802) which underscores the potential of employing procarbazine, lomustine, and vincristine (PCV) in tandem with radiotherapy, particularly in the context of recurrent LGGs post-radiotherapy. In this investigation, individuals who received a combined regimen of PCV and radiotherapy exhibited more favorable outcomes in terms of progression-free survival (PFS). Nevertheless, there was no statistically significant disparity in overall survival, thereby suggesting that PCV may serve as a potent adjunct both as a secondary intervention and when administered concomitantly with radiotherapy. It is imperative to note, however, that there exists a dearth of consensus regarding the optimal timing of surgery and its overarching impact on LGG management, necessitating further comprehensive exploration through prospective studies, mirroring the scrutiny accorded to the timing of radiotherapy in the treatment of LGGs [91].

It is paramount to acknowledge that radiotherapy stands as the sole therapeutic modality validated through a randomized controlled trial to confer certain advantages upon patients grappling with LGGs. Nonetheless, the optimal utilization of radiotherapy remains a topic of incessant deliberation. The EORTC 22845 study has proffered insights into this discourse, demonstrating that individuals subjected to early radiotherapy (54 Gy) experienced prolonged intervals devoid of disease progression (PFS) and exhibited superior seizure control relative to those subjected to delayed radiotherapy. Concretely, the progression-free survival stretched to 5.3 years for the early treatment cohort as opposed to 3.4 years for their delayed treatment counterparts ($p < 0.0001$). Furthermore, a noteworthy 75% of individuals in the early treatment cohort achieved seizure control in comparison to 59% in the delayed treatment cohort ($p = 0.0329$). Despite these discernible benefits, there was no marked discrepancy in overall survival between the two cohorts, with values of 7.4 years for the early cohort and 7.2 years for the delayed cohort. Given the absence of definitive data regarding quality of life, researchers have proffered the contention that it may be reasonable to defer radiotherapy for LGG patients who are in robust health. This hesitation emanates from the ambiguous equilibrium between the advantages inherent to extended progression-free survival and seizure control and the potential merits associated with overall survival. Additionally, it is worth noting that 35% of patients slated for deferred radiotherapy ultimately circumvented its necessity, thereby mitigating potential side effects [92].

Recent studies have cast a focused spotlight upon the evaluation of quality of life post-radiotherapy to gain deeper insights into its ramifications for individuals afflicted by LGGs. A phenomenon known as radiation leukoencephalopathy, which may manifest months or even years subsequent to cranial radiotherapy, is typified by a gradual decline in multifarious domains, including personality, equilibrium, urinary continence, attention, memory, and higher-order cognitive faculties [93]. To ameliorate these deleterious sequelae, select studies proffer the notion that through meticulous adjustments of total dosage, sessional dose, and irradiation field, it is feasible to uphold treatment efficacy while concurrently attenuating associated risks [94]. Nevertheless, in light of the relatively protracted overall survival (OS) rates observed among LGG patients, the potential of encountering these complications remains palpable. A recent comprehensive inquiry conducted by Douw et al. [95] undertook an exhaustive analysis of cognitive and quality of life outcomes among 65 LGG patients, with half having undergone radiotherapy. Over an average observation period spanning 12 years, the study unearthed that 27% of non-irradiated patients manifested substantive cognitive impairments in at least 5 of the 18 evaluated parameters. In stark contrast, this proportion burgeoned to 53% for those who had received radiotherapy. Predominant deficits were observed in the realms of cognitive processing and attention, with other noticeable, albeit statistically non-significant, declines detected in information processing speed, motor dexterity, and working memory [91,95].

In the sphere of pediatric neuro-oncology, the emergence of molecularly targeted treatments tailored for pediatric low-grade gliomas (pLGGs) has been greeted with considerable enthusiasm. These therapeutic interventions, with a specific focus on the dysregulated Ras-MAPK pathway, exemplified by RAF inhibitors and MEK inhibitors, are either receiving validation from the FDA or undergoing rigorous clinical evaluations for their applicability in the context of pLGGs [96,97]. However, it is of paramount significance to underscore that first-generation Type 1 BRAF inhibitors are not recommended for pLGGs characterized by BRAF rearrangements due to their proclivity to incite the paradoxical activation of the MAPK pathway via heightened RAF dimerization [98].

The PNOC001 phase II study, which embarked upon an investigation into the efficacy of the mTOR pathway inhibitor everolimus in cases of recurrent or progressive pLGG, charted pioneering territory by mandating a prerequisite for tissue diagnosis [99]. Subsequently, PNOC014 emerged as the inaugural trial tasked with scrutinizing the safety profile of a Pan-RAF inhibitor among pediatric patients grappling with LGG. The auspicious findings gleaned from the initial cohort of patients have expedited the progression to PNOC026/Day101-001—a phase II study singularly dedicated to appraising the oral Pan-RAF inhibitor (Day101) in individuals afflicted by recurrent or progressive pLGGs characterized by BRAF alterations [100]. Furthermore, therapeutic agents designed specifically to target the BRAF V600E mutation, such as dabrafenib and vemurafenib, have demonstrated encouraging outcomes in early-phase clinical trials involving patients with pLGGs. A recent revelation stemming from the phase II trial presented by Bouffet et al. at the American Society of Clinical Oncology (ASCO) Annual Meeting unveiled a noteworthy overall response rate (ORR) for the combination therapy of dabrafenib and trametinib (47%), signifying a substantial enhancement in comparison to the ORR associated with the conventional chemotherapy regimen employing carboplatin and vincristine (11%) [101].

It merits mention that therapeutic agents custom-tailored to target aberrant cellular pathways in pediatric low-grade gliomas (pLGGs) exhibit a toxicity spectrum that diverges markedly from that encountered with traditional chemotherapeutic regimens. Traditional chemotherapy regimens for pLGGs, while efficacious, are often accompanied by a constellation of adverse effects, encompassing myelosuppression, alopecia, ototoxicity—particularly notable with the utilization of carboplatin—and, although less frequently observed, perturbations in fertility potential, notably associated with procarbazine [102]. Conversely, targeted therapeutic modalities such as MEK and BRAF inhibitors give rise to a distinct set of side effects, which encompass dermatological toxicities, elevations in creatine phosphokinase (CPK), cardiovascular complications, and ocular adverse events [103].

7. Conclusions

The landscape of LGG treatment is undergoing a transformative shift. Emerging strategies challenge traditional methods, questioning the risks of a less dynamic approach and the direct implications of radiotherapy while highlighting the merits of proactive measures like comprehensive surgical removal and initial chemotherapy. Given the current data, a compelling approach might be to prioritize extensive surgery when feasible and reserve radiotherapy for the point of disease advancement. Ongoing clinical trials hold the promise of redefining LGG treatment, particularly spotlighting the potential role of temozolomide, which might even negate the necessity for radiotherapy in the future. It is imperative that future research delves deeper, leveraging advanced imaging and molecular markers to decode prognoses more accurately.

Funding: This research received no external funding.

Institutional Review Board Statement: Not applicable.

Informed Consent Statement: Not applicable.

Data Availability Statement: All data are available online on libraries such as PubMed.

Conflicts of Interest: The authors declare no conflict of interest.

References

1. Forst, D.A.; Nahed, B.V.; Loeffler, J.S.; Batchelor, T.T. Low-Grade Gliomas. *Oncologist* **2014**, *19*, 403–413. [CrossRef]
2. Sanai, N.; Chang, S.; Berger, M.S. Low-grade gliomas in adults: A review. *J. Neurosurg.* **2011**, *115*, 948–965. [CrossRef]
3. Louis, D.N.; Perry, A.; Burger, P.; Ellison, D.W.; Reifenberger, G.; von Deimling, A.; Aldape, K.; Brat, D.; Collins, V.P.; Eberhart, C.; et al. International Society of Neuropathology-Haarlem Consensus Guidelines for Nervous System Tumor Classification and Grading. *Brain Pathol.* **2014**, *24*, 429–435. [CrossRef]

4. Louis, D.N.; Perry, A.; Reifenberger, G.; Von Deimling, A.; Figarella-Branger, D.; Cavenee, W.K.; Ohgaki, H.; Wiestler, O.D.; Kleihues, P.; Ellison, D.W. The 2016 World Health Organization Classification of Tumors of the Central Nervous System: A summary. *Acta Neuropathol.* **2016**, *131*, 803–820. [CrossRef] [PubMed]
5. Ostrom, Q.T.; Gittleman, H.; Xu, J.; Kromer, C.; Wolinsky, Y.; Kruchko, C.; Barnholtz-Sloan, J.S. CBTRUS Statistical Report: Primary Brain and Other Central Nervous System Tumors Diagnosed in the United States in 2009–2013. *Neuro-Oncology* **2016**, *18*, v1–v75. [CrossRef] [PubMed]
6. Schiff, D. Low-grade Gliomas. *Contin. Lifelong Learn. Neurol.* **2017**, *23*, 1564–1579. [CrossRef]
7. Qaddoumi, I.; Orisme, W.; Wen, J.; Santiago, T.; Gupta, K.; Dalton, J.D.; Tang, B.; Haupfear, K.; Punchihewa, C.; Easton, J.; et al. Genetic alterations in uncommon low-grade neuroepithelial tumors: BRAF, FGFR1, and MYB mutations occur at high frequency and align with morphology. *Acta Neuropathol.* **2016**, *131*, 833–845. [CrossRef]
8. Ostrom, Q.T.; de Blank, P.M.; Kruchko, C.; Petersen, C.M.; Liao, P.; Finlay, J.L.; Stearns, D.S.; Wolff, J.E.; Wolinsky, Y.; Letterio, J.J.; et al. Alex's Lemonade Stand Foundation Infant and Childhood Primary Brain and Central Nervous System Tumors Diagnosed in the United States in 2007–2011. *Neuro-Oncology* **2015**, *16* (Suppl. 10), x1–x36. [CrossRef]
9. Ostrom, Q.T.; Patil, N.; Cioffi, G.; Waite, K.; Kruchko, C.; Barnholtz-Sloan, J.S. CBTRUS Statistical Report: Primary Brain and Other Central Nervous System Tumors Diagnosed in the United States in 2013–2017. *Neuro-Oncology* **2020**, *22* (Suppl. 1), iv1–iv96. [CrossRef]
10. Louis, D.N.; Perry, A.; Wesseling, P.; Brat, D.J.; Cree, I.A.; Figarella-Branger, D.; Hawkins, C.; Ng, H.K.; Pfister, S.M.; Reifenberger, G.; et al. The 2021 WHO Classification of Tumors of the Central Nervous System: A summary. *Neuro-Oncology* **2021**, *23*, 1231–1251. [CrossRef]
11. Fouke, S.J.; Benzinger, T.; Gibson, D.; Ryken, T.C.; Kalkanis, S.N.; Olson, J.J. The role of imaging in the management of adults with diffuse low grade glioma: A systematic review and evidence-based clinical practice guideline. *J. Neurooncol.* **2015**, *125*, 457–479. [CrossRef]
12. Schomas, D.A.; Laack, N.N.I.; Rao, R.D.; Meyer, F.B.; Shaw, E.G.; O'Neill, B.P.; Giannini, C.; Brown, P.D. Intracranial low-grade gliomas in adults: 30-year experience with long-term follow-up at Mayo Clinic. *Neuro-Oncology* **2009**, *11*, 437–445. [CrossRef]
13. Choi, C.; Raisanen, J.M.; Ganji, S.K.; Zhang, S.; McNeil, S.S.; An, Z.; Madan, A.; Hatanpaa, K.J.; Vemireddy, V.; Sheppard, C.A.; et al. Prospective Longitudinal Analysis of 2-Hydroxyglutarate Magnetic Resonance Spectroscopy Identifies Broad Clinical Utility for the Management of Patients with IDH -Mutant Glioma. *J. Clin. Oncol.* **2016**, *34*, 4030–4039. [CrossRef] [PubMed]
14. Van Den Bent, M.J. Interobserver variation of the histopathological diagnosis in clinical trials on glioma: A clinician's perspective. *Acta Neuropathol.* **2010**, *120*, 297–304. [CrossRef] [PubMed]
15. Bourne, T.D.; Schiff, D. Update on molecular findings, management and outcome in low-grade gliomas. *Nat. Rev. Neurol.* **2010**, *6*, 695–701. [CrossRef] [PubMed]
16. Schiff, D.; Brown, P.D.; Giannini, C. Outcome in adult low-grade glioma: The impact of prognostic factors and treatment. *Neurology* **2007**, *69*, 1366–1373. [CrossRef] [PubMed]
17. Balss, J.; Meyer, J.; Mueller, W.; Korshunov, A.; Hartmann, C.; Von Deimling, A. Analysis of the IDH1 codon 132 mutation in brain tumors. *Acta Neuropathol.* **2008**, *116*, 597–602. [CrossRef] [PubMed]
18. Yan, H.; Parsons, D.W.; Jin, G.; McLendon, R.; Rasheed, B.A.; Yuan, W.; Kos, I.; Batinic-Haberle, I.; Jones, S.; Riggins, G.J.; et al. IDH1 and IDH2 Mutations in Gliomas. *N. Engl. J. Med.* **2009**, *360*, 765–773. [CrossRef] [PubMed]
19. Dang, L.; White, D.W.; Gross, S.; Bennett, B.D.; Bittinger, M.A.; Driggers, E.M.; Fantin, V.R.; Jang, H.G.; Jin, S.; Keenan, M.C.; et al. Cancer-associated IDH1 mutations produce 2-hydroxyglutarate. *Nature* **2009**, *462*, 739–744. [CrossRef]
20. Brat, D.J.; Aldape, K.; Colman, H.; Figrarella-Branger, D.; Fuller, G.N.; Giannini, C.; Holland, E.C.; Jenkins, R.B.; Kleinschmidt-DeMasters, B.; Komori, T.; et al. cIMPACT-NOW update 5: Recommended grading criteria and terminologies for IDH-mutant astrocytomas. *Acta Neuropathol.* **2022**, *139*, 603–608. [CrossRef]
21. Komori, T. Grading of adult diffuse gliomas according to the 2021 WHO Classification of Tumors of the Central Nervous System. *Lab. Investig.* **2022**, *102*, 126–133. [CrossRef]
22. Gritsch, S.; Batchelor, T.T.; Castro, L.N.G. Diagnostic, therapeutic, and prognostic implications of the 2021 World Health Organization classification of tumors of the central nervous system. *Cancer* **2022**, *128*, 47–58. [CrossRef]
23. The Cancer Genome Atlas Research Network. Comprehensive, Integrative Genomic Analysis of Diffuse Lower-Grade Gliomas. *N. Engl. J. Med.* **2015**, *372*, 2481–2498. [CrossRef]
24. Tesileanu, C.M.S.; Dirven, L.; Wijnenga, M.M.J.; Koekkoek, J.A.F.; E Vincent, A.J.P.; Dubbink, H.J.; Atmodimedjo, P.N.; Kros, J.M.; Van Duinen, S.G.; Smits, M.; et al. Survival of diffuse astrocytic glioma, IDH1/2 wildtype, with molecular features of glioblastoma, WHO grade IV: A confirmation of the cIMPACT-NOW criteria. *Neuro-Oncology* **2020**, *22*, 515–523. [CrossRef] [PubMed]
25. Nabors, L.B.; Portnow, J.; Ahluwalia, M.; Baehring, J.; Brem, H.; Brem, S.; Butowski, N.; Campian, J.L.; Clark, S.W.; Fabiano, A.J.; et al. Central Nervous System Cancers, Version 3.2020, NCCN Clinical Practice Guidelines in Oncology. *J. Natl. Compr. Cancer Netw.* **2020**, *18*, 1537–1570. [CrossRef]
26. Plass, C.; Pfister, S.M.; Lindroth, A.M.; Bogatyrova, O.; Claus, R.; Lichter, P. Mutations in regulators of the epigenome and their connections to global chromatin patterns in cancer. *Nat. Rev. Genet.* **2013**, *14*, 765–780. [CrossRef] [PubMed]
27. Fontebasso, A.M.; Gayden, T.; Nikbakht, H.; Neirinck, M.; Papillon-Cavanagh, S.; Majewski, J.; Jabado, N. Epigenetic dysregulation: A novel pathway of oncogenesis in pediatric brain tumors. *Acta Neuropathol.* **2014**, *128*, 615–627. [CrossRef]

28. Lu, C.; Ward, P.S.; Kapoor, G.S.; Rohle, D.; Turcan, S.; Abdel-Wahab, O.; Edwards, C.R.; Khanin, R.; Figueroa, M.E.; Melnick, A.; et al. IDH mutation impairs histone demethylation and results in a block to cell differentiation. *Nature* **2012**, *483*, 474–478. [CrossRef]
29. Turcan, S.; Rohle, D.; Goenka, A.; Walsh, L.A.; Fang, F.; Yilmaz, E.; Campos, C.; Fabius, A.W.M.; Lu, C.; Ward, P.S.; et al. IDH1 mutation is sufficient to establish the glioma hypermethylator phenotype. *Nature* **2012**, *483*, 479–483. [CrossRef]
30. Lewis, P.W.; Müller, M.M.; Koletsky, M.S.; Cordero, F.; Lin, S.; Banaszynski, L.A.; Garcia, B.A.; Muir, T.W.; Becher, O.J.; Allis, C.D. Inhibition of PRC2 Activity by a Gain-of-Function H3 Mutation Found in Pediatric Glioblastoma. *Science* **2013**, *340*, 857–861. [CrossRef]
31. De Blank, P.; Fouladi, M.; Huse, J.T. Molecular markers and targeted therapy in pediatric low-grade glioma. *J. Neurooncol.* **2020**, *150*, 5–15. [CrossRef]
32. Capper, D.; Jones, D.T.W.; Sill, M.; Hovestadt, V.; Schrimpf, D.; Sturm, D.; Koelsche, C.; Sahm, F.; Chavez, L.; Reuss, D.E.; et al. DNA methylation-based classification of central nervous system tumours. *Nature* **2018**, *555*, 469–474. [CrossRef] [PubMed]
33. Banerjee, A.; Jakacki, R.I.; Onar-Thomas, A.; Wu, S.; Nicolaides, T.; Poussaint, T.Y.; Fangusaro, J.; Phillips, J.; Perry, A.; Turner, D.; et al. A phase I trial of the MEK inhibitor selumetinib (AZD6244) in pediatric patients with recurrent or refractory low-grade glioma: A Pediatric Brain Tumor Consortium (PBTC) study. *Neuro-Oncology* **2017**, *19*, 1135–1144. [CrossRef] [PubMed]
34. Fangusaro, J.; Onar-Thomas, A.; Poussaint, T.Y.; Wu, S.; Ligon, A.H.; Lindeman, N.; Banerjee, A.; Packer, R.J.; Kilburn, L.B.; Goldman, S.; et al. Selumetinib in paediatric patients with BRAF-aberrant or neurofibromatosis type 1-associated recurrent, refractory, or progressive low-grade glioma: A multicentre, phase 2 trial. *Lancet Oncol.* **2019**, *20*, 1011–1022. [CrossRef]
35. Bouffet, E.; Kieran, M.; Hargrave, D.; Roberts, S.; Aerts, I.; Broniscer, A.; Geoerger, B.; Dasgupta, K.; Tseng, L.; Russo, M.; et al. LGG-46. Trametinib Therapy in Pediatric Patients with Low-Grade Gliomas (Lgg) with Braf Gene Fusion; A Disease-Specific Cohort in the First Pediatric Testing of Trametinib. *Neuro-Oncology* **2018**, *20* (Suppl. 2), i114. [CrossRef]
36. Robison, N.; Pauly, J.; Malvar, J.; Gruber-Filbin, M.; de Mola, R.L.; Dorris, K.; Bendel, A.; Bowers, D.; Bornhorst, M.; Gauvain, K.; et al. LGG-44. A Phase I Dose Escalation Trial of the Mek1/2 Inhibitor Mek162 (Binimetinib) in Children with Low-Grade Gliomas and Other Ras/Raf Pathway-Activated Tumors. *Neuro-Oncology* **2018**, *20* (Suppl. 2), i114. [CrossRef]
37. Cabanillas, M.E.; Patel, A.; Danysh, B.P.; Dadu, R.; Kopetz, S.; Falchook, G. BRAF Inhibitors: Experience in Thyroid Cancer and General Review of Toxicity. *Horm. Cancer* **2015**, *6*, 21–36. [CrossRef] [PubMed]
38. Bavle, A.; Jones, J.; Lin, F.Y.; Malphrus, A.; Adesina, A.; Su, J. Dramatic clinical and radiographic response to BRAF inhibition in a patient with progressive disseminated optic pathway glioma refractory to MEK inhibition. *Pediatr. Hematol. Oncol.* **2017**, *34*, 254–259. [CrossRef]
39. Lassaletta, A.; Stucklin, A.G.; Ramaswamy, V.; Zapotocky, M.; McKeown, T.; Hawkins, C.; Bouffet, E.; Tabori, U. Profound clinical and radiological response to BRAF inhibition in a 2-month-old diencephalic child with hypothalamic/chiasmatic glioma. *Pediatr. Blood Cancer* **2016**, *63*, 2038–2041. [CrossRef]
40. Karajannis, M.A.; Legault, G.; Fisher, M.J.; Milla, S.S.; Cohen, K.J.; Wisoff, J.H.; Harter, D.H.; Goldberg, J.D.; Hochman, T.; Merkelson, A.; et al. Phase II study of sorafenib in children with recurrent or progressive low-grade astrocytomas. *Neuro-Oncology* **2014**, *16*, 1408–1416. [CrossRef]
41. Wright, K.D.; Zimmerman, M.A.; Fine, E.; Aspri, T.; Kieran, M.W.; Chi, S. LGG-26. Type II Braf Inhibitor Tak-580 Shows Promise for Upcoming Clinal Trial as Evidenced by Single Patient Ind Study. *Neuro-Oncology* **2018**, *20* (Suppl. 2), i110. [CrossRef]
42. Selt, F.; van Tilburg, C.M.; Bison, B.; Sievers, P.; Harting, I.; Ecker, J.; Pajtler, K.W.; Sahm, F.; Bahr, A.; Simon, M.; et al. Response to trametinib treatment in progressive pediatric low-grade glioma patients. *J. Neurooncol.* **2020**, *149*, 499–510. [CrossRef] [PubMed]
43. Louis, D.N.; von Deimling, A. Grading of diffuse astrocytic gliomas: Broders, Kernohan, Zülch, the WHO... and Shakespeare. *Acta Neuropathol.* **2017**, *134*, 517–520. [CrossRef] [PubMed]
44. Louis, D.N.; Wesseling, P.; Aldape, K.; Brat, D.J.; Capper, D.; Cree, I.A.; Eberhart, C.; Figarella-Branger, D.; Fouladi, M.; Fuller, G.N.; et al. cIMPACT-NOW update 6: New entity and diagnostic principle recommendations of the cIMPACT-Utrecht meeting on future CNS tumor classification and grading. *Brain Pathol.* **2020**, *30*, 844–856. [CrossRef] [PubMed]
45. Sievers, P.; Sill, M.; Schrimpf, D.; Stichel, D.; E Reuss, D.; Sturm, D.; Hench, J.; Frank, S.; Krskova, L.; Vicha, A.; et al. A subset of pediatric-type thalamic gliomas share a distinct DNA methylation profile, H3K27me3 loss and frequent alteration of EGFR. *Neuro-Oncology* **2021**, *23*, 34–43. [CrossRef]
46. Clarke, M.; Mackay, A.; Ismer, B.; Pickles, J.C.; Tatevossian, R.G.; Newman, S.; Bale, T.A.; Stoler, I.; Izquierdo, E.; Temelso, S.; et al. Infant High-Grade Gliomas Comprise Multiple Subgroups Characterized by Novel Targetable Gene Fusions and Favorable Outcomes. *Cancer Discov.* **2020**, *10*, 942–963. [CrossRef] [PubMed]
47. Ellison, D.W.; Hawkins, C.; Jones, D.T.; Onar-Thomas, A.; Pfister, S.M.; Reifenberger, G.; Louis, D.N. cIMPACT-NOW update 4: Diffuse gliomas characterized by MYB, MYBL1, or FGFR1 alterations or BRAF V600E mutation. *Acta Neuropathol.* **2019**, *137*, 683–687. [CrossRef]
48. Johnson, D.R.; Kaufmann, T.J.; Patel, S.H.; Chi, A.S.; Snuderl, M.; Jain, R. There is an exception to every rule—T2-FLAIR mismatch sign in gliomas. *Neuroradiology* **2019**, *61*, 225–227. [CrossRef]
49. Wisoff, J.H.; Sanford, R.; Heier, L.; Sposto, R.; Burger, P.C.; Yates, A.J.; Holmes, E.J.; E Kun, L. Primary neurosurgery for pediatric low-grade gliomas: A prospective multi-institutional study from the Children's Oncology Group. *Neurosurgery* **2011**, *68*, 1548–1555. [CrossRef]

50. Phi, J.H.; Kim, S.-K. Clinical pearls and advances in molecular researches of epilepsy-associated tumors. *J. Korean Neurosurg. Soc.* **2019**, *62*, 313–320. [CrossRef]
51. Chiang, J.; Harreld, J.H.; Tinkle, C.L.; Moreira, D.C.; Li, X.; Acharya, S.; Qaddoumi, I.; Ellison, D.W. A single-center study of the clinicopathologic correlates of gliomas with a MYB or MYBL1 alteration. *Acta Neuropathol.* **2019**, *138*, 1091–1092. [CrossRef]
52. Shakur, S.F.; McGirt, M.J.; Johnson, M.W.; Burger, P.C.; Ahn, E.; Carson, B.S.; Jallo, G.I. Angiocentric glioma: A case series: Clinical article. *J. Neurosurgery: Pediatr.* **2009**, *3*, 197–202. [CrossRef]
53. Wang, M.; Tihan, T.; Rojiani, A.M.; Bodhireddy, S.R.; Prayson, R.A.; Iacuone, J.J.; Alles, A.J.; Donahue, D.J.; Hessler, R.B.; Kim, J.H.; et al. Monomorphous angiocentric glioma: A distinctive epileptogenic neoplasm with features of infiltrating astrocytoma and ependymoma. *J. Neuropathol. Exp. Neurol.* **2005**, *64*, 875–881. [CrossRef]
54. Kurokawa, R.; Baba, A.; Emile, P.; Kurokawa, M.; Ota, Y.; Kim, J.; Capizzano, A.; Srinivasan, A.; Moritani, T. Neuroimaging features of angiocentric glioma: A case series and systematic review. *J. Neuroimaging* **2022**, *32*, 389–399. [CrossRef]
55. D'Aronco, L.; Rouleau, C.; Gayden, T.; Crevier, L.; Décarie, J.C.; Perreault, S.; Jabado, N.; Bandopadhayay, P.; Ligon, K.L.; Ellezam, B. Brainstem angiocentric gliomas with MYB–QKI rearrangements. *Acta Neuropathol.* **2017**, *134*, 667–669. [CrossRef]
56. Pearson, G.; Robinson, F.; Beers Gibson, T.; Xu, B.E.; Karandikar, M.; Berman, K.; Cobb, M.H. Mitogen-activated protein (MAP) kinase pathways: Regulation and physiological functions. *Endocr. Rev.* **2001**, *22*, 153–183. [PubMed]
57. Guo, Y.J.; Pan, W.W.; Liu, S.B.; Shen, Z.F.; Xu, Y.; Hu, L.L. ERK/MAPK signalling pathway and tumorigenesis. *Exp. Ther. Med.* **2020**, *19*, 1997–2007. [CrossRef] [PubMed]
58. Zhang, W.; Liu, H.T. MAPK signal pathways in the regulation of cell proliferation in mammalian cells. *Cell Res.* **2002**, *12*, 9–18. [CrossRef]
59. Orton, R.J.; Sturm, O.E.; Vyshemirsky, V.; Calder, M.; Gilbert, D.R.; Kolch, W. Computational modelling of the receptor-tyrosine-kinase-activated MAPK pathway. *Biochem. J.* **2005**, *392*, 249–261. [CrossRef]
60. Huse, J.T.; Snuderl, M.; Jones, D.T.W.; Brathwaite, C.D.; Altman, N.; Lavi, E.; Saffery, R.; Sexton-Oates, A.; Blumcke, I.; Capper, D.; et al. Polymorphous low-grade neuroepithelial tumor of the young (PLNTY): An epileptogenic neoplasm with oligodendroglioma-like components, aberrant CD34 expression, and genetic alterations involving the MAP kinase pathway. *Acta Neuropathol.* **2017**, *133*, 417–429. [CrossRef] [PubMed]
61. Johnson, D.R.; Giannini, C.; Jenkins, R.B.; Kim, D.K.; Kaufmann, T.J. Plenty of calcification: Imaging characterization of polymorphous low-grade neuroepithelial tumor of the young. *Neuroradiology* **2019**, *61*, 1327–1332. [CrossRef]
62. Lelotte, J.; Duprez, T.; Raftopoulos, C.; Michotte, A. Polymorphous low-grade neuroepithelial tumor of the young: Case report of a newly described histopathological entity. *Acta Neurol. Belg.* **2020**, *120*, 729–732. [CrossRef] [PubMed]
63. Gupta, V.R.; Giller, C.; Kolhe, R.; Forseen, S.E.; Sharma, S. Polymorphous low-grade neuroepithelial tumor of the young: A case report with genomic findings. *World Neurosurg.* **2019**, *132*, 347–355. [CrossRef] [PubMed]
64. Fabbri, V.P.; Caporalini, C.; Asioli, S.; Bucciero, A. Paediatric-type diffuse low-grade gliomas: A clinically and biologically distinct group of tumours with a favourable outcome. *Pathologica* **2022**, *114*, 410–421. [CrossRef] [PubMed]
65. Ryall, S.; Tabori, U.; Hawkins, C. Pediatric low-grade glioma in the era of molecular diagnostics. *Acta Neuropathol. Commun.* **2020**, *8*, 30. [CrossRef] [PubMed]
66. Fisher, P.G.; Tihan, T.; Goldthwaite, P.T.; Wharam, M.D.; Carson, B.S.; Weingart, J.D.; Repka, M.X.; Cohen, K.J.; Burger, P.C. Outcome analysis of childhood low-grade astrocytomas. *Pediatr. Blood Cancer* **2008**, *51*, 245–250. [CrossRef] [PubMed]
67. Listernick, R.; Ferner, R.E.; Liu, G.T.; Gutmann, D.H. Optic pathway gliomas in neurofibromatosis-1: Controversies and recommendations. *Ann. Neurol.* **2007**, *61*, 189–198. [CrossRef]
68. Sievert, A.J.; Fisher, M.J. Pediatric Low-Grade Gliomas. *J. Child Neurol.* **2009**, *24*, 1397–1408. [CrossRef]
69. Gajjar, A.; Sanford, R.; Heideman, R.; Jenkins, J.J.; Walter, A.; Li, Y.; Langston, J.W.; Muhlbauer, M.; Boyett, J.M.; Kun, L. Low-grade astrocytoma: A decade of experience at St. Jude Children's Research Hospital. *J. Clin. Oncol.* **1997**, *15*, 2792–2799. [CrossRef]
70. Jaunmuktane, Z.; Capper, D.; Jones, D.T.W.; Schrimpf, D.; Sill, M.; Dutt, M.; Suraweera, N.; Pfister, S.M.; von Deimling, A.; Brandner, S. Methylation array profiling of adult brain tumours: Diagnostic outcomes in a large, single centre. *Acta Neuropathol. Commun.* **2019**, *7*, 24. [CrossRef]
71. Capper, D.; Stichel, D.; Sahm, F.; Jones, D.T.W.; Schrimpf, D.; Sill, M.; Schmid, S.; Hovestadt, V.; Reuss, D.E.; Koelsche, C.; et al. Practical implementation of DNA methylation and copy-number-based CNS tumor diagnostics: The Heidelberg experience. *Acta Neuropathol.* **2018**, *136*, 181–210. [CrossRef] [PubMed]
72. Castro, L.N.G.; Wesseling, P. The cIMPACT-NOW updates and their significance to current neuro-oncology practice. *Neuro-Oncol. Pract.* **2021**, *8*, 4–10. [CrossRef] [PubMed]
73. Pignatti, F.; Bent, M.v.D.; Curran, D.; Debruyne, C.; Sylvester, R.; Therasse, P.; Áfra, D.; Cornu, P.; Bolla, M.; Vecht, C.; et al. Prognostic Factors for Survival in Adult Patients with Cerebral Low-Grade Glioma. *J. Clin. Oncol.* **2002**, *20*, 2076–2084. [CrossRef] [PubMed]
74. Pouratian, N.; Mut, M.; Jagannathan, J.; Lopes, M.B.; Shaffrey, M.E.; Schiff, D. Low-grade gliomas in older patients: A retrospective analysis of prognostic factors. *J. Neurooncol.* **2008**, *90*, 341–350. [CrossRef] [PubMed]
75. Schomas, D.A.; Laack, N.N.; Brown, P.D. Low-grade gliomas in older patients: Long-term follow-up from Mayo Clinic. *Cancer* **2009**, *115*, 3969–3978. [CrossRef] [PubMed]

76. Smith, J.S.; Chang, E.F.; Lamborn, K.R.; Chang, S.M.; Prados, M.D.; Cha, S.; Tihan, T.; VandenBerg, S.; McDermott, M.W.; Berger, M.S. Role of Extent of Resection in the Long-Term Outcome of Low-Grade Hemispheric Gliomas. *J. Clin. Oncol.* **2008**, *26*, 1338–1345. [CrossRef] [PubMed]
77. McGirt, M.J.; Chaichana, K.L.; Attenello, F.J.; Weingart, J.D.; Than, K.; Burger, P.C.; Olivi, A.; Brem, H.; Quiñones-Hinojosa, A. Extent of Surgical Resection Is Independently Associated with Survival in Patients with Hemispheric Infiltrating Low-Grade Gliomas. *Neurosurgery* **2008**, *63*, 700–708. [CrossRef]
78. Patel, S.; Bansal, A.; Young, E.; Batchala, P.; Patrie, J.; Lopes, M.; Jain, R.; Fadul, C.; Schiff, D. Extent of Surgical Resection in Lower-Grade Gliomas: Differential Impact Based on Molecular Subtype. *AJNR Am. J. Neuroradiol.* **2019**, *40*, 1149–1155. [CrossRef]
79. Cairncross, G.; Wang, M.; Shaw, E.; Jenkins, R.; Brachman, D.; Buckner, J.; Fink, K.; Souhami, L.; Laperriere, N.; Curran, W.; et al. Phase III Trial of Chemoradiotherapy for Anaplastic Oligodendroglioma: Long-Term Results of RTOG 9402. *J. Clin. Oncol.* **2013**, *31*, 337–343. [CrossRef]
80. Ceccarelli, M.; Barthel, F.P.; Malta, T.M.; Sabedot, T.S.; Salama, S.R.; Murray, B.A.; Morozova, O.; Newton, Y.; Radenbaugh, A.; Pagnotta, S.M.; et al. Molecular Profiling Reveals Biologically Discrete Subsets and Pathways of Progression in Diffuse Glioma. *Cell* **2016**, *164*, 550–563. [CrossRef]
81. Patel, E.D.; Bander, E.D.; A Venn, R.; Powell, T.; Cederquist, G.Y.-M.; Schaefer, P.M.; A Puchi, L.; Akhmerov, A.; Ogilvie, S.; Reiner, A.S.; et al. The Role of Extent of Resection in IDH1 Wild-Type or Mutant Low-Grade Gliomas. *Neurosurgery* **2018**, *82*, 808–814. [CrossRef] [PubMed]
82. Schei, S.; Solheim, O.; Salvesen, Ø.; Hansen, T.I.; Sagberg, L.M. Patient-reported cognitive function before and after glioma surgery. *Acta Neurochir.* **2022**, *164*, 2009–2019. [CrossRef] [PubMed]
83. Wefel, J.S.; Noll, K.R.; Rao, G.; Cahill, D.P. Neurocognitive function varies by IDH1 genetic mutation status in patients with malignant glioma prior to surgical resection. *Neuro-Oncology* **2016**, *18*, 1656–1663. [CrossRef] [PubMed]
84. Gehring, K.; Taphoorn, M.J.; Sitskoorn, M.M.; Aaronson, N.K. Predictors of subjective versus objective cognitive functioning in patients with stable grades II and III glioma. *Neuro-Oncol. Pract.* **2015**, *2*, 20–31. [CrossRef] [PubMed]
85. Duffau, H.; Lopes, M.; Arthuis, F.; Bitar, A.; Sichez, J.-P.; Van Effenterre, R.; Capelle, L. Contribution of intraoperative electrical stimulations in surgery of low grade gliomas: A comparative study between two series without (1985–1996) and with (1996–2003) functional mapping in the same institution. *J. Neurol. Neurosurg. Psychiatry* **2005**, *76*, 845. [CrossRef] [PubMed]
86. Duffau, H. Surgery of low-grade gliomas: Towards a 'functional neurooncology'. *Curr. Opin. Oncol.* **2009**, *21*, 543–549. [CrossRef]
87. Liu, R.; Solheim, K.; Polley, M.-Y.; Lamborn, K.R.; Page, M.; Fedoroff, A.; Rabbitt, J.; Butowski, N.; Prados, M.; Chang, S.M. Quality of life in low-grade glioma patients receiving temozolomide. *Neuro-Oncology* **2009**, *11*, 59–68. [CrossRef]
88. Shaw, E.G.; Berkey, B.; Coons, S.W.; Brachman, D.; Buckner, J.C.; Stelzer, K.J.; Barger, G.R.; Brown, P.D.; Gilbert, M.R.; Mehta, M. Initial report of Radiation Therapy Oncology Group (RTOG) 9802: Prospective studies in adult low-grade glioma (LGG). *J. Clin. Oncol.* **2006**, *24*, 1500. [CrossRef]
89. Duffau, H.; Taillandier, L.; Capelle, L. Radical surgery after chemotherapy: A new therapeutic strategy to envision in grade II glioma. *J. Neurooncol.* **2006**, *80*, 171–176. [CrossRef]
90. Gururangan, S.; Fisher, M.J.; Allen, J.C.; Herndon, J.E.; Quinn, J.A.; Reardon, D.A.; Vredenburgh, J.J.; Desjardins, A.; Phillips, P.C.; Watral, M.A.; et al. Temozolomide in Children with progressive low-grade glioma1. *Neuro-Oncology* **2007**, *9*, 161–168. [CrossRef]
91. Pouratian, N.; Schiff, D. Management of Low-Grade Glioma. *Curr. Neurol. Neurosci. Rep.* **2010**, *10*, 224–231. [CrossRef] [PubMed]
92. Van den Bent, M.J.; Afra, D.; De Witte, O.; Hassel, M.B.; Schraub, S.; Hoang-Xuan, K.; Malmström, P.-O.; Collette, L.; Piérart, M.; Mirimanoff, R.; et al. Long-term efficacy of early versus delayed radiotherapy for low-grade astrocytoma and oligodendroglioma in adults: The EORTC 22845 randomised trial. *Lancet* **2005**, *366*, 985–990. [CrossRef] [PubMed]
93. Surma-Aho, O.; Niemela, M.; Vilkki, J.; Kouri, M.; Brander, A.; Salonen, O.; Paetau, A.; Kallio, M.; Pyykkonen, L.J.; Jaaskelainen, J. Adverse long-term effects of brain radiotherapy in adult low-grade glioma patients. *Neurology* **2001**, *56*, 1285–1290. [CrossRef] [PubMed]
94. Baumert, B.G.; Stupp, R. Low-grade glioma: A challenge in therapeutic options: The role of radiotherapy. *Ann. Oncol.* **2008**, *19*, vii217–vii222. [CrossRef] [PubMed]
95. Douw, L.; Klein, M.; Fagel, S.S.; van den Heuvel, J.; Taphoorn, M.J.; Aaronson, N.K.; Postma, T.J.; Vandertop, W.P.; Mooij, J.J.; Boerman, R.H.; et al. Cognitive and radiological effects of radiotherapy in patients with low-grade glioma: Long-term follow-up. *Lancet Neurol.* **2009**, *8*, 810–818. [CrossRef]
96. Zhao, Y.; Adjei, A.A. The clinical development of MEK inhibitors. *Nat. Rev. Clin. Oncol.* **2014**, *11*, 385–400. [CrossRef]
97. Nicolaides, T.; Nazemi, K.J.; Crawford, J.; Kilburn, L.; Minturn, J.; Gajjar, A.; Gauvain, K.; Leary, S.; Dhall, G.; Aboian, M.; et al. Phase I study of vemurafenib in children with recurrent or progressive BRAFV600E mutant brain tumors: Pacific Pediatric Neuro-Oncology Consortium study (PNOC-002). *Oncotarget* **2020**, *11*, 1942–1952. [CrossRef]
98. Sievert, A.J.; Lang, S.-S.; Boucher, K.L.; Madsen, P.J.; Slaunwhite, E.; Choudhari, N.; Kellet, M.; Storm, P.B.; Resnick, A.C. Paradoxical activation and RAF inhibitor resistance of BRAF protein kinase fusions characterizing pediatric astrocytomas. *Proc. Natl. Acad. Sci. USA* **2013**, *110*, 5957–5962. [CrossRef]
99. Mueller, S.; Aboian, M.; Nazemi, K.; Gauvain, K.; Yoon, J.; Minturn, J.; Leary, S.; AbdelBaki, M.S.; Goldman, S.; Elster, J.; et al. LGG-53. PNOC001 (NCT01734512): A Phase II Study of Everolimus for Recurrent or Progressive Pediatric Low-Grade Gliomas (pLGG). *Neuro-Oncology* **2020**, *22* (Suppl. S3), iii376. [CrossRef]

100. Wright, K.; Krzykwa, E.; Greenspan, L.; Chi, S.; Yeo, K.K.; Prados, M.; Mueller, S.; Haas-Kogan, D. CTNI-19. Phase I Trial of Day101 in Pediatric Patients with Radiographically Recurrent or Progressive Low-Grade Glioma (LGG). *Neuro-Oncology* **2020**, *22* (Suppl. 2), ii46. [CrossRef]
101. Bouffet, E.; Hansford, J.; Garré, M.L.; Hara, J.; Plant-Fox, A.; Aerts, I.; Locatelli, F.; Van der Lugt, J.; Papusha, L.; Sahm, F.; et al. Primary analysis of a phase II trial of dabrafenib plus trametinib (dab + tram) in BRAF V600–mutant pediatric low-grade glioma (pLGG). *J. Clin. Oncol.* **2020**, *40*, LBA2002. [CrossRef]
102. Ater, J.L.; Zhou, T.; Holmes, E.; Mazewski, C.M.; Booth, T.N.; Freyer, D.R.; Lazarus, K.H.; Packer, R.J.; Prados, M.; Sposto, R.; et al. Randomized Study of Two Chemotherapy Regimens for Treatment of Low-Grade Glioma in Young Children: A Report from the Children's Oncology Group. *J. Clin. Oncol.* **2012**, *30*, 2641–2647. [CrossRef] [PubMed]
103. Egan, G.; Hamilton, J.; McKeown, T.; Bouffet, E.; Tabori, U.; Dirks, P.; Bartels, U. Trametinib Toxicities in Patients with Low-grade Gliomas and Diabetes Insipidus: Related Findings? *J. Pediatr. Hematol. Oncol.* **2020**, *42*, e248–e250. [CrossRef] [PubMed]

Disclaimer/Publisher's Note: The statements, opinions and data contained in all publications are solely those of the individual author(s) and contributor(s) and not of MDPI and/or the editor(s). MDPI and/or the editor(s) disclaim responsibility for any injury to people or property resulting from any ideas, methods, instructions or products referred to in the content.

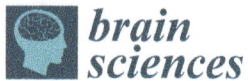

Review

Exploring Monocytes-Macrophages in Immune Microenvironment of Glioblastoma for the Design of Novel Therapeutic Strategies

Matías Daniel Caverzán [1,2], Lucía Beaugé [1,3], Paula Martina Oliveda [3], Bruno Cesca González [3], Eugenia Micaela Bühler [3,4] and Luis Exequiel Ibarra [3,4,*]

1. Instituto de Investigaciones en Tecnologías Energéticas y Materiales Avanzados (IITEMA), Universidad Nacional de Rio Cuarto (UNRC) y Consejo Nacional de Investigaciones Científicas y Técnicas (CONICET), Río Cuarto X5800BIA, Argentina
2. Departamento de Patología Animal, Facultad de Agronomía y Veterinaria, Universidad Nacional de Rio Cuarto, Rio Cuarto X5800BIA, Argentina
3. Departamento de Biología Molecular, Facultad de Ciencias Exactas, Fisicoquímicas y Naturales, Universidad Nacional de Rio Cuarto, Rio Cuarto X5800BIA, Argentina
4. Instituto de Biotecnología Ambiental y Salud (INBIAS), Universidad Nacional de Rio Cuarto (UNRC) y Consejo Nacional de Investigaciones Científicas y Técnicas (CONICET), Rio Cuarto X5800BIA, Argentina
* Correspondence: libarra@exa.unrc.edu.ar

Citation: Caverzán, M.D.; Beaugé, L.; Oliveda, P.M.; Cesca González, B.; Bühler, E.M.; Ibarra, L.E. Exploring Monocytes-Macrophages in Immune Microenvironment of Glioblastoma for the Design of Novel Therapeutic Strategies. *Brain Sci.* 2023, *13*, 542. https://doi.org/10.3390/brainsci13040542

Academic Editor: Álmos Klekner

Received: 7 February 2023
Revised: 20 March 2023
Accepted: 22 March 2023
Published: 24 March 2023

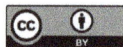

Copyright: © 2023 by the authors. Licensee MDPI, Basel, Switzerland. This article is an open access article distributed under the terms and conditions of the Creative Commons Attribution (CC BY) license (https://creativecommons.org/licenses/by/4.0/).

Abstract: Gliomas are primary malignant brain tumors. These tumors seem to be more and more frequent, not only because of a true increase in their incidence, but also due to the increase in life expectancy of the general population. Among gliomas, malignant gliomas and more specifically glioblastomas (GBM) are a challenge in their diagnosis and treatment. There are few effective therapies for these tumors, and patients with GBM fare poorly, even after aggressive surgery, chemotherapy, and radiation. Over the last decade, it is now appreciated that these tumors are composed of numerous distinct tumoral and non-tumoral cell populations, which could each influence the overall tumor biology and response to therapies. Monocytes have been proved to actively participate in tumor growth, giving rise to the support of tumor-associated macrophages (TAMs). In GBM, TAMs represent up to one half of the tumor mass cells, including both infiltrating macrophages and resident brain microglia. Infiltrating macrophages/monocytes constituted ~ 85% of the total TAM population, they have immune functions, and they can release a wide array of growth factors and cytokines in response to those factors produced by tumor and non-tumor cells from the tumor microenvironment (TME). A brief review of the literature shows that this cell population has been increasingly studied in GBM TME to understand its role in tumor progression and therapeutic resistance. Through the knowledge of its biology and protumoral function, the development of therapeutic strategies that employ their recruitment as well as the modulation of their immunological phenotype, and even the eradication of the cell population, can be harnessed for therapeutic benefit. This revision aims to summarize GBM TME and localization in tumor niches with special focus on TAM population, its origin and functions in tumor progression and resistance to conventional and experimental GBM treatments. Moreover, recent advances on the development of TAM cell targeting and new cellular therapeutic strategies based on monocyte/macrophages recruitment to eradicate GBM are discussed as complementary therapeutics.

Keywords: glioblastoma; macrophages; monocytes; tumor microenvironment; targeted therapy; cell-based therapy

1. Introduction

Brain and other nervous system cancers are among the most fatal cancers in several countries around the world [1–3]. In 2019, there were 347,992 global cases of brain and

Central Nervous System (CNS) cancers, which showed a significant increase in its incidence (94.35%) from the period between 1990 to 2019 [4]. An estimated 251,329 people passed away from primary cancerous brain and central nervous system (CNS) tumors in 2020 [5]. Among brain tumors, malignant brain tumor incidence rates are slightly decreasing over the last decade; however, mortality rates increased in the same period of time [1]. Specifically, in the malignant brain tumor group, 5-year glioblastoma (GBM) survival only increased from 4% to 7% during the last years [1]. However, survival rates vary widely and depend on several factors, including the degree of malignancy and cellular and molecular distinctive features.

Over the years, the identification of distinct genetic and epigenetic profiles in various brain tumors has improved the classification of more than 100 cancerous diseases that can appear in this preferential location and allows the discovery of new diagnostic, prognostic, and predictive molecular biomarkers to improve the prediction of response to treatment and therapeutic outcome [6]. The classification of brain tumors has experienced numerous changes over the past half century. The World Health Organization (WHO) has played a key role in the effort to split malignancies according to clinical and histological profiles from the first classification launched in 1979 [7]. This increased complexity as reflected in the last classification in 2021 summarizes the current understanding of the clinical, histologic, and molecular features of CNS tumors and paves the way for further precision in tumor classification and a shift towards increased use of targeted therapeutics [8].

Among malignant gliomas, GBM is one of the most aggressive malignancies, accounting for 14.5% of all central nervous system tumors and 48.6% of malignant central nervous system tumors [9]. The median overall survival (OS) of GBM patients is only 15 months, which highlights the failure with conventional treatments applied so far [10]. The ongoing effort to identify potential new molecular or cellular targets for the development of effective clinical therapies has not yet led to significant improvements in survival rate, with most patients surviving not more than a few years. In this sense, the understanding of the molecular interactions among not only tumor cells but also other types of non-tumor cells that reside into tumors has made it possible to improve therapeutic targeting [11]. Nevertheless, the majority of studies related to GBM treatments over the last decades has focused on eradication of tumor cells, whereas more recent efforts have been placed on understanding the microenvironment surrounding tumor cells, the interaction between these cellular and acellular components in different preformed tumor niches, and how to design new treatment options that target these components in a multi-attack approach [12,13]. Tumor-associated macrophages (TAMs) play an essential role in the GBM microenvironment since this non-tumoral cell population represents up to 50% of tumor mass and specific treatments to eliminate these cells have been proposed in the past [14,15]. In this review, updated research on the components of the tumor microenvironment (TME) in GBM is presented, with a special focus on the main non-tumor cell population represented by macrophages and their location into GBM tumor niches. The main aspects included in the analysis are related to the origin of these cells, their recruitment within the GBM, their participation in the gliomagenesis process as well as in the resistance to the main treatments used. Moreover, the main findings related to the therapeutic targeting of macrophages based on their recruitment, polarization, and functions for GBM therapy are presented.

2. Search Strategy and Selection Criteria

The original published research studies in peer-reviewed journals cited in this review were published between 2014 and 2023, with a major focus on the years 2018 to 2022. The PubMed, Scopus, Google Academic, and the US National Institutes of Health Clinical Trials Registry (http://www.clinicaltrials.gov, accessed on 10 December 2022) databases were used to search relevant studies with the following keywords: "malignant gliomas", "glioblastoma", "tumor microenvironment", "macrophages", "targeting macrophages", "microglia", "monocyte recruitment" in different combinations. Duplicates and articles in languages other than English were excluded. Full articles with restricted access were also excluded. All references were cited to the content-related parts of the review.

3. Classification, Biological Features, and Tumor Niches of GBMs

Tumors generated from different glial cells in the CNS are known as gliomas. To unify the diagnostic criteria, WHO proposed a CNS tumor classification and nomenclature guide based on the combination of parameters such as tumor mass extension into the brain tissue, the proliferation of the microvasculature, genetic alterations, presence of necrotic areas, and cell proliferation index [16]. Low-grade gliomas (LGG) (grades 1 and 2) are less invasive while high-grade gliomas (3 and 4) represent the most challenging brain tumors. WHO Classification of Tumors of the CNS (WHO CNS5), revised recently, has suffered substantial changes by moving further to advance the role of molecular and genetic biomarkers' identification in the diagnostics of CNS tumor classification but remaining rooted in other established approaches to tumor characterization, including histology and immunohistochemistry [8]. In addition, the number denoted in the gradation is now Arabic instead of a Roman numeral. This classification would have an impact in the correct diagnosis, treatment definition, and prognosis of the disease. For example, the identification of mutations in isocitrate dehydrogenase (IDH) defines gliomas with the best prognosis independently of their tumor grade [17]. IDH mutation in GBM is frequently associated with TP53 mutation, and it has a generally better prognosis than IDH-wildtype glioblastoma.

Among malignant gliomas, grade 4 tumors or GBM are the most aggressive, and they possess high levels of intratumoral and intertumoral heterogeneity. Apart from containing different genetic signatures, GBMs present different transcriptomic profiles, which have recently originated a new classification: classical, mesenchymal, neural, and proneural tumors [18]. However, this classification does not impose a different therapeutic approach, so it is not routinely performed in the clinic [11]. For this reason, the WHO classification includes GBM as part of the diffuse astrocytic and oligodendroglial tumors group and they are divided into three subgroups based on IDH mutations: (1) glioblastoma, IDH-wildtype, clinically identified as primary GBM and predominant in patients over 55 years of age, (2) glioblastoma, IDH-mutant, clinically identified as secondary GBM and more common in younger patients, and (3) glioblastoma NOS (not otherwise specified), which does not fit into the other categories and is not well defined [9].

During the gliomagenesis process, different genetic abnormalities signatures lead to GBM malignant cell transformation; however, tumors masses formed need a great amount of genetic, epigenetic, and metabolic changes in order to continue proliferation and expansion to the surrounding healthy brain tissue, including changes in energetic metabolism, invasive capacity, remodeling of the extracellular matrix (ECM), cell migration and promotion of angiogenesis [9]. The detachment of invading tumor cells from the primary tumor mass accompanied by decreased expression of Cx43 and increased CD44 expression, followed by the anchored and degradation of ECM by overexpressed MMP-9 and MMP-2, allow the colonization of tumor cells into normal brain tissues such as brain parenchyma, leptomeningeal space, white matter tracts of corpus callosum, and perivascular space [19,20]. GBM cells also attract non-tumoral cells such as microglia, astrocytes, and endothelial cells that secrete proteases to enhance migration [14]. In this migration movement, tumor cells in immediate proximity of pre-existing and degenerated vessels begin to die, forming foci of necrosis. These foci become surrounded by tumor cells, which eventually form pseudopalisade and upregulate the expression of vascular endothelial growth factor (VEGF), leading to vascular hyperplasia, distinguishing glomeruloid vascular proliferation areas. Different niches within the tumor mass will be created, which contemplate the coexistence of tumor cells and non-tumor cells in different areas such as the hypoxic/necrotic niche, invasive front, and perivascular zones that not only define different cell constituents [21], but are also characterized by cell plasticity, heterogeneity, and resistance to radiotherapy and chemotherapy [12].

4. Tumor Microenvironment (TME) in GBM Niches

TME plays an essential role in cancer development. Various non-tumor cells participate in the TME, collaborating in growth, survival, invasion, and metastasis of tumor cells [22]. Tumor cells structure the tumor parenchyma and non-tumor cells, which are part of the stroma, have a cellular heterogeneity. Normal and reactive astrocytes, fibroblasts, immune cells, microglia, macrophages, endothelial cells, and vascular pericytes are part of the microenvironment of the GBM. Furthermore, proteins and non-protein biomolecules (polysaccharides, hormones, nitric oxide, etc.) are produced by all the cell types to promote neoplastic growth, and they are also main components of the TME [23]. More importantly, glioma stem cells (GSCs) have the capacity to generate new tumor cells and support cancer growth and regrowth even after the majority of treatments employed [22]. The location of GSCs into the tumor has been discussed, but they can be found in different niches of GBM close to central necrosis [22].

Perivascular niches are composed of blood vessels such as capillaries or arterioles, and GSCs have close contact with them [24]. Furthermore, reactive astrocytes presented in these areas generate angiopoietins 1 and 2 (Ang-1 or Ang-2) and VEGF, which are important cytokines for tumor cells that use the perivascular space for invasion and co-opt existing vessels as satellite tumors [25]. VEGF induced Ang-1 pericytes' recruitment to improve vascular stability. Moreover, these molecules also participate in the recruitment of myeloid cell populations into GBM [26,27]. Around necrotic zone, Ang-1 is absent because hypoxia down-regulates Ang-1 expression; nevertheless, Ang-1 is more perceived in the tumor periphery [28].

The main molecular inductor of angiogenesis in perinecrotic areas is hypoxia-inducible factor 1 (HIF-1), which intensifies VEGF expression after translocation to nuclei [28]. On the other hand, perinecrotic niches are considered zones of high tumor cell proliferation and low endothelial cell development. An important feature in necrotic foci is the appearance of GSC around them [28].

Moreover, other non-cellular components belonging to ECM are upregulated into TME, such as hyaluronan, vitronectin, osteopontin, tenascin-C, SPARC, and BEHAB with an impact on the GBM progression. Their overexpression is correlated with poor prognosis [29]. This is of particular interest because hyaluronan helps in the progression of malignant gliomas by facilitating primary brain tumor invasion in and migration through its two cellular receptors, CD44 and RHAMM [29]. CD44 is the major receptor for hyaluronan and it contributes to cell–matrix interactions, cell migration, and regulation of tumor growth [29]. Tight junctions between ECM components and integrins of neoplastic cells lead to an increment in apoptotic resistance, proliferation, and migration [30]. Other overexpressed proteins such as fibronectin, which has the ability to regulate cell adhesion and migration, have been proposed as promoters of tumor invasion [31]. The overexpression of TGF-β, TGF-α, EGF, VEGF, and TNF-α promote both survival and tumor proliferation of GBM [32]. Many GBMs present EGFR amplification and/or mutation, and to a lesser extent they overexpress PDGF receptors. Those EGFR-dependent tumors would develop drug treatment resistance [33,34].

TAMs play an essential role in the GBM microenvironment. These cells can come from two different tissue origins. Microglia cells are derived from primitive hematopoiesis in the fetal yolk sac and take up residence in the brain during early fetal development [35]. Microglia differentiation and proliferation requires colony-stimulating factor 1 (CSF1), CD34, and the transcription factor PU.1 [35]. Under normal physiological conditions, the brain is only occupied by resident microglia, and the presence of other bone-marrow-derived macrophages (BMDM) are associated with the diseased brain. Microglia are long-lived and have self-renewal capacity compared with BMDM [36]. In addition, peripheral macrophages driven by inflammatory factors from GBM tumor cells and other TME cell populations promote the infiltration of circulating BMDM derived from hematopoietic stem cells that can migrate to tumor tissue; they penetrate the blood–brain tumor barrier (BBTB), and probably the intact blood–brain barrier (BBB), where they differentiate into monocyte-derived macrophages and promote tumor progression [14,37]. The BBB provides both a physical and a physiological barrier between the brain parenchyma and the bloodstream restricting the entry of various components such as peptides and proteins, due to tight junctions [38] and also limits the permeability of immune cells from blood [39]. Upon brain injury produced by GBM tumorigenesis, the BBB becomes compromised (forming the BTBB) leading to significant influx of circulating BMDM and other immunological cells [40]. Moreover, Wang L.J. reported through immune landscape analysis that the risk score was significantly related to TME, specifically taking into account the macrophage cell population in malignant gliomas. Authors demonstrated the value of TAMs-related signature in predicting the prognosis of glioma, and they provided potential targeted therapy for glioma by in silico analysis [41]. Pinto L. et al. analyzed and characterized myeloid and lymphoid infiltrate in grade 2, 3, and 4 gliomas human samples by multicolor flow cytometry, along with the composition of the cell subsets of circulating myeloid cells [40]. They described that the infiltration by BMDM reached the highest percentages in GBM, and it increased from the periphery to the center of the lesion, where it exerted a strong immunosuppression that was absent in marginal areas instead. Chen et al. in 2017 agreed that BMDMs predominate within the GBM parenchyma, while microglia reside at the tumor periphery, so TAMs are represented by ~85% of infiltrating BMDM and ~15% of microglia [15].

Thus, the majority of immune cells in GBM includes a vast diversity of myeloid and lymphoid cells, which comprise BMDMs, myeloid-derived suppressor cells (MDSCs), DCs, lymphocytes, natural killer (NK), neutrophils, etc. [42]. However, the complex cell–cell interactions provide a unique physiological advantage for glioma cells that establishes an immune-suppressive and tumor-development-permissive microenvironment that is featured with high resident and recruited myeloid cell substances, hyporesponsive, and exhausted tumor infiltrating lymphocyte (TIL), which makes malignant glioma known as an immunologically "cold" tumor [43,44]. In addition, some studies indicated that reducing the number of MDSCs recruitment may slow the progression of glioma tumor cells [45]. Lymphoid cells are presented in GBM, but they are infrequent and they represent less than 2% of the tumor mass [46]. A representative scheme of different cell components of GBM TME is summarized in Figure 1. Principal functions of GBM cellular components are listed in Table 1.

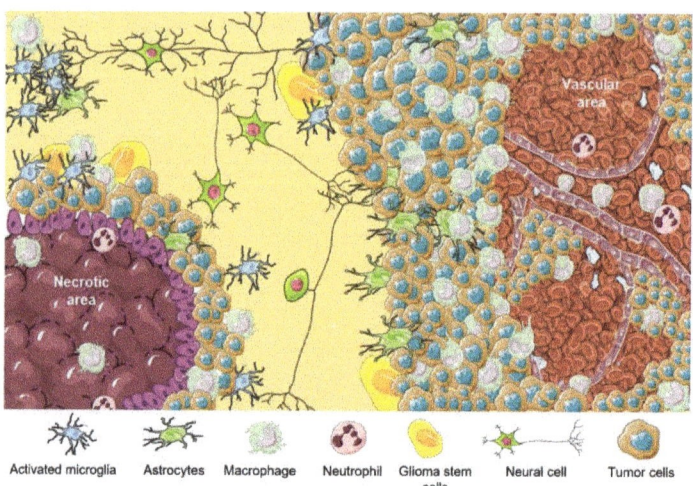

Figure 1. TME in GBM. Representative scheme of different GBM tumor areas. TAMs are associated with perinecrotic core centers, perivascular areas, and tumor front invasion zones. This figure was created using Servier Medical Art templates, which are licensed under a Creative Commons Attribution 3.0 Unported License; https://smart.servier.com (accessed on 1 February 2023).

Table 1. Main functions of cellular components of TME of GBM.

TME Cellular Components	Functions
Astrocytes	Homeostasis regulation
Endothelial cells	Angiogenesis and BBB formation
Microglia	Immune regulation
M1-like macrophages	Proinflammatory
M2-like Macrophages	Anti-inflammatory and tumor progression promoter
Neurons	Receive, process, and transmit information
Pericytes	Angiogenesis and BBB formation
GSCs	Tumor perpetuation and resistance

As we mentioned previously, the prominent genomic feature that mostly distinguishes LGG from malignant gliomas, such as GBM, is the mutational status of the two genes encoding the cytoplasmatic IDH1 and/or the mitochondrial IDH2, where ~80% of LGGs present IDH mutations, compared to only ~5% of GBMs. Interestingly, IDH mutations are an independent prognostic factor in gliomas and they are associated with increased survival in all types, including GBM [17,47]. IDH status also denote TME cell components differences between tumors with the wild-type isoform and those with the mutated IDH [48]. Unlike GBMs with IDH-wildtype, GBMs with the IDH mutation have been shown to have less M2 macrophage infiltration and fewer PD-1-expressing T cells [49]. A study based on samples from patients with GBM showed that there is less infiltration of TAMs in GBM with IDH mutation, being more proinflammatory, which could reflect a better prognosis for these patients, and the fact that microglia in mutated IDH also have a proinflammatory role [50].

5. Monocyte Recruitment as Main Source of TAMs in GBM

It is well-known that numerous types of circulating cells are recruited into tumor tissues. After migration from the bone marrow into the peripheral blood, monocytes enter different tissues, and they differentiate into macrophages. There is increasing evidence that monocytes, in particular, migrate into GBM, where they differentiate into macrophages and they accumulate in distinct zones of the TME depending on the pattern of chemokine expression and secretion [51].

It has not been long since it has been recognized that TAMs from GBMs have a monocyte origin besides microglial origin and that the recruitment of different types of monocytes from the bloodstream is closely related to the GBM microenvironment and its different areas, and the BBB does not necessarily have to be disrupted [52,53]. Monocytes are not a homogeneous population, but they rather vary in phenotype and function. Based on this, monocytes from mice can be divided into two main subsets based on the expression of *LY6C* and *CX3CR1* genes which have been termed classical and non-classical monocytes [15,54]. Human monocytes are commonly divided into three subsets based on CD14 and CD16 expression, and the recent incorporation of 6-sulfo LacNac (SLAN) expression allows a better differentiation between subtypes [53]: classical monocytes (CD14+ CD16− SLAN−), intermediate monocytes (CD14+ CD16+ SLAN−), and non-classical monocytes (CD14low/− CD16+ SLAN+) [55]. Classical monocytes, similar to those of mouse $LY6C^{HI}$ monocytes, highly express CCR2; they are the most prevalent monocyte subset in human blood, and they are recruited in inflamed environments [52].

As previously mentioned, when monocytes extravasate and reach the GBM tumor mass, they begin to differentiate into mature macrophages. In this step, tumor-derived chemokines and monocyte chemokine receptors play a critical role in monocyte/macrophage recruitment (Figure 2). Over the last century, it has been shown that various receptor–ligand pairs can regulate monocyte/macrophage recruitment into specific tumor microenvironments. Among the receptor-ligand pairs, the ligands of CD62L/CD62L, CCR2/CCL2, CX3CR1/CX3CL1, and VEGFR1/VEGF-A have been the most significantly implicated in monocyte/macrophage recruitment into specific TME areas. Ligands for these receptors are produced in the TME by GBM tumor cells, leukocytes, endothelial cells, and infiltrating fibroblasts, and their expression has been shown to positively correlate with the number of macrophages in tumors [15,56,57].

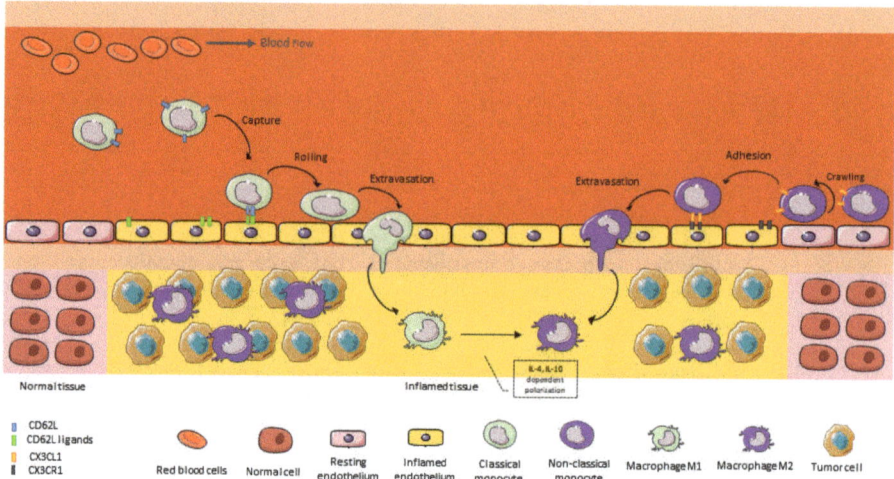

Figure 2. BMDM recruitment into inflamed brain tissue. An activated endothelium allows the recruitment of cells from the bloodstream through a well-orchestrated and coordinated mechanism. This figure was created using Servier Medical Art templates, which are licensed under a Creative Commons Attribution 3.0 Unported License; https://smart.servier.com (accessed on 1 February 2023).

CCL2, also known as monocyte chemotactic protein-1 (MCP-1) or small inducible cytokine A2 (SCYA2), is a highly potent chemoattractant of monocytes/macrophages to areas of tissue injury and inflammation, as well as to tumor areas. Many studies have made it clear that CCL2 is the primary cytokine in monocyte recruitment into the inflamed CNS [40,53,58,59]. Moreover, the extent of CCL2 expression is associated with glioma grade [60]. In the setting of murine GBM, research has shown that neoplastic cells in GBM express high levels of CCL2, which contributes to the directional infiltration of CCR2^{Hi} inflammatory monocytes into the tumor [61]. CCL7 also mediates the recruitment of BMDMs via binding to CCR2 [62]. Loss of CCL2 or CCL7 can significantly reduce the recruitment of BMDMs (40–50% reduction) during inflammation processes and it enhances therapeutic response [63]. Additionally, it was shown with orthotopic GSC xenografts that periostin secreted by tumor cells specifically supported the recruitment of anti-inflammatory and consequently pro-tumor monocyte-derived macrophages, a result validated with immunohistochemistry on human GBM tissue, which showed more CCR2+ cells in the tumor infiltrate [64].

GBM tumor niches could recruit different subtypes of monocytes. For instance, due to reduced oxygen supply, the central regions of GBM tumors show high levels of hypoxia and in this hypoxic region, hypoxia-inducible chemokines that attract monocytes/macrophages, such as VEGF-A, SDF-1 are enriched compared to the peritumoral region [28,65–67]. On the other hand, CX3CL1/CX3CR1 chemokine axis elicited adhesion and migration of TAMs, they increased the expression of matrix metalloproteinase (MMP) 2, MMP9, and MMP14 enzymes that degrade ECM, and they are concerned in tumor invasiveness [68]. For this reason, this axis is more implicated in the non-classical monocyte recruitment into the perivascular area. CX3CR1 signaling enhances accumulation of BMDMs and angiogenesis during malignant transformation of LGG [69]. In another study, the expression of CX3CL1 was inversely correlated with patient overall survival with the uppermost scores of CX3CL1 expression in grades 3–4 tumors: oligodendrogliomas, anaplastic astrocytomas, and GBM [70]. In concordance, a recent study demonstrated that the transcripts of seven chemokines, including CCL2, CCL8, CCL18, CCL28, CXCL1, CXCL5, and CXCL13 were highly expressed in GBM, which was also evidenced with a large immune cell infiltrate and it was accompanied by worse GBM patient outcomes [71]. $CCR2^{Hi}$ inflammatory monocytes are rapidly recruited to sites of inflammation and sites of tissue remodeling as well, and they have been shown to be the major source of TAMs in GBM [15,72]. These monocytes will be homed in perivascular and perinecrotic/hypoxic areas [72]. For instance, Chen et al. demonstrated that CCR2+ inflammatory monocytes are rapidly recruited into a GBM orthotopic mouse model and they are highly motile cells to reach different zones, but they also could rapidly change to a stationary $CX3CR1^{hi}CCR2^{lo}$ and $CX3CR1^{hi}CCR2-$ TAM profile in perivascular areas adjacent to endothelial cells and pericytes [73].

Another important chemoattractant axis for TAM recruitment is CXCL12/CXCR4 axis. As it was previously mentioned, CXCL12, also known as SDF-1 is enriched in hypoxic areas and it is related to glioma progression, cancer cell–TME interaction, cellular invasion, and tumor angiogenesis [67,74,75]. Angiogenesis is one of the key hallmarks of GBM, and CXCL12 binding to CXCR4 participates in this process via boosting VEGF release [67,76]. It has been reported that high CXCL12 levels in GBM may attract CXCR4-positive vascular and inflammatory cells such as TAMs that, once within the tumor, secrete tumor-promoting cytokines as well as growth and pro-angiogenic factors [77,78]. CXCR4 high levels of expression have been related to negative prognostic significance in malignant glioma patients [79]. Some of these ligand–receptor axes will be discussed later as targets to decrease TAM recruitment.

6. Macrophages Functions in Malignant Gliomas

Macrophages have been classified as M1 and M2 subtypes. These immune cells have clout in tumors due to M1 having better prognosis in patients than the infiltrating of M2 [80]. Macrophage subtypes have many differences, M1 cells have a proinflammatory phenotype that generate interleukin-1 (IL-1), IL-12, IL-23, IL-6, Tumor Necrosis Factor α (TNF-α), and ROS. In counterpart, M2 TAMs have an anti-inflammatory and tumor progression promoter phenotype, they generate IL-10, IL-4, IL5, VEGF, and they cause immune suppression promoting transforming growth factor β (TGF-β). Additionally, M2 helps recruit Th2 helper T cells, which release IL-4, IL-5, and IL-10 [81]. On the other hand, TAMs with an M2-like phenotype participate in the proliferation, survival, and migration of tumor cells [82]. It is known that TAMs release IL-6 and IL-1β that activate various cell proliferation pathways [83]. IL-6 secretion by macrophages is highly correlated with the poor prognosis of GBM patients, and its quantification in the cerebrospinal fluid was proposed as a prognostic marker [84].

In GBM, there is a predisposition for BMDMs to be found in the tumor nucleus in a greater proportion; however, microglia-derived TAMs are found in the periphery of the tumor [15]. In this regard, a study demonstrated that M2-like TAMs represented by macrophages CD204+ were correlated with poor prognosis in GBM and they expressed markers from both M1 and M2 activation profiles. Furthermore, these TAMs were located around blood vessels and perinecrotic areas, where a protumoral interaction with GSCs is postulated [85]. Perivascular TAMs (with a more M2 phenotype) are proangiogenic and protumoral, because they present a variety of markers such as VEGFA, CCR2, and Tie2 [86]. It has been reported that microglia/macrophages cells present proangiogenic factors such as CXCL2 and CD13 that act independently of VEGF. This could explain the recurrence of GBM and the failure of antiangiogenic therapies against VEGF [87].

Although the GBM TME exhibits proangiogenic characteristics through VEGF and other molecules, it is also characterized by the secretion of TGF-β by TAMs that acts by suppressing the function and proliferation of cytotoxic T cells [88]. Moreover, an important lymphocyte depletion is initiated in GBM due to the large presence of macrophages, with a suppressed Th1 profile and a higher M2 response [89]. The immunosuppressive effects of GBM can be attributed to the elevated levels of TGF-β, since it promotes the stimulation of the M2 phenotype in macrophages with release of the immunosuppressive cytokine

IL-10. In addition, TGF-β decreases the production of molecules such as granzyme A/B, interferon gamma, and perforin, which are fundamental molecules in cytotoxicity mediated by NK and T cells [90]. Moreover, M2 macrophages express chemokines that increase the recruitment of regulatory T cells (Tregs), such as chemokine C-C ligand 2 (CCL2), CCL5, CCL20, and CCL22. These chemokines also inhibit the activity of CD4+ and CD8+ effector cells, NK cells, and DCs [40,91].

Microglia cells promote the invasion of neoplastic cells through the secretion of TGF-β, which promotes the release of MMP2 that degrades components of the ECM, such as gelatins, collagen, and elastin [31]. Additionally, TAMs release other invasion-promoting molecules such as CCL5 and CCL8, which degrade the ECM [92]. CCL5 of microglia/macrophages favors glioma tumor progression through the CC5 receptor (CCR5), therefore GBM patients who overexpress CCR5 have a worse prognosis. CCL5/CCR5 interaction triggers MMP invasion and intracellular calcium cascade [93]. Together with MMPs, ADAM (A Disintegrin and Metalloprotease) metalloendopeptidases are related to the progression of GBM. ADAM8 is expressed in both M1 and M2 macrophages, while MMP9 and MMP14 are associated with M2 and related with poor patient prognosis. MMP14 inhibition improved survival in experimental animals with GBM, and may be a possible therapeutic target [94]. On the other hand, the M1 phenotype of macrophages is allied with the expression of ADAM10 and ADAM17, resulting in a better prognosis for patients with GBM [95]. Different protumoral functions with principal molecules involved with microglia and BMDMs TAMs are summarized in Figure 3.

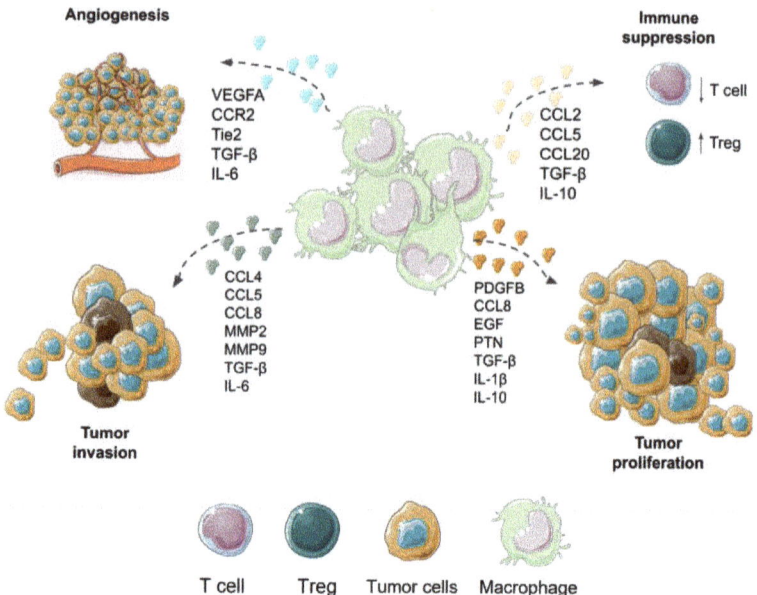

Figure 3. Macrophage functions supporting GBM malignancy. The role of TAMs in different biological events such as angiogenesis, proliferation, invasion, and immune suppression. This figure was created using Servier Medical Art templates, which are licensed under a Creative Commons Attribution 3.0 Unported License; https://smart.servier.com (accessed on 1 February 2023).

7. Conventional and Alternative Treatment Modalities for GBM

The current standard of care coordinates patients with newly diagnosed GBM to be treated with maximal safe resection surgery, followed by a course of radiotherapy (RT) with a simultaneous dose of temozolomide (TMZ), and then adjuvant chemotherapy of several maintenance cycles with TMZ (Stupp protocol). Post-surgery, the treatment regimen consists of 6 weeks of RT to the surgical cavity, followed by adjuvant chemotherapy, consisting of a total of six cycles of treatment with TMZ at a dose of 150–200 mg/m^2 for 5 days for every 28-day cycle [10,96]. After this standard first-line treatment, the progression of the disease is highly heterogeneous with a median survival of 14.6 months, with only a 10% to 15% of patients reaching 3 years of life during the current standard-of-care period [97]. According to a systematic review of randomized clinical trials, RT plus TMZ provides better survival outcomes than RT alone [98]. However, long-term administration of TMZ generally generates resistance, limiting its efficacy. The contribution of macrophages to the therapeutic resistance of TMZ was also reported [99].

New therapeutic schemes include tumor-treating fields (TTFields) with low-intensity, alternating electric fields delivered by transducer arrays applied to the scalp over the regions of the brain where tumors are localized. The use of TTFields produces mitosis inhibition and cell cycle arrest, disturbs DNA repair, interrupts cell migration, and thus suppresses tumor growth and invasion [100,101]. The effectiveness and safety of TTFields in GBMs management have been confirmed in various randomized clinical studies, and it has been established as the fourth treatment option in addition to surgery, RT, and chemotherapy [102]. Nevertheless, TTFields given during maintenance TMZ still fails to improve the median overall survival (OS) for more than 21 months [13]. However, a benefit is the promotion of the production of immune-stimulating proinflammatory environment with recruitment of proinflammatory cells from blood such as monocytes [103].

Molecular targeting approach is another therapeutic strategy greatly explored in GBM. Most molecular therapies have been developed to specifically inhibit tumor angiogenesis [104,105] or to block ligand-independent and dependent signaling pathways, such as dual-targeted of PI3K/mTOR signaling with PDGFR and VEGFR inhibitors [57,106].

From an immunotherapy approach, treatments with immune checkpoint inhibitors such as anti-CTLA-4 mAb, PD-1 and PD-L1 inhibitors demonstrated improved OS in some patients with malignant gliomas, suggesting that immunotherapy is a potential treatment option for CNS tumors, mainly in combination modalities [107]. Despite this, a persistent challenge remains for immunotherapy in the treatment of GBM due to the existence of redundant mechanisms of tumor-mediated immune suppression from its environment. Dendritic cell (DC) immunotherapy is an alternative emerging strategy for the treatment of GBM. Recently, phase I and II clinical trials testing DC vaccines in patients with newly diagnosed and recurrent GBM were conducted. The results demonstrated that DC immunotherapy enhanced progression-free survival (PFS) in GBM patients and elevated numbers of tumor-infiltrating CD8+ lymphocytes [108]. Accordingly, Iurlaro R. and colleagues recently engineered T-cell bispecific antibodies (TCB) that bind both the T-cell receptor and tumor-specific antigens [109]. The tumor-specific antigen proposed by the group was the epidermal growth factor receptor variant III (EGFRvIII), which is expressed on the surface of tumor cells; it is not expressed in normal tissues, and it represents a common mutation event in GBM patients. EGFRvIII-TCB showed specificity for EGFRvIII and promoted tumor cell killing as well as T-cell activation. In addition, EGFRvIII-TCB promoted T-cell recruitment into GBM animal models [109]. Advantages and limitations for conventional treatments are shown in Figure 4.

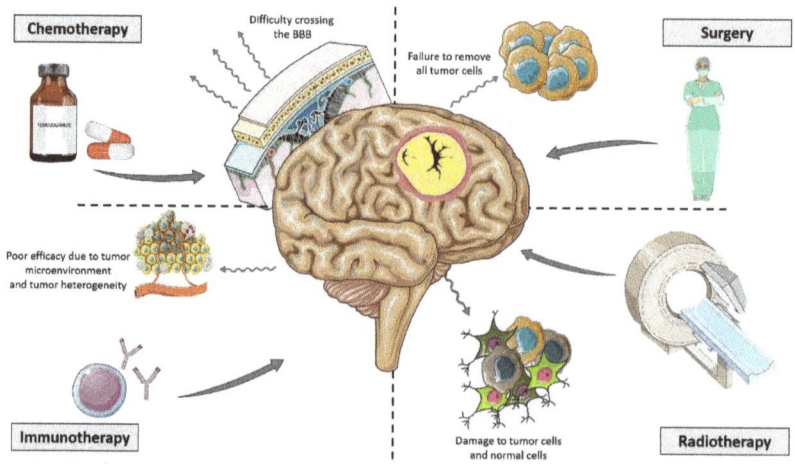

Figure 4. Conventional treatment modalities for GBM. Main treatment options for GBM patients are represented by solid straight lines. Limitations for these main treatments are schematized as refractory lines. This figure was created using Servier Medical Art templates, which are licensed under a Creative Commons Attribution 3.0 Unported License; https://smart.servier.com (accessed on 1 February 2023).

Alternative treatment modalities such as photo-assisted therapies have extensively been validated for newly diagnosed and recurrent GBM [110–112]. When glioma cells absorb a molecule called photosensitizer (PS), exposure to high intensity laser light will be able to kill tumor cells by light activable reactive oxygen species (ROS) reactions in the photodynamic therapy (PDT) [113,114]. Clinical trials with classical PS have been conducted in a few countries such as Australia, France, and Japan, where results in newly diagnosed HGG patients indicate greater success (NCT01966809, NCT01148966, NCT04391062, JMA-IIA00026) [115,116]. PDT approach not only involves direct tumor cell destruction, but also the mechanisms of ROS-mediated activation can promote other antitumoral effects such as the activation of immune response [117], a vascular supply reduction [118], and also the opening of the BBB to enhance drug permeability into brain tissue [111]. Photoactivation of PSs also allows the emission of fluorescence and phosphorescence that can be used in the diagnosis of remaining tumor cells and/or delimitation of surgical margins [119,120]. A challenge for some photo-assisted therapies is the requirement of all the elements needed in the tumor site. In this sense, devices to activate sensitizers are not found everywhere. Alternative treatment modalities in preclinical and clinical trials are shown in Figure 5. Other limitations for these new therapies come from TME such as the presence of endothelial cells of the BBB, macrophages engulfing therapeutic nanoparticles, hypoxia developed by tumor growth, etc. [121]. PDT and sonodynamic therapy (SDT) need the consumption of oxygen to generate ROS and induce cancer cell death. Under a hypoxia environment, the reduced oxygen supply is a challenge for both PDT and SDT. However, TME components could offer therapeutic strategies that can be applied with nanotechnology to achieve higher specificity for target cells and avoid damage to nearby healthy tissue. For instance, nanoparticle surfaces have been functionalized with various targeting moieties for molecular recognition of tumoral and non-tumoral cells [122]. In another approach, nanoparticles have been developed to employ tumor hypoxia or oxidative stress to accomplish a therapeutic effect [121].

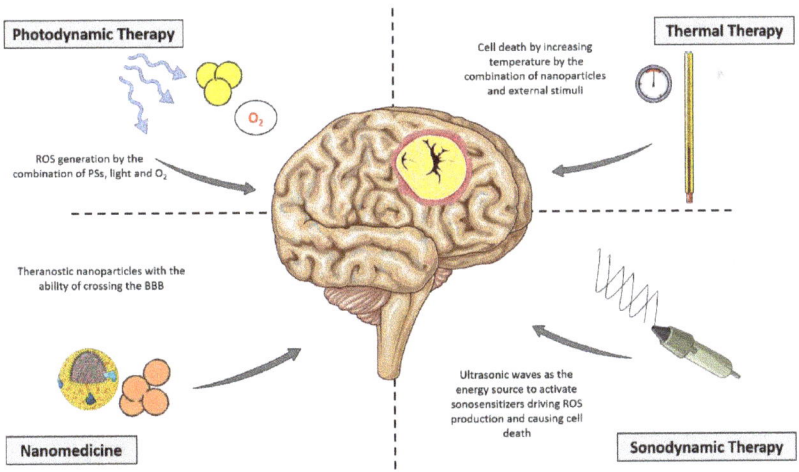

Figure 5. Alternative treatment modalities for GBM. Non-standard treatment options for GBM patients with the main mechanisms of action are represented by solid straight lines. This figure was created using Servier Medical Art templates, which are licensed under a Creative Commons Attribution 3.0 Unported License; https://smart.servier.com (accessed on 1 February 2023).

As it can be seen, the therapeutic approach for GBM requires a multiple attack towards several molecular targets with the help of surrounding cells. This highlights the importance of studying the intercellular relationships between tumor cells and other types of non-tumor cells inhabiting the tumor mass. From this point of view, the principal non-tumoral cell population represented by TAMs could help to improve the efficacy of different treatments modalities. In the following section, a brief examination of treatments that focus on TAMs and that can be used in combination with the above treatments will be discussed.

8. Therapeutic Strategies Focused on TAMs of GBM

The overwhelming evidence of the presence of TAMs in the immune infiltrate of both murine and human malignant gliomas has raised awareness of the persuasive role these cells may have on several biological events to develop an immunosuppressive environment, enabling the glioma cell progression and invasion and the contribution to the resistance to many treatment interventions. Understanding the phenotype, function, and the cell programming or plasticity of these cells is of great importance since the focus on glioma therapy is shifted towards targeting the microenvironment cells as well as the tumor cells.

8.1. Strategies to Deplete Macrophages or Inhibit Monocyte Recruitment into GBMs

Macrophages of malignant glioma TME are characterized by their plasticity and heterogeneity; however, in a dichotomy approach where two extreme types of macrophage phenotypes co-exist in gliomas' TME, pro-tumoral M2 macrophages with low expression of IL-12, IL-23, and a high expression of IL-10 and TGF-β have become an attractive therapeutic target to help eradicate this type of tumor. Furthermore, M2 macrophages also have high levels of arginase 1, mannose receptors, and scavenger receptors that serve to classify these cells in the context of several tumors. Studies have shown that TAMs are highly implicated in suppressing anti-tumor immune functions of T cells and directly facilitate tumor cell immune escape [123]. For these reasons, as the higher macrophage infiltration in the TME of GBM is often correlated with poor treatment outcomes and prognosis [27], depleting them by specifically targeting and killing them is an attractive strategy that was evaluated in the recent past.

One of main strategies to deplete TAMs is to target the colony-stimulating factor 1 receptor (CSF-1R). CSF-1R belongs to a type III protein kinase receptor family and binds to two ligands, CSF-1 and IL-34. After binding, ligands induce homodimerization of CSF-1R and activation of receptor signaling, which is crucial for the differentiation and survival of macrophages in tissues [124]. Gabrusiewicz K. et al. modeled in vivo GBM using intracranial GL261-bearing CSF-1R–GFP+ macrophage Fas-induced apoptosis transgenic mice [125]. In their mice, transitory macrophage population ablation was achieved by exposure to AP20187, a ligand which induces Fas-mediated apoptosis through activation of the caspase-8 pathway in myeloid lineage cells; and afterward, tumors showed lower mitotic index, microvascular density, and a reduction in tumor growth [124]. In order to achieve depletion of TAMs by CSF-1R, small molecule inhibitors and monoclonal antibodies were developed in the last decade with a few of them reaching clinical trials for the GBM treatment as monotherapy or in combination with other drugs [126,127]. For instance, cabiralizumab, a recombinant monoclonal antibody to CSF-1R, is in a phase 1a/1b doses-escalation study alone and in combination with nivolumab, another monoclonal antibody anti-PD-1 for advanced solid tumors including malignant gliomas (NCT02526017). An example of a small molecule against CSF-1R is PLX3397, a potent CSF-1R and c-Kit inhibitor [128], which is also in clinical trials for recurrent GBMs (NCT01349036, phase 2 study—terminated) and also for newly diagnosed GBMs in combination with TMZ and RT (NCT01790503). These drugs demonstrated outstanding results in preclinical mice models [128,129]; however, their efficacy in human GBM is still under investigation.

Another strategy to deplete TAMs, which is currently under evaluation is to target CXCR4 with antagonists. CXCR4 is overexpressed in numerous human cancers including glioma, and it has been shown to promote tumor growth, invasion, angiogenesis, metastasis, relapse, and therapeutic resistance [56]. In addition to being overexpressed in tumor cells and GSCs, it is also found in TAMs. AMD3100, USL311, and POL5551 have been used to deplete TAMs in GBM in combination with chemotherapy, RT, and antivascular therapy [65,130,131]. Gagner J.P. et al. demonstrated that the combination of POL5551 and B20-4.1.1, an anti-VEGF antibody, reduced tumor invasiveness, vascular density, and reduced Iba1-positive microglia TAM population within tumors compared to antivascular therapy alone in preclinical GBM mouse models [65]. It is known that the action of antiangiogenic agents in malignant gliomas is not very effective and leads to a greater accumulation of immunosuppressive myeloid populations in hypoxic areas [132]. Their findings raise the possibility that CXCR4 antagonists may interfere with the microglial mechanism of escape of GBM to anti-VEGF therapy. A clinical trial, which has already ended, evaluated USL311 as a single agent and in combination with lomustine for advanced and recurrent GBM through a phase $\frac{1}{2}$ dose-escalation study in order to determine treatment modality and regimen of administration (NCT02765165). A common feature among these therapies is that they are ineffective when applied alone and require a combinatory modality to succeed.

8.2. Strategies to Reprogramme TAMs to an Antitumoral and Phagocitic Profile

Although TAMs with a M2-like phenotype play an important role in tumor development and progression, M1 TAMs have been shown to effectively eliminate cancer cells [133,134]. Reprograming TAMs from their tumor supporting phenotype (M2) towards an anti-tumor phenotype (M1) can therefore inhibit tumor growth and enhance an anti-cancer immune signaling. To achieve this, several molecules have been reported in TAM or in glioma cells from which molecular interactions with TAM perpetuate the M2 phenotype and could be therapeutic targets. Experimental studies have revealed a macrophage-mediated drug resistance mechanism in which the TME undergoes adaptation in response to macrophage-targeted CSF1R inhibition therapy in gliomas. As we previously mentioned, CSF1R targeting not only diminishes TAM population but also its blockage could revert polarization to a M1 phenotype [129]. Sun et al. demonstrated how macrophage phenotype could be exploited to exert anti-tumor effects by treating macrophages with an inhibitor of the CSF1R, thus making them switch from M2 to M1 phenotype and stimulating phagocytosis of tumor cells. However, after prolonged treatment with CSF1R inhibitors, IL4 accumulated from other TME cell types stimulated TAMs to secrete insulin-like growth factor 1 (IGF1), which in turn sustains the survival and growth of glioma cells [135]. For this reason, a combined treatment modality with CSFR inhibition and IGF1 receptor (IGF1R) inhibition will be the goal of designing more effective therapies for gliomas [135]. In another approach to reprogram TAMs, Mukherjee S. et al. developed novel liposomal formulation of TriCurin (TrLp). TriCurin is a mixed of curcumin with two other polyphenols, epicatechin gallate from green tea and resveratrol from red grapes. These TrLp liposomes were able to produce a major stimulation of the innate immune system by repolarizing TAM to the tumoricidal M1-like phenotype and also triggering intra-tumor recruitment of NK cells from the bloodstream into GBM GL261 mouse model [136].

Toll-like receptors (TLRs) are essential in the recognition of molecular patterns enhanced by a broad spectrum of infectious agents, and they stimulate a variety of inflammatory responses. Among them, TLR9 is expressed intracellularly in innate immune cells within the endosomal compartments, and it is activated by its binding to DNA rich in CpG motifs. A recent study has shown that fungal polymer Schizophyllan (SPG)-based nanoparticles (well-known ligand for Dectin-1 receptors) entrapping short DNA CpG ODN 1826 activated the signal transducer and activator of transcription 1 (STAT1) within GBM TAMs, which in turn promotes the synthesis of Th1-type cytokines such as IL-1β, IFN-γ, iNOS, and TNF-α and further restricts tumor growth [137]. Another receptor evaluated to reprogram M2 TAMs was H1 histamine receptor (Hrh1), which is significantly upregulated in the M2-like compared M1-like TAMs. Chryplewicz et al. demonstrated that imipramine, a re-purposed tricyclic antidepressant reprogrammed TAMs into a pro-inflammatory M1 phenotype, and these cells were responsible for the recruitment of T cells, in part by expressing the chemokines CXCL9 and CXCL10 [138].

As well as the activation of STAT-1 is associated with the transcription of genes related with the M1 profile in TAMs, the activation of STAT-3 has an opposite effect, activating genes related to anti-inflammatory proteins and therefore polarizing macrophages towards an M2 profile. STAT3 is a cytoplasmic transcription factor that regulates cell proliferation, differentiation, apoptosis, angiogenesis, inflammation, and immune responses [139]. Aberrant STAT3 activation triggers tumor progression through oncogenic gene expression in numerous cancer types including malignant gliomas [140,141]. Moreover, STAT3 activation in immune cells causes elevation of immunosuppressive factors [142]. One of the first studies that validated STAT3 inhibition as a repolarization strategy towards an M1 profile in GBM TAMs with a beneficial outcome was presented by Zhang L. et al. in 2009 [143]. In this study, CPA-7, an inhibitor of Stat3 dimerization, and STAT3 siRNA were used efficiently to reverse the immune profile of TAMs and cause tumor growth inhibition in the GL261 GBM mouse model [143]. The effect of TAM with active STAT3 leads to the secretion of interleukin (IL)-1β, which promote GBM growth by also allowing the activation of STAT3 and nuclear factor-kappa B (NF-kB) signaling in tumor cells [144]. In a recent study, STAT3 activation in GBM cells stimulated by TGF-β and released by M2 TAMs allows GSCs maintenance and self-renewal as a main tumor growth mechanism [145]. Furthermore, noncoding RNAs were postulated to play an important role in upstream signals to regulate the expression and activation of STAT3 in TME cells [146]. For example, it was proposed that miR-1246, derived from hypoxic glioma cells, induced M2 TAM polarization by targeting TERF2IP to activate the STAT3 signaling pathway [147]. Targeting this microRNA may contribute to antitumor immunotherapy in GBM patients.

CD40 is expressed on several antigen presenting cells including TAMs. CD40 has been proposed as a molecular target to reprogram M2 TAMs to an antitumoral phenotype in GBM management. In order to accomplish this, agonistic CD40 monoclonal antibody (mAb) has been used [148,149]. In fact, some studies have shown efficacy combining these mAB with other molecular treatments to increase therapeutic success, such as COX-2 and

IL-6 inhibitions [150,151]. Therefore, re-education of TAMs rather than depletion may represent a more effective strategy as monotherapy or in a combination modality.

8.3. Cell-Based Therapy Using Monocytes-Macrophages for GBM

Taking into account that mononuclear phagocytes are in constant traffic into tumors, macrophages have been explored on their own as therapeutic agents in the TME of different type of cancers [37,152,153]. In the new era, the use of biological agents as medicinal products is revolutionizing the field of medicine. These products are obtained from living organisms or their tissues, which include viruses, serum, toxins, antitoxins, vaccines, blood components or derivatives, allergenic products, hormones, cytokines, antibodies, among others. Somatic cell therapy involves the use of cells collected from patients that must have undergone "more than minimal manipulation" (propagation, expansion, selection, or pharmacologically treated to alter the biological characteristics of the naïve cells) to accomplish a therapeutic action. In this sense, monocytes–macrophages could serve as advanced therapy medicinal products (ATMPs) and they are been explored for several diseases [153–155].

Strategies for macrophage cell therapy are based on the fact that monocytes are capable to act as Trojan horses, delivering small molecules such as cytokines, miRNA [156,157], or nanoparticles to the TME [158,159], and it is also possible to modify these cells with engineered receptors to achieve a better homing performance into tumors [160]. In concordance, cell delivery with other cells such as mesenchymal stem cells, monocytes, and neutrophils has been also used in the targeted delivery of a wide variety of anticancer agents, including nanoparticles, chemotherapeutics, proteins, suicide genes, and viruses [161–164]. Unlike other anticancer agents, these cells migrate to and infiltrate tumors through an active process despite high interstitial pressures and stromal barriers. This "tumor-homing" capacity is achieved through cytokine gradients, growth factors, ECM remodeling enzymes, and chemokines [37]. Recently, monocytes have been used as carriers of conjugated polymer nanoparticle for improving PDT management of GBM in vitro e in vivo [161]. In this study, inflammatory activated monocytes engulfed huge amounts of nanoparticles without affecting cell viability or chemotactic ability towards GBM orthotopic tumors. In addition, circulating monocyte-derived macrophages loaded with phototherapeutic nanoparticles were able to penetrate deeper GBM spheroids by increasing the spatial distribution of the nanoparticles in these three-dimensional models achieving an improved PDT outcome [161]. Another study used primary M1 macrophages as multifunctional carriers combined with PLGA nanoparticles to deliver doxorubicin for glioma therapy with success, and it demonstrated the ability of migration, infiltration, and good drug loading characteristic of the M1 phenotype, besides reflecting the strong phagocytic ability of these cells [165].

In a recent study, it was demonstrated that nanoparticle properties such as elasticity, composition, surface charge, and size influence transendothelial migration of monocytes in a human BBB model [166]. The study revealed that 200-nm-sized protein-based particles increased the migration of loaded monocytes by two-fold, whereas a much bigger poly-(methyl methacrylate) (PMMA, 500 nm in size) reduced the migration by half. These results were confirmed by the evaluation of expression of transmigration genes by RNAseq in loaded monocytes, where different leukocyte migration genes including CXCL10, VCAM1, and ITGAM were highly upregulated in both protein-based nanoparticle loaded monocytes versus PMMA-500 loaded monocytes [166]. In another recent study, Gardell et al. created engineered human monocyte-derived macrophages to secrete a bispecific T cell engager (BiTE) specific to the mutated EGFRvIII expressed by some GBM tumors. They proved that transduced human macrophages were capable to secrete a lentivirally encoded functional EGFRvIII-targeted BiTE protein capable of inducing T cell activation, proliferation, degranulation, and killing of antigen-specific GBM tumor cells [167]. Furthermore, BiTE secreting macrophages reduced early tumor burden in both subcutaneous and intracranial mouse models of GBM, a response which was enhanced using macrophages that were dual transduced to secrete both the BiTE protein and IL-12, preventing tumor growth in an aggressive GBM model [167].

Of particular interest is the observation that TAMs localize mostly to poorly vascularized hypoxic regions of tumors, which are highly resistant to conventional treatments such as chemotherapy and RT [132,168–172]. Therefore, TAMs may be especially useful for the treatment of tumors with significant hypoxic regions, such as GBM.

On the other hand, macrophages have also been tested as an adoptive cell therapy with chimeric antigen receptor (CAR) immunotherapy. Since macrophages can efficiently infiltrate solid tumors, they are major immune regulators and abundantly present in TME; their therapeutic effect could be beneficial for the activation of immature dendritic cells and CD8+ T cells [173–175]. In a recent study by Chen Chen et al., macrophages present in GBM were exploited with CAR technology for tumor recurrency post-surgery in a GBM GL261 syngeneic orthotopic mouse model [176]. CAR gene-loaded nanoparticles in a hydrogel were able to introduce GSC-targeted CAR genes into TAM nuclei after intracavity delivery to generate CAR-macrophages. The resulting CAR-macrophages were able to seek and engulf GSCs and clear residual GSCs by stimulating an adaptive antitumor immune response and preventing postoperative glioma relapse by inducing long-term antitumor immunity [176].

9. Conclusions

Despite the advances in GBM research, there is an emerging need for identifying reliable targets in order to improve the drastic survival rates of GBM patients. The understanding of the biological and molecular behavior of different GBM subtypes, such as specific mutations in IDH, have contributed to deciphering the prognosis of disease, and design new therapeutic opportunities. However, studies should not focus solely on the tumor cells. The GBM tumor development environment plays an essential role in the progression of the disease, in which non-tumor cells intervene, collaborating in the progression and resistance to therapies. Different tumor niches are developed into GBM tissue where TAMs represent the most abundant immune cells of the TEM contributing with molecular signaling for tumor progression and resistance to conventional therapies. Therefore, TAMs may be appropriate candidates to target or to use as cellular therapy, taking advantage of its "home to" capacity through the recruitment of monocyte precursors from bloodstream. The molecular targeting strategies to deplete or reprogram TAMs in GBM tumor niches has generated several new drugs that are at best in clinical investigation for recurrent GBM with a modest efficiency increasing OS. From the analysis of these new molecular targets, it a better performance can be appreciated when combined with other therapeutic approaches. New therapeutic challenges must focus on multiple combinations of treatments to eradicate or improve survival in patients with GBM due to molecular targeting focus in TAMs selectivity, not significantly improve GBM survival by itself. This multiple approach may come from new alternative therapies under investigation, such as photo-assisted therapies that have the advantage of being able to be combined with other treatments without adding adverse secondary effects. On the other hand, the role of these alternative treatments on the TME and specifically on the macrophage population in GBM requires further studies to determine a possible synergistic action.

Author Contributions: Conceptualization, L.E.I.; data curation, M.D.C., L.B., P.M.O., B.C.G., E.M.B. and L.E.I.; formal analysis, M.D.C., L.B., P.M.O., B.C.G., E.M.B. and L.E.I.; visualization, M.D.C., L.B. and L.E.I.; Funding acquisition, L.E.I.; Investigation, M.D.C., L.B., P.M.O., B.C.G., E.M.B. and L.E.I.; project administration, L.E.I.; Supervision, L.E.I.; writing—original draft, M.D.C., L.B., P.M.O., B.C.G., E.M.B. and L.E.I.; writing—review and editing, L.E.I. All authors have read and agreed to the published version of the manuscript.

Funding: This research was funded by grants from Agencia Nacional de Promoción Científica y Tecnológica (PICT) (PICT-2020-SERIEA-00051) and CONICET (PIBAA 2022-2023 28720210100004CO) to L.E.I.

Institutional Review Board Statement: Not applicable.

Informed Consent Statement: Not applicable.

Data Availability Statement: Not applicable.

Acknowledgments: M.D.C.: L.B. and E.M.B. thank CONICET for PhD scholarships. L.E.I. is a member of the Scientific Researcher Career at CONICET and faculty at UNRC.

Conflicts of Interest: The authors declare no conflict of interest.

Abbreviations

ADAM: A Disintegrin and Metalloprotease, Ang-1: Angiopoietin-1, anti-CTLA-4 mAb: monoclonal antibody against CTL antigen 4, APC: antigen presenting cell, Arg1: arginase 1, ATMPs: advanced therapy medicinal products, ATRX: alpha-thalassemia/mental retardation, X-linked, BBB: blood brain barrier, BBTB: blood–brain tumor barrier, BEHAB: brain-enriched hyaluronan binding, BiTE: bispecific T cell engager, BMDM: bone-marrow-derived macrophages, c-Kit: tyrosine–protein kinase Kit, CAR: chimeric antigen receptor, CCL: chemokine C-C ligand 5, CCR: C-C chemokine receptor, CD: cluster of differentiation, CD62L: L-selectin, CNS: central nervous system, COX-2: cyclooxygenase 2, CSF-1R: colony-stimulating factor 1 receptor, CSF1: colony-stimulating factor 1, CSF1R: receptor of the colony-stimulating factor-1, CX3CL1: chemokine (C-X3-C motif) ligand 1, CX3CR1: CX3C motif chemokine receptor 1, Cx43: connexin43, CXCL: C-X-C motif chemokine ligand, CXCR4: chemokine receptor C-X-C type 4, DC: dendritic cell, DNA: deoxyribonucleic acid, EC: endothelial cells, ECM: extracellular matrix, EGF: epidermal growth factor, EGFR: epidermal growth factor receptor, EGFRvIII: epidermal growth factor receptor variant III, GBM: glioblastomas, GSCs: glioma stem cells, HIF-1: hypoxia-inducible factor 1, Hrh1: H1 histamine receptor, IDH: isocitrate dehydrogenase, IFN-γ: interferon-γ, IGF1: insulin-like growth factor 1, IGF1R: insulin-like growth factor receptor 1, IL: interleukin, iNOS: nitric oxide synthase, LGG: low-grade gliomas, LY6C: lymphocyte antigen 6 complex, locus C1, M-CSF: Colony stimulating factor Macrophages, M1: macrophage subtype 1, M2: macrophage subtype 2, MAPK: mitogen-activated protein kinase, MCP-1: monocyte chemotactic protein-1, MDSCs: myeloid-derived suppressor cells, miRNA: microRNA, MMP: matrix metalloproteinase, mTOR: mammalian target of rapamycin, NF-kB: nuclear factor-kappa B, NF1: neurofibromin 1, NK: natural killer, NOS: not otherwise specified, OS: overall survival, PD-1: programmed death-1, PD-L1: programmed cell death-ligand 1, PDGF: platelet derived growth factor, PDGFR: receptor platelet derived growth factor, PDT: photodynamic therapy, PFS: progression-free survival, PI3K: phosphatidylinositol-3-kinase, PS: photosensitizer, RHAMM: receptor for hyaluronan-mediated motility, RNA: ribonucleic acid, ROS: reactive oxygen species, RT: radiotherapy, SCYA2: small inducible cytokine A2, SDF-1: factor 1 derived cell stroma, SLAN: 6-sulfo LacNac, SPARC: secreted protein acidic and rich in cysteine, STAT3: signal transducer and activator of transcription 3, TAMs: tumor-associated macrophages, TCB: T-cell bispecific antibodies, TGF-α: transforming growth factor α, TGF-β: transforming growth factor β, Tie2: tyrosine-protein kinase, TIL: tumor infiltrating lymphocyte, TLRs: toll-like receptors, TME: tumor microenvironment, TMZ: temozolomide, TNF-α: tumor necrosis factor α, TP53: tumor protein p53, Tregs: regulatory T cells, TrLp: TriCurin, TTFields: tumor-treating fields, VCAM1: vascular cell adhesion molecule 1, VEGF-A: vascular endothelial growth factor A, VEGF: vascular endothelial growth factor, VEGFR1: vascular endothelial growth factor receptor-1, WHO: World Health Organization.

References

1. Miller, K.D.; Ostrom, Q.T.; Kruchko, C.; Patil, N.; Tihan, T.; Cioffi, G.; Fuchs, H.E.; Waite, K.A.; Jemal, A.; Siegel, R.L.; et al. Brain and other central nervous system tumor statistics, 2021. *CA Cancer J. Clin.* **2021**, *71*, 381–406. [CrossRef] [PubMed]
2. Brain, Other CNS and Intracranial Tumours Mortality Statistics. Cancer Research UK. Available online: https://www.cancerresearchuk.org/health-professional/cancer-statistics/statistics-by-cancer-type/brain-other-cns-and-intracranial-tumours/mortality (accessed on 6 March 2023).
3. Khazaei, Z.; Goodarzi, E.; Borhaninejad, V.; Iranmanesh, F.; Mirshekarpour, H.; Mirzaei, B.; Naemi, H.; Bechashk, S.M.; Darvishi, I.; Ershad Sarabi, R.; et al. The association between incidence and mortality of brain cancer and human development index (HDI): An ecological study. *BMC Public Health* **2020**, *20*, 1696. [CrossRef] [PubMed]

4. Fan, Y.; Zhang, X.; Gao, C.; Jiang, S.; Wu, H.; Liu, Z.; Dou, T. Burden and trends of brain and central nervous system cancer from 1990 to 2019 at the global, regional, and country levels. *Arch. Public Health* **2022**, *80*, 209. [CrossRef] [PubMed]
5. Sung, H.; Ferlay, J.; Siegel, R.L.; Laversanne, M.; Soerjomataram, I.; Jemal, A.; Bray, F. Global Cancer Statistics 2020: GLOBOCAN Estimates of Incidence and Mortality Worldwide for 36 Cancers in 185 Countries. *CA Cancer J. Clin.* **2021**, *71*, 209–249. [CrossRef] [PubMed]
6. Park, S.H. The Role of Epigenetics in Brain and Spinal Cord Tumors. *Adv. Exp. Med. Biol.* **2023**, *1394*, 119–136. [CrossRef] [PubMed]
7. Scheithauer, B.W.; Clinic, M. Development of the WHO Classification of Tumors of the Central Nervous System: A Historical Perspective. *Brain Pathol.* **2009**, *19*, 551–564. [CrossRef] [PubMed]
8. Louis, D.N.; Perry, A.; Wesseling, P.; Brat, D.J.; Cree, I.A.; Figarella-Branger, D.; Hawkins, C.; Ng, H.K.; Pfister, S.M.; Reifenberger, G.; et al. The 2021 WHO Classification of Tumors of the Central Nervous System: A summary. *Neuro. Oncol.* **2021**, *23*, 1231–1251. [CrossRef] [PubMed]
9. Delgado-Martín, B.; Medina, M.Á. Advances in the Knowledge of the Molecular Biology of Glioblastoma and Its Impact in Patient Diagnosis, Stratification, and Treatment. *Adv. Sci.* **2020**, *7*, 1902971. [CrossRef]
10. Kirby, A.J.; Finnerty, G.T. New strategies for managing adult gliomas. *J. Neurol.* **2020**, *268*, 3666–3674. [CrossRef]
11. Gargini, R.; Segura-Collar, B.; Sánchez-Gómez, P. Cellular plasticity and tumor microenvironment in gliomas: The struggle to hit a moving target. *Cancers* **2020**, *12*, 1622. [CrossRef]
12. Jung, E.; Osswald, M.; Ratliff, M.; Dogan, H.; Xie, R.; Weil, S.; Hoffmann, D.C.; Kurz, F.T.; Kessler, T.; Heiland, S.; et al. Tumor cell plasticity, heterogeneity, and resistance in crucial microenvironmental niches in glioma. *Nat. Commun.* **2021**, *12*, 1014. [CrossRef]
13. Tan, A.C.; Ashley, D.M.; López, G.Y.; Malinzak, M.; Friedman, H.S.; Khasraw, M. Management of glioblastoma: State of the art and future directions. *CA. Cancer J. Clin.* **2020**, *70*, 299–312. [CrossRef] [PubMed]
14. Hambardzumyan, D.; Gutmann, D.H.; Kettenmann, H. The role of microglia and macrophages in glioma maintenance and progression. *Nat. Neurosci.* **2015**, *19*, 20–27. [CrossRef] [PubMed]
15. Chen, Z.; Feng, X.; Herting, C.J.; Garcia, V.A.; Nie, K.; Pong, W.W.; Rasmussen, R.; Dwivedi, B.; Seby, S.; Wolf, S.A.; et al. Cellular and molecular identity of tumor-associated macrophages in glioblastoma. *Cancer Res.* **2017**, *77*, 2266–2278. [CrossRef]
16. Louis, D.N.; Perry, A.; Reifenberger, G.; von Deimling, A.; Figarella-Branger, D.; Cavenee, W.K.; Ohgaki, H.; Wiestler, O.D.; Kleihues, P.; Ellison, D.W. The 2016 World Health Organization Classification of Tumors of the Central Nervous System: A summary. *Acta Neuropathol.* **2016**, *131*, 803–820. [CrossRef]
17. Miller, J.J.; Gonzalez Castro, L.N.; McBrayer, S.; Weller, M.; Cloughesy, T.; Portnow, J.; Andronesi, O.; Barnholtz-Sloan, J.S.; Baumert, B.G.; Berger, M.S.; et al. Isocitrate dehydrogenase (IDH) mutant gliomas: A Society for Neuro-Oncology (SNO) consensus review on diagnosis, management, and future directions. *Neuro-Oncology* **2022**, *25*, 4–25. [CrossRef]
18. Zhang, P.; Xia, Q.; Liu, L.; Li, S.; Dong, L. Current Opinion on Molecular Characterization for GBM Classification in Guiding Clinical Diagnosis, Prognosis, and Therapy. *Front. Mol. Biosci.* **2020**, *7*, 562798. [CrossRef]
19. de Gooijer, M.C.; Guillén Navarro, M.; Bernards, R.; Wurdinger, T.; van Tellingen, O. An Experimenter's Guide to Glioblastoma Invasion Pathways. *Trends Mol. Med.* **2018**, *24*, 763–780. [CrossRef]
20. Vollmann-Zwerenz, A.; Leidgens, V.; Feliciello, G.; Klein, C.A.; Hau, P. Tumor cell invasion in glioblastoma. *Int. J. Mol. Sci.* **2020**, *21*, 1932. [CrossRef] [PubMed]
21. Hambardzumyan, D.; Bergers, G. Glioblastoma: Defining Tumor Niches. *Trends Cancer* **2015**, *1*, 252–265. [CrossRef]
22. Schiffer, D.; Annovazzi, L.; Casalone, C.; Corona, C.; Mellai, M. Glioblastoma: Microenvironment and Niche Concept. *Cancers* **2018**, *11*, 5. [CrossRef] [PubMed]
23. Lathia, J.D.; Mack, S.C.; Mulkearns-Hubert, E.E.; Valentim, C.L.L.; Rich, J.N. Cancer stem cells in glioblastoma. *Genes Dev.* **2015**, *29*, 1203–1217. [CrossRef]
24. Calabrese, C.; Poppleton, H.; Kocak, M.; Hogg, T.L.; Fuller, C.; Hamner, B.; Oh, E.Y.; Gaber, M.W.; Finklestein, D.; Allen, M.; et al. A Perivascular Niche for Brain Tumor Stem Cells. *Cancer Cell* **2007**, *11*, 69–82. [CrossRef]
25. Watkins, S.; Robel, S.; Kimbrough, I.F.; Robert, S.M.; Ellis-Davies, G.; Sontheimer, H. Disruption of astrocyte–vascular coupling and the blood–brain barrier by invading glioma cells. *Nat. Commun.* **2014**, *5*, 4196. [CrossRef]
26. Scholz, A.; Harter, P.N.; Cremer, S.; Yalcin, B.H.; Gurnik, S.; Yamaji, M.; Di Tacchio, M.; Sommer, K.; Baumgarten, P.; Bähr, O.; et al. Endothelial cell-derived angiopoietin-2 is a therapeutic target in treatment-naive and bevacizumab-resistant glioblastoma. *EMBO Mol. Med.* **2016**, *8*, 39–57. [CrossRef] [PubMed]
27. Lin, Y.J.; Wu, C.Y.J.; Wu, J.Y.; Lim, M. The Role of Myeloid Cells in GBM Immunosuppression. *Front. Immunol.* **2022**, *13*, 2407. [CrossRef]
28. Schiffer, D.; Mellai, M.; Bovio, E.; Bisogno, I.; Casalone, C.; Annovazzi, L. Glioblastoma niches: From the concept to the phenotypical reality. *Neurol. Sci.* **2018**, *39*, 1161–1168. [CrossRef] [PubMed]
29. Bellail, A.C.; Hunter, S.B.; Brat, D.J.; Tan, C.; Van Meir, E.G. Microregional extracellular matrix heterogeneity in brain modulates glioma cell invasion. *Int. J. Biochem. Cell Biol.* **2004**, *36*, 1046–1069. [CrossRef]
30. Chamberlain, M.C.; Cloughsey, T.; Reardon, D.A.; Wen, P.Y. A novel treatment for glioblastoma: Integrin inhibition. *Expert Rev. Neurother.* **2014**, *12*, 421–435. [CrossRef]
31. Brandao, M.; Simon, T.; Critchley, G.; Giamas, G. Astrocytes, the rising stars of the glioblastoma microenvironment. *Glia* **2019**, *67*, 779–790. [CrossRef]

32. Zhu, V.F.; Yang, J.; LeBrun, D.G.; Li, M. Understanding the role of cytokines in Glioblastoma Multiforme pathogenesis. *Cancer Lett.* **2012**, *316*, 139–150. [CrossRef]
33. Furnari, F.B.; Cloughesy, T.F.; Cavenee, W.K.; Mischel, P.S. Heterogeneity of epidermal growth factor receptor signalling networks in glioblastoma. *Nat. Rev. Cancer* **2015**, *15*, 302–310. [CrossRef] [PubMed]
34. Saleem, H.; Kulsoom Abdul, U.; Küçükosmanoglu, A.; Houweling, M.; Cornelissen, F.M.G.; Heiland, D.H.; Hegi, M.E.; Kouwenhoven, M.C.M.; Bailey, D.; Würdinger, T.; et al. The TICking clock of EGFR therapy resistance in glioblastoma: Target Independence or target Compensation. *Drug Resist. Updat.* **2019**, *43*, 29–37. [CrossRef] [PubMed]
35. Saijo, K.; Glass, C.K. Microglial cell origin and phenotypes in health and disease. *Nat. Rev. Immunol.* **2011**, *11*, 775–787. [CrossRef]
36. Herold-Mende, C.; Linder, B.; Andersen, J.K.; Miletic, H.; Hossain, J.A. Tumor-Associated Macrophages in Gliomas—Basic Insights and Treatment Opportunities. *Cancers* **2022**, *14*, 1319. [CrossRef]
37. Ibarra, L.E. Cellular Trojan horses for delivery of nanomedicines to brain tumors: Where do we stand and what is next? *Nanomedicine* **2021**, *16*, 517–522. [CrossRef] [PubMed]
38. Jena, L.; McErlean, E.; McCarthy, H. Delivery across the blood-brain barrier: Nanomedicine for glioblastoma multiforme. *Drug Deliv. Transl. Res.* **2020**, *10*, 304–318. [CrossRef] [PubMed]
39. Muldoon, L.L.; Alvarez, J.I.; Begley, D.J.; Boado, R.J.; Del Zoppo, G.J.; Doolittle, N.D.; Engelhardt, B.; Hallenbeck, J.M.; Lonser, R.R.; Ohlfest, J.R.; et al. Immunologic Privilege in the Central Nervous System and the Blood–Brain Barrier. *J. Cereb. Blood Flow Metab.* **2012**, *33*, 13–21. [CrossRef]
40. Pinton, L.; Masetto, E.; Vettore, M.; Solito, S.; Magri, S.; D'Andolfi, M.; Del Bianco, P.; Lollo, G.; Benoit, J.P.; Okada, H.; et al. The immune suppressive microenvironment of human gliomas depends on the accumulation of bone marrow-derived macrophages in the center of the lesion. *J. Immunother. Cancer* **2019**, *7*, 58. [CrossRef] [PubMed]
41. Wang, L.J.; Xue, Y.; Lou, Y. Tumor-associated macrophages related signature in glioma. *Aging* **2022**, *14*, 2720–2735. [CrossRef]
42. De Leo, A.; Ugolini, A.; Veglia, F. Myeloid Cells in Glioblastoma Microenvironment. *Cells* **2020**, *10*, 18. [CrossRef] [PubMed]
43. D'Alessio, A.; Proietti, G.; Sica, G.; Scicchitano, B.M. Pathological and molecular features of glioblastoma and its peritumoral tissue. *Cancers* **2019**, *11*, 469. [CrossRef] [PubMed]
44. Tong, N.; He, Z.; Ma, Y.; Wang, Z.; Huang, Z.; Cao, H.; Xu, L.; Zou, Y.; Wang, W.; Yi, C.; et al. Tumor Associated Macrophages, as the Dominant Immune Cells, Are an Indispensable Target for Immunologically Cold Tumor—Glioma Therapy? *Front. Cell Dev. Biol.* **2021**, *9*, 1952. [CrossRef]
45. Zhang, X.; Liu, Y.; Dai, L.; Shi, G.; Deng, J.; Luo, Q.; Xie, Q.; Cheng, L.; Li, C.; Lin, Y.; et al. BATF2 prevents glioblastoma multiforme progression by inhibiting recruitment of myeloid-derived suppressor cells. *Oncogene* **2021**, *40*, 1516–1530. [CrossRef]
46. González-Tablas Pimenta, M.; Otero, Á.; Arandia Guzman, D.A.; Pascual-Argente, D.; Ruíz Martín, L.; Sousa-Casasnovas, P.; García-Martin, A.; Roa Montes de Oca, J.C.; Villaseñor-Ledezma, J.; Torres Carretero, L.; et al. Tumor cell and immune cell profiles in primary human glioblastoma: Impact on patient outcome. *Brain Pathol.* **2021**, *31*, 365–380. [CrossRef]
47. Han, S.; Liu, Y.; Cai, S.J.; Qian, M.; Ding, J.; Larion, M.; Gilbert, M.R.; Yang, C. IDH mutation in glioma: Molecular mechanisms and potential therapeutic targets. *Br. J. Cancer* **2020**, *122*, 1580–1589. [CrossRef] [PubMed]
48. Gonzalez, N.; Asad, A.S.; Gómez Escalante, J.; Peña Agudelo, J.A.; Nicola Candia, A.J.; García Fallit, M.; Seilicovich, A.; Candolfi, M. Potential of IDH mutations as immunotherapeutic targets in gliomas: A review and meta-analysis. *Expert Opin. Ther. Targets* **2022**, *25*, 1045–1060. [CrossRef]
49. Wang, X.; Wang, X.; Li, J.; Liang, J.; Ren, X.; Yun, D.; Liu, J.; Fan, J.; Zhang, Y.; Zhang, J.; et al. PDPN contributes to constructing immunosuppressive microenvironment in IDH wildtype glioma. *Cancer Gene Ther.* **2023**, *30*, 345–357. [CrossRef]
50. Poon, C.C.; Gordon, P.M.K.; Liu, K.; Yang, R.; Sarkar, S.; Mirzaei, R.; Ahmad, S.T.; Hughes, M.L.; Yong, V.W.; Kelly, J.J.P.; et al. Differential microglia and macrophage profiles in human IDH-mutant and -wild type glioblastoma. *Oncotarget* **2019**, *10*, 3129–3143. [CrossRef]
51. Lee, H.W.; Choi, H.J.; Ha, S.J.; Lee, K.T.; Kwon, Y.G. Recruitment of monocytes/macrophages in different tumor microenvironments. *Biochim. Biophys. Acta Rev. Cancer* **2013**, *1835*, 170–179. [CrossRef]
52. Xu, C.; Xiao, M.; Li, X.; Xin, L.; Song, J.; Zhan, Q.; Wang, C.; Zhang, Q.; Yuan, X.; Tan, Y.; et al. Origin, activation, and targeted therapy of glioma-associated macrophages. *Front. Immunol.* **2022**, *13*, 5996. [CrossRef] [PubMed]
53. Lehman, N.; Kowalska, W.; Zarobkiewicz, M.; Mazurek, M.; Mrozowska, K.; Bojarska-Junak, A.; Rola, R. Pro- vs. Anti-Inflammatory Features of Monocyte Subsets in Glioma Patients. *Int. J. Mol. Sci.* **2023**, *24*, 1879. [CrossRef] [PubMed]
54. Francke, A.; Herold, J.; Weinert, S.; Strasser, R.H.; Braun-Dullaeus, R.C. Generation of mature murine monocytes from heterogeneous bone marrow and description of their properties. *J. Histochem. Cytochem.* **2011**, *59*, 813–825. [CrossRef]
55. Boyette, L.B.; MacEdo, C.; Hadi, K.; Elinoff, B.D.; Walters, J.T.; Ramaswami, B.; Chalasani, G.; Taboas, J.M.; Lakkis, F.G.; Di Metes, M. Phenotype, function, and differentiation potential of human monocyte subsets. *PLoS ONE* **2017**, *12*, e0176460. [CrossRef] [PubMed]
56. Urbantat, R.M.; Vajkoczy, P.; Brandenburg, S. Advances in Chemokine Signaling Pathways as Therapeutic Targets in Glioblastoma. *Cancers* **2021**, *13*, 2983. [CrossRef]
57. Popescu, A.M.; Alexandru, O.; Brindusa, C.; Purcaru, S.O.; Tache, D.E.; Tataranu, L.G.; Taisescu, C.; Dricu, A. Targeting the VEGF and PDGF signaling pathway in glioblastoma treatment. *Int. J. Clin. Exp. Pathol.* **2015**, *8*, 7825.
58. Chang, A.L.; Miska, J.; Wainwright, D.A.; Dey, M.; Rivetta, C.V.; Yu, D.; Kanojia, D.; Pituch, K.C.; Qiao, J.; Pytel, P.; et al. CCL2 produced by the glioma microenvironment is essential for the recruitment of regulatory t cells and myeloid-derived suppressor cells. *Cancer Res.* **2016**, *76*, 5671–5682. [CrossRef]

59. Vakilian, A.; Khorramdelazad, H.; Heidari, P.; Sheikh Rezaei, Z.; Hassanshahi, G. CCL2/CCR2 signaling pathway in glioblastoma multiforme. *Neurochem. Int.* **2017**, *103*, 1–7. [CrossRef]
60. Kuratsu, J.I.; Yoshizato, K.; Yoshimura, T.; Leonard, E.J.; Takeshima, H.; Ushio, Y. Quantitative Study of Monocyte Chemoattractant Protein-1 (MCP-1) in Cerebrospinal Fluid and Cyst Fluid from Patients with Malignant Glioma. *JNCI J. Natl. Cancer Inst.* **1993**, *85*, 1836–1839. [CrossRef] [PubMed]
61. Feng, X.; Szulzewsky, F.; Yerevanian, A.; Chen, Z.; Heinzmann, D.; Rasmussen, R.D.; Alvarez-Garcia, V.; Kim, Y.; Wang, B.; Tamagno, I.; et al. Loss of CX3CR1 increases accumulation of inflammatory monocytes and promotes gliomagenesis. *Oncotarget* **2015**, *6*, 15077–15094. [CrossRef]
62. Tsou, C.L.; Peters, W.; Si, Y.; Slaymaker, S.; Aslanian, A.M.; Weisberg, S.P.; Mack, M.; Charo, I.F. Critical roles for CCR2 and MCP-3 in monocyte mobilization from bone marrow and recruitment to inflammatory sites. *J. Clin. Investig.* **2007**, *117*, 902–909. [CrossRef]
63. Tu, M.M.; Abdel-Hafiz, H.A.; Jones, R.T.; Jean, A.; Hoff, K.J.; Duex, J.E.; Chauca-Diaz, A.; Costello, J.C.; Dancik, G.M.; Tamburini, B.A.J.; et al. Inhibition of the CCL2 receptor, CCR2, enhances tumor response to immune checkpoint therapy. *Commun. Biol.* **2020**, *3*, 720. [CrossRef] [PubMed]
64. Zhou, W.; Ke, S.Q.; Huang, Z.; Flavahan, W.; Fang, X.; Paul, J.; Wu, L.; Sloan, A.E.; McLendon, R.E.; Li, X.; et al. Periostin secreted by glioblastoma stem cells recruits M2 tumour-associated macrophages and promotes malignant growth. *Nat. Cell Biol.* **2015**, *17*, 170–182. [CrossRef] [PubMed]
65. Gagner, J.P.; Sarfraz, Y.; Ortenzi, V.; Alotaibi, F.M.; Chiriboga, L.A.; Tayyib, A.T.; Douglas, G.J.; Chevalier, E.; Romagnoli, B.; Tuffin, G.; et al. Multifaceted C-X-C Chemokine Receptor 4 (CXCR4) Inhibition Interferes with Anti–Vascular Endothelial Growth Factor Therapy–Induced Glioma Dissemination. *Am. J. Pathol.* **2017**, *187*, 2080–2094. [CrossRef]
66. Guo, X.; Xue, H.; Shao, Q.; Wang, J.; Guo, X.; Zhang, J.; Xu, S.; Li, T.; Zhang, P.; Gao, X.; et al. Hypoxia promotes glioma-associated macrophage infiltration via periostin and subsequent M2 polarization by upregulating TGF-beta and M-CSFR. *Oncotarget* **2016**, *7*, 80521–80542. [CrossRef] [PubMed]
67. Wang, S.C.; Hong, J.H.; Hsueh, C.; Chiang, C.S. Tumor-secreted SDF-1 promotes glioma invasiveness and TAM tropism toward hypoxia in a murine astrocytoma model. *Lab. Investig.* **2012**, *92*, 151–162. [CrossRef] [PubMed]
68. Held-Feindt, J.; Hattermann, K.; Müerköster, S.S.; Wedderkopp, H.; Knerlich-Lukoschus, F.; Ungefroren, H.; Mehdorn, H.M.; Mentlein, R. CX3CR1 promotes recruitment of human glioma-infiltrating microglia/macrophages (GIMs). *Exp. Cell Res.* **2010**, *316*, 1553–1566. [CrossRef]
69. Lee, S.; Latha, K.; Manyam, G.; Yang, Y.; Rao, A.; Rao, G. Role of CX3CR1 signaling in malignant transformation of gliomas. *Neuro. Oncol.* **2020**, *22*, 1463–1473. [CrossRef]
70. Erreni, M.; Solinas, G.; Brescia, P.; Osti, D.; Zunino, F.; Colombo, P.; Destro, A.; Roncalli, M.; Mantovani, A.; Draghi, R.; et al. Human glioblastoma tumours and neural cancer stem cells express the chemokine CX3CL1 and its receptor CX3CR1. *Eur. J. Cancer* **2010**, *46*, 3383–3392. [CrossRef]
71. Gao, W.; Li, Y.; Zhang, T.; Lu, J.; Pan, J.; Qi, Q.; Dong, S.; Chen, X.; Su, Z.; Li, J. Systematic Analysis of Chemokines Reveals CCL18 is a Prognostic Biomarker in Glioblastoma. *J. Inflamm. Res.* **2022**, *15*, 2731–2743. [CrossRef]
72. Friedmann-Morvinski, D.; Hambardzumyan, D. Monocyte-neutrophil entanglement in glioblastoma. *J. Clin. Investig.* **2023**, *133*, e163451. [CrossRef] [PubMed]
73. Chen, Z.; Ross, J.L.; Hambardzumyan, D. Intravital 2-photon imaging reveals distinct morphology and infiltrative properties of glioblastoma-associated macrophages. *Proc. Natl. Acad. Sci. USA* **2019**, *116*, 14254–14259. [CrossRef] [PubMed]
74. Zagzag, D.; Lukyanov, Y.; Lan, L.; Ali, M.A.; Esencay, M.; Mendez, O.; Yee, H.; Voura, E.B.; Newcomb, E.W. Hypoxia-inducible factor 1 and VEGF upregulate CXCR4 in glioblastoma: Implications for angiogenesis and glioma cell invasion. *Lab. Investig.* **2006**, *86*, 1221–1232. [CrossRef] [PubMed]
75. Kenig, S.; Alonso, M.B.D.; Mueller, M.M.; Lah, T.T. Glioblastoma and endothelial cells cross-talk, mediated by SDF-1, enhances tumour invasion and endothelial proliferation by increasing expression of cathepsins B, S, and MMP-9. *Cancer Lett.* **2010**, *289*, 53–61. [CrossRef]
76. Codrici, E.; Popescu, I.D.; Tanase, C.; Enciu, A.M. Friends with Benefits: Chemokines, Glioblastoma-Associated Microglia/Macrophages, and Tumor Microenvironment. *Int. J. Mol. Sci.* **2022**, *23*, 2509. [CrossRef]
77. Yang, S.X.; Chen, J.H.; Jiang, X.F.; Wang, Q.L.; Chen, Z.Q.; Zhao, W.; Feng, Y.H.; Xin, R.; Shi, J.Q.; Bian, X.W. Activation of chemokine receptor CXCR4 in malignant glioma cells promotes the production of vascular endothelial growth factor. *Biochem. Biophys. Res. Commun.* **2005**, *335*, 523–528. [CrossRef]
78. Salmaggi, A.; Gelati, M.; Pollo, B.; Frigerio, S.; Eoli, M.; Silvani, A.; Broggi, G.; Ciusani, E.; Croci, D.; Boiardi, A.; et al. CXCL12 in malignant glial tumors: A possible role in angiogenesis and cross-talk between endothelial and tumoral cells. *J. Neurooncol.* **2004**, *67*, 305–317. [CrossRef]
79. Gagliardi, F.; Narayanan, A.; Reni, M.; Franzin, A.; Mazza, E.; Boari, N.; Bailo, M.; Zordan, P.; Mortini, P. The role of CXCR4 in highly malignant human gliomas biology: Current knowledge and future directions. *Glia* **2014**, *62*, 1015–1023. [CrossRef]
80. Cendrowicz, E.; Sas, Z.; Bremer, E.; Rygiel, T.P. The role of macrophages in cancer development and therapy. *Cancers* **2021**, *13*, 1946. [CrossRef]
81. Zheng, X.; Turkowski, K.; Mora, J.; Brüne, B.; Seeger, W.; Weigert, A.; Savai, R. Redirecting tumor-associated macrophages to become tumoricidal effectors as a novel strategy for cancer therapy. *Oncotarget* **2017**, *8*, 48436–48452. [CrossRef]

82. Wei, J.; Chen, P.; Gupta, P.; Ott, M.; Zamler, D.; Kassab, C.; Bhat, K.P.; Curran, M.A.; De Groot, J.F.; Heimberger, A.B. Immune biology of glioma-associated macrophages and microglia: Functional and therapeutic implications. *Neuro. Oncol.* **2020**, *22*, 180–194. [CrossRef]
83. Lu, J.; Xu, Z.; Duan, H.; Ji, H.; Zhen, Z.; Li, B.; Wang, H.; Tang, H.; Zhou, J.; Guo, T.; et al. Tumor-associated macrophage interleukin-β promotes glycerol-3-phosphate dehydrogenase activation, glycolysis and tumorigenesis in glioma cells. *Cancer Sci.* **2020**, *111*, 1979–1990. [CrossRef] [PubMed]
84. Hori, T.; Sasayama, T.; Tanaka, K.; Koma, Y.I.; Nishihara, M.; Tanaka, H.; Nakamizo, S.; Nagashima, H.; Maeyama, M.; Fujita, Y.; et al. Tumor-associated macrophage related interleukin-6 in cerebrospinal fluid as a prognostic marker for glioblastoma. *J. Clin. Neurosci.* **2019**, *68*, 281–289. [CrossRef] [PubMed]
85. Sørensen, M.D.; Kristensen, B.W. Tumour-associated CD204+ microglia/macrophages accumulate in perivascular and perinecrotic niches and correlate with an interleukin-6-enriched inflammatory profile in glioblastoma. *Neuropathol. Appl. Neurobiol.* **2022**, *48*, e12772. [CrossRef] [PubMed]
86. Erbani, J.; Boon, M.; Akkari, L. Therapy-induced shaping of the glioblastoma microenvironment: Macrophages at play. *Semin. Cancer Biol.* **2022**, *86*, 41–56. [CrossRef] [PubMed]
87. Blank, A.; Kremenetskaia, I.; Urbantat, R.M.; Acker, G.; Turkowski, K.; Radke, J.; Schneider, U.C.; Vajkoczy, P.; Brandenburg, S. Microglia/macrophages express alternative proangiogenic factors depending on granulocyte content in human glioblastoma. *J. Pathol.* **2021**, *253*, 160–173. [CrossRef]
88. Cui, X.; Morales, R.T.T.; Qian, W.; Wang, H.; Gagner, J.P.; Dolgalev, I.; Placantonakis, D.; Zagzag, D.; Cimmino, L.; Snuderl, M.; et al. Hacking macrophage-associated immunosuppression for regulating glioblastoma angiogenesis. *Biomaterials* **2018**, *161*, 164–178. [CrossRef] [PubMed]
89. Pires-Afonso, Y.; Niclou, S.P.; Michelucci, A. Revealing and Harnessing Tumour-Associated Microglia/Macrophage Heterogeneity in Glioblastoma. *Int. J. Mol. Sci.* **2020**, *21*, 689. [CrossRef]
90. Birch, J.L.; Coull, B.J.; Spender, L.C.; Watt, C.; Willison, A.; Syed, N.; Chalmers, A.J.; Hossain-Ibrahim, M.K.; Inman, G.J. Multifaceted transforming growth factor-beta (TGFβ) signalling in glioblastoma. *Cell. Signal.* **2020**, *72*, 109638. [CrossRef]
91. Wang, G.; Zhong, K.; Wang, Z.; Zhang, Z.; Tang, X.; Tong, A.; Zhou, L. Tumor-associated microglia and macrophages in glioblastoma: From basic insights to therapeutic opportunities. *Front. Immunol.* **2022**, *13*, 4077. [CrossRef]
92. Andersen, R.S.; Anand, A.; Harwood, D.S.L.; Kristensen, B.W. Tumor-Associated Microglia and Macrophages in the Glioblastoma Microenvironment and Their Implications for Therapy. *Cancers* **2021**, *13*, 4255. [CrossRef] [PubMed]
93. Yu-Ju Wu, C.; Chen, C.H.; Lin, C.Y.; Feng, L.Y.; Lin, Y.C.; Wei, K.C.; Huang, C.Y.; Fang, J.Y.; Chen, P.Y. CCL5 of glioma-associated microglia/macrophages regulates glioma migration and invasion via calcium-dependent matrix metalloproteinase 2. *Neuro. Oncol.* **2020**, *22*, 253–266. [CrossRef]
94. Ulasov, I.V.; Mijanovic, O.; Savchuk, S.; Gonzalez-Buendia, E.; Sonabend, A.; Xiao, T.; Timashev, P.; Lesniak, M.S. TMZ regulates GBM stemness via MMP14-DLL4-Notch3 pathway. *Int. J. Cancer* **2020**, *146*, 2218–2228. [CrossRef] [PubMed]
95. Gjorgjevski, M.; Hannen, R.; Carl, B.; Li, Y.; Landmann, E.; Buchholz, M.; Bartsch, J.W.; Nimsky, C. Molecular profiling of the tumor microenvironment in glioblastoma patients: Correlation of microglia/macrophage polarization state with metalloprotease expression profiles and survival. *Biosci. Rep.* **2019**, *39*, 20182361. [CrossRef]
96. Manrique-Guzmán, S.; Herrada-Pineda, T.; Revilla-Pacheco, F. Surgical Management of Glioblastoma. In *Glioblastoma*; De Vleeschouwer, S., Ed.; Exon Publications: Brisbane City, QLD, Australia, 2017; pp. 243–261. [CrossRef]
97. Rayfield, C.A.; Grady, F.; De Leon, G.; Rockne, R.; Carrasco, E.; Jackson, P.; Vora, M.; Johnston, S.K.; Hawkins-Daarud, A.; Clark-Swanson, K.R.; et al. Distinct Phenotypic Clusters of Glioblastoma Growth and Response Kinetics Predict Survival. *JCO Clin. Cancer Informatics* **2018**, *2*, 1–14. [CrossRef]
98. Yang, L.J.; Zhou, C.F.; Lin, Z.X. Temozolomide and Radiotherapy for Newly Diagnosed Glioblastoma Multiforme: A Systematic Review. *Cancer Investig.* **2014**, *32*, 31–36. [CrossRef] [PubMed]
99. Zhang, G.; Tao, X.; Ji, B.; Gong, J. Hypoxia-Driven M2-Polarized Macrophages Facilitate Cancer Aggressiveness and Temozolomide Resistance in Glioblastoma. *Oxid. Med. Cell. Longev.* **2022**, *2022*, 1614336. [CrossRef]
100. Lassman, A.B.; Joanta-Gomez, A.E.; Pan, P.C.; Wick, W. Current usage of tumor treating fields for glioblastoma. *Neuro-Oncology Adv.* **2020**, *2*, vdaa069. [CrossRef] [PubMed]
101. Voloshin, T.; Schneiderman, R.S.; Volodin, A.; Shamir, R.R.; Kaynan, N.; Zeevi, E.; Koren, L.; Klein-Goldberg, A.; Paz, R.; Giladi, M.; et al. Tumor Treating Fields (TTFields) Hinder Cancer Cell Motility through Regulation of Microtubule and Actin Dynamics. *Cancers* **2020**, *12*, 3016. [CrossRef]
102. Guo, X.; Yang, X.; Wu, J.; Yang, H.; Li, Y.; Li, J.; Liu, Q.; Wu, C.; Xing, H.; Liu, P.; et al. Tumor-Treating Fields in Glioblastomas: Past, Present, and Future. *Cancers* **2022**, *14*, 3669. [CrossRef]
103. Chen, D.; Le, S.B.; Hutchinson, T.E.; Calinescu, A.A.; Sebastian, M.; Jin, D.; Liu, T.; Ghiaseddin, A.; Rahman, M.; Tran, D.D. Tumor Treating Fields dually activate STING and AIM2 inflammasomes to induce adjuvant immunity in glioblastoma. *J. Clin. Investig.* **2022**, *132*, e149258. [CrossRef] [PubMed]
104. Ameratunga, M.; Pavlakis, N.; Wheeler, H.; Grant, R.; Simes, J.; Khasraw, M.; Ameratunga, M.; Pavlakis, N.; Wheeler, H.; Grant, R.; et al. Anti-angiogenic therapy for high-grade glioma (Review). *Cochrane Database Syst. Rev.* **2018**, *11*, CD008218. [CrossRef] [PubMed]

105. Hyman, D.M.; Rizvi, N.; Natale, R.; Armstrong, D.K.; Birrer, M.; Recht, L.; Dotan, E.; Makker, V.; Kaley, T.; Kuruvilla, D.; et al. Phase I study of MEDI3617, a selective angiopoietin-2 inhibitor alone and combined with carboplatin/paclitaxel, paclitaxel, or bevacizumab for advanced solid tumors. *Clin. Cancer Res.* **2018**, *24*, 2749–2757. [CrossRef]
106. Lin, F.; De Gooijer, M.C.; Hanekamp, D.; Chandrasekaran, G.; Buil, L.C.M.; Thota, N.; Sparidans, R.W.; Beijnen, J.H.; Wurdinger, T.; Van Tellingen, O. PI3K-mTOR Pathway inhibition exhibits efficacy against high-grade glioma in clinically relevant mouse models. *Clin. Cancer Res.* **2017**, *23*, 1286–1298. [CrossRef]
107. Persico, P.; Lorenzi, E.; Dipasquale, A.; Pessina, F.; Navarria, P.; Politi, L.S.; Santoro, A.; Simonelli, M. Checkpoint Inhibitors as High-Grade Gliomas Treatment: State of the Art and Future Perspectives. *J. Clin. Med.* **2021**, *10*, 1367. [CrossRef]
108. Wen, P.Y.; Reardon, D.A.; Armstrong, T.S.; Phuphanich, S.; Aiken, R.D.; Landolfi, J.C.; Curry, W.T.; Zhu, J.J.; Glantz, M.; Peereboom, D.M.; et al. A randomized double-blind placebo-controlled phase II trial of dendritic cell vaccine ICT-107 in newly diagnosed patients with glioblastoma. *Clin. Cancer Res.* **2019**, *25*, 5799–5807. [CrossRef]
109. Iurlaro, R.; Waldhauer, I.; Planas-Rigol, E.; Bonfill-Teixidor, E.; Arias, A.; Nicolini, V.; Freimoser-Grundschober, A.; Cuartas, I.; Martínez-Moreno, A.; Martínez-Ricarte, F.; et al. A Novel EGFRvIII T-Cell Bispecific Antibody for the Treatment of Glioblastoma. *Mol. Cancer Ther.* **2022**, *21*, 1499–1509. [CrossRef] [PubMed]
110. Akimoto, J. Photodynamic therapy for malignant brain tumors. *Neurol. Med. Chir.* **2016**, *56*, 151–157. [CrossRef]
111. Ibarra, L.E.; Vilchez, M.L.; Caverzán, M.D.; Milla Sanabria, L.N. Understanding the glioblastoma tumor biology to optimize photodynamic therapy: From molecular to cellular events. *J. Neurosci. Res.* **2021**, *99*, 1024–1047. [CrossRef]
112. Mahmoudi, K.; Garvey, K.L.; Bouras, A.; Cramer, G.; Stepp, H.; Jesu Raj, J.G.; Bozec, D.; Busch, T.M.; Hadjipanayis, C.G. 5-aminolevulinic acid photodynamic therapy for the treatment of high-grade gliomas. *J. Neurooncol.* **2019**, *141*, 595–607. [CrossRef]
113. Caverzán, M.D.; Beaugé, L.; Chesta, C.A.; Palacios, R.E.; Ibarra, L.E. Photodynamic therapy of Glioblastoma cells using doped conjugated polymer nanoparticles: An in vitro comparative study based on redox status. *J. Photochem. Photobiol. B Biol.* **2020**, *212*, 112045. [CrossRef] [PubMed]
114. Foresto, E.; Gilardi, P.; Ibarra, L.E.; Cogno, I.S. Light-activated green drugs: How we can use them in photodynamic therapy and mass-produce them with biotechnological tools. *Phytomedicine Plus* **2021**, *1*, 100044. [CrossRef]
115. Alsaab, H.O.; Alghamdi, M.S.; Alotaibi, A.S.; Alzhrani, R.; Alwuthaynani, F.; Althobaiti, Y.S.; Almalki, A.H.; Sau, S.; Iyer, A.K. Progress in Clinical Trials of Photodynamic Therapy for Solid Tumors and the Role of Nanomedicine. *Cancers* **2020**, *12*, 2793. [CrossRef]
116. Leroy, H.A.; Baert, G.; Guerin, L.; Delhem, N.; Mordon, S.; Reyns, N.; Vignion-Dewalle, A.S. Interstitial Photodynamic Therapy for Glioblastomas: A Standardized Procedure for Clinical Use. *Cancers* **2021**, *13*, 5754. [CrossRef] [PubMed]
117. Tan, L.; Shen, X.; He, Z.; Lu, Y. The Role of Photodynamic Therapy in Triggering Cell Death and Facilitating Antitumor Immunology. *Front. Oncol.* **2022**, *12*, 2234. [CrossRef]
118. Bartusik-Aebisher, D.; Żołyniak, A.; Barnaś, E.; Machorowska-Pieniążek, A.; Oleś, P.; Kawczyk-Krupka, A.; Aebisher, D. The Use of Photodynamic Therapy in the Treatment of Brain Tumors—A Review of the Literature. *Molecules* **2022**, *27*, 6847. [CrossRef] [PubMed]
119. Eljamel, M.S.; Goodman, C.; Moseley, H. ALA and Photofrin®Fluorescence-guided resection and repetitive PDT in glioblastoma multiforme: A single centre Phase III randomised controlled trial. *Lasers Med. Sci.* **2008**, *23*, 361–367. [CrossRef]
120. Arias-Ramos, N.; Ibarra, L.E.; Serrano-Torres, M.; Yagüe, B.; Caverzán, M.D.; Chesta, C.A.; Palacios, R.E.; López-Larrubia, P. Iron Oxide Incorporated Conjugated Polymer Nanoparticles for Simultaneous Use in Magnetic Resonance and Fluorescent Imaging of Brain Tumors. *Pharmaceutics* **2021**, *13*, 1258. [CrossRef] [PubMed]
121. Li, X.; Geng, X.; Chen, Z.; Yuan, Z. Recent advances in glioma microenvironment-response nanoplatforms for phototherapy and sonotherapy. *Pharmacol. Res.* **2022**, *179*, 106218. [CrossRef]
122. Sorrin, A.J.; Kemal Ruhi, M.; Ferlic, N.A.; Karimnia, V.; Polacheck, W.J.; Celli, J.P.; Huang, H.C.; Rizvi, I. Photodynamic Therapy and the Biophysics of the Tumor Microenvironment. *Photochem. Photobiol.* **2020**, *96*, 232–259. [CrossRef]
123. Vidyarthi, A.; Agnihotri, T.; Khan, N.; Singh, S.; Tewari, M.K.; Radotra, B.D.; Chatterjee, D.; Agrewala, J.N. Predominance of M2 macrophages in gliomas leads to the suppression of local and systemic immunity. *Cancer Immunol. Immunother.* **2019**, *68*, 1995–2004. [CrossRef]
124. Coniglio, S.J.; Segall, J.E. Review: Molecular mechanism of microglia stimulated glioblastoma invasion. *Matrix Biol.* **2013**, *32*, 372–380. [CrossRef] [PubMed]
125. Gabrusiewicz, K.; Hossain, M.B.; Cortes-Santiago, N.; Fan, X.; Kaminska, B.; Marini, F.C.; Fueyo, J.; Gomez-Manzano, C. Macrophage Ablation Reduces M2-Like Populations and Jeopardizes Tumor Growth in a MAFIA-Based Glioma Model. *Neoplasia* **2015**, *17*, 374–384. [CrossRef] [PubMed]
126. Barca, C.; Foray, C.; Hermann, S.; Herrlinger, U.; Remory, I.; Laoui, D.; Schäfers, M.; Grauer, O.M.; Zinnhardt, B.; Jacobs, A.H. The Colony Stimulating Factor-1 Receptor (CSF-1R)-Mediated Regulation of Microglia/Macrophages as a Target for Neurological Disorders (Glioma, Stroke). *Front. Immunol.* **2021**, *12*, 5200. [CrossRef] [PubMed]
127. Przystal, J.M.; Becker, H.; Canjuga, D.; Tsiami, F.; Anderle, N.; Keller, A.L.; Pohl, A.; Ries, C.H.; Schmittnaegel, M.; Korinetska, N.; et al. Targeting csf1r alone or in combination with pd1 in experimental glioma. *Cancers* **2021**, *13*, 2400. [CrossRef] [PubMed]
128. Yan, D.; Kowal, J.; Akkari, L.; Schuhmacher, A.J.; Huse, J.T.; West, B.L.; Joyce, J.A. Inhibition of colony stimulating factor-1 receptor abrogates microenvironment-mediated therapeutic resistance in gliomas. *Oncogene* **2017**, *36*, 6049–6058. [CrossRef] [PubMed]

129. Pyonteck, S.M.; Akkari, L.; Schuhmacher, A.J.; Bowman, R.L.; Sevenich, L.; Quail, D.F.; Olson, O.C.; Quick, M.L.; Huse, J.T.; Teijeiro, V.; et al. CSF-1R inhibition alters macrophage polarization and blocks glioma progression. *Nat. Med.* **2013**, *19*, 1264–1272. [CrossRef]
130. Rios, A.; Hsu, S.H.; Blanco, A.; Buryanek, J.; Day, A.; McGuire, M.F.; Brown, R.E. Durable response of glioblastoma to adjuvant therapy consisting of temozolomide and a weekly dose of AMD3100 (plerixafor), a CXCR4 inhibitor, together with lapatinib, metformin and niacinamide. *Oncoscience* **2016**, *3*, 156–163. [CrossRef]
131. Giordano, F.A.; Link, B.; Glas, M.; Herrlinger, U.; Wenz, F.; Umansky, V.; Martin Brown, J.; Herskind, C. Targeting the Post-Irradiation Tumor Microenvironment in Glioblastoma via Inhibition of CXCL12. *Cancers* **2019**, *11*, 272. [CrossRef]
132. Piao, Y.; Liang, J.; Holmes, L.; Zurita, A.J.; Henry, V.; Heymach, J.V.; De Groot, J.F. Glioblastoma resistance to anti-VEGF therapy is associated with myeloid cell infiltration, stem cell accumulation, and a mesenchymal phenotype. *Neuro. Oncol.* **2012**, *14*, 1379–1392. [CrossRef]
133. Aminin, D.; Wang, Y.M. Macrophages as a "weapon" in anticancer cellular immunotherapy. *Kaohsiung J. Med. Sci.* **2021**, *37*, 749–758. [CrossRef]
134. Guerra, A.D.; Yeung, O.W.H.; Qi, X.; Kao, W.J.; Man, K. The Anti-Tumor Effects of M1 Macrophage-Loaded Poly (ethylene glycol) and Gelatin-Based Hydrogels on Hepatocellular Carcinoma. *Theranostics* **2017**, *7*, 3732–3744. [CrossRef] [PubMed]
135. Zheng, Y.; Bao, J.; Zhao, Q.; Zhou, T.; Sun, X. A spatio-temporal model of macrophage-mediated drug resistance in glioma immunotherapy. *Mol. Cancer Ther.* **2018**, *17*, 814–824. [CrossRef] [PubMed]
136. Mukherjee, S.; Baidoo, J.N.E.; Sampat, S.; Mancuso, A.; David, L.; Cohen, L.S.; Zhou, S.; Banerjee, P. Liposomal TriCurin, A Synergistic Combination of Curcumin, Epicatechin Gallate and Resveratrol, Repolarizes Tumor-Associated Microglia/Macrophages, and Eliminates Glioblastoma (GBM) and GBM Stem Cells. *Molecules* **2018**, *23*, 201. [CrossRef]
137. Tiwari, R.K.; Singh, S.; Gupta, C.L.; Pandey, P.; Singh, V.K.; Sayyed, U.; Shekh, R.; Bajpai, P. Repolarization of glioblastoma macrophage cells using non-agonistic Dectin-1 ligand encapsulating TLR-9 agonist: Plausible role in regenerative medicine against brain tumor. *Int. J. Neurosci.* **2020**, *131*, 591–598. [CrossRef]
138. Chryplewicz, A.; Scotton, J.; Tichet, M.; Zomer, A.; Shchors, K.; Joyce, J.A.; Homicsko, K.; Hanahan, D. Cancer cell autophagy, reprogrammed macrophages, and remodeled vasculature in glioblastoma triggers tumor immunity. *Cancer Cell* **2022**, *40*, 1111–1127.e9. [CrossRef]
139. Lee, H.; Jeong, A.J.; Ye, S.K. Highlighted STAT3 as a potential drug target for cancer therapy. *BMB Rep.* **2019**, *52*, 415–423. [CrossRef]
140. Remy, J.; Linder, B.; Weirauch, U.; Day, B.W.; Stringer, B.W.; Herold-Mende, C.; Aigner, A.; Krohn, K.; Kögel, D. STAT3 Enhances Sensitivity of Glioblastoma to Drug-Induced Autophagy-Dependent Cell Death. *Cancers* **2022**, *14*, 339. [CrossRef]
141. West, A.J.; Tsui, V.; Stylli, S.S.; Nguyen, H.P.T.; Morokoff, A.P.; Kaye, A.H.; Luwor, R.B. The role of interleukin-6-STAT3 signalling in glioblastoma. *Oncol. Lett.* **2018**, *16*, 4095–4104. [CrossRef] [PubMed]
142. Piperi, C.; Papavassiliou, K.A.; Papavassiliou, A.G. Pivotal Role of STAT3 in Shaping Glioblastoma Immune Microenvironment. *Cells* **2019**, *8*, 1398. [CrossRef]
143. Zhang, L.; Alizadeh, D.; van Handel, M.; Kortylewski, M.; Yu, H.; Badie, B. Stat3 inhibition activates tumor macrophages and abrogates glioma growth in mice. *Glia* **2009**, *57*, 1458–1467. [CrossRef] [PubMed]
144. Kai, K.; Komohara, Y.; Esumi, S.; Fujiwara, Y.; Yamamoto, T.; Uekawa, K.; Ohta, K.; Takezaki, T.; Kuroda, J.; Shinojima, N.; et al. Macrophage/microglia-derived IL-1β induces glioblastoma growth via the STAT3/NF-κB pathway. *Hum. Cell* **2022**, *35*, 226–237. [CrossRef] [PubMed]
145. Peng, P.; Zhu, H.; Liu, D.; Chen, Z.; Zhang, X.; Guo, Z.; Dong, M.; Wan, L.; Zhang, P.; Liu, G.; et al. TGFBI secreted by tumor-associated macrophages promotes glioblastoma stem cell-driven tumor growth via integrin αvβ5-Src-Stat3 signaling. *Theranostics* **2022**, *12*, 4221–4236. [CrossRef] [PubMed]
146. Bian, Z.; Ji, W.; Xu, B.; Huo, Z.; Huang, H.; Huang, J.; Jiao, J.; Shao, J.; Zhang, X. Noncoding RNAs involved in the STAT3 pathway in glioma. *Cancer Cell Int.* **2021**, *21*, 445. [CrossRef]
147. Qian, M.; Wang, S.; Guo, X.; Wang, J.; Zhang, Z.; Qiu, W.; Gao, X.; Chen, Z.; Xu, J.; Zhao, R.; et al. Hypoxic glioma-derived exosomes deliver microRNA-1246 to induce M2 macrophage polarization by targeting TERF2IP via the STAT3 and NF-κB pathways. *Oncogene* **2019**, *39*, 428–442. [CrossRef]
148. Shoji, T.; Saito, R.; Chonan, M.; Shibahara, I.; Sato, A.; Kanamori, M.; Sonoda, Y.; Kondo, T.; Ishii, N.; Tominaga, T. Local convection-enhanced delivery of an anti-CD40 agonistic monoclonal antibody induces antitumor effects in mouse glioma models. *Neuro. Oncol.* **2016**, *18*, 1120–1128. [CrossRef]
149. Helleberg Madsen, N.; Schnack Nielsen, B.; Larsen, J.; Gad, M. In vitro 2D and 3D cancer models to evaluate compounds that modulate macrophage polarization. *Cell. Immunol.* **2022**, *378*, 104574. [CrossRef]
150. Kosaka, A.; Ohkuri, T.; Okada, H. Combination of an agonistic anti-CD40 monoclonal antibody and the COX-2 inhibitor celecoxib induces anti-glioma effects by promotion of type-1 immunity in myeloid cells and T-cells. *Cancer Immunol. Immunother.* **2014**, *63*, 847–857. [CrossRef]
151. Yang, F.; He, Z.; Duan, H.; Zhang, D.; Li, J.; Yang, H.; Dorsey, J.F.; Zou, W.; Ali Nabavizadeh, S.; Bagley, S.J.; et al. Synergistic immunotherapy of glioblastoma by dual targeting of IL-6 and CD40. *Nat. Commun.* **2021**, *12*, 3424. [CrossRef]
152. Mantovani, A.; Allavena, P.; Marchesi, F.; Garlanda, C. Macrophages as tools and targets in cancer therapy. *Nat. Rev. Drug Discov.* **2022**, *21*, 799–820. [CrossRef]

153. Mass, E.; Lachmann, N. From macrophage biology to macrophage-based cellular immunotherapies. *Gene Ther.* **2021**, *28*, 473–476. [CrossRef] [PubMed]
154. Iglesias-López, C.; Agustí, A.; Obach, M.; Vallano, A. Regulatory framework for advanced therapy medicinal products in Europe and United States. *Front. Pharmacol.* **2019**, *10*, 921. [CrossRef] [PubMed]
155. Lee, S.; Kivimäe, S.; Dolor, A.; Szoka, F.C. Macrophage-based cell therapies: The long and winding road. *J. Control. Release* **2016**, *240*, 527–540. [CrossRef]
156. Zhang, J.; Shan, W.F.; Jin, T.T.; Wu, G.Q.; Xiong, X.X.; Jin, H.Y.; Zhu, S.M. Propofol exerts anti-hepatocellular carcinoma by microvesicle-mediated transfer of miR-142-3p from macrophage to cancer cells. *J. Transl. Med.* **2014**, *12*, 279. [CrossRef]
157. Zhou, X.; Chen, B.; Zhang, Z.; Huang, Y.; Li, J.; Wei, Q.; Cao, D.; Ai, J. Crosstalk between Tumor-Associated Macrophages and MicroRNAs: A Key Role in Tumor Microenvironment. *Int. J. Mol. Sci.* **2022**, *23*, 13258. [CrossRef]
158. Wang, H.F.; Liu, Y.; Yang, G.; Zhao, C.X. Macrophage-mediated cancer drug delivery. *Mater. Today Sustain.* **2021**, *11*, 100055. [CrossRef]
159. Feng, S.; Cui, S.; Jin, J.; Gu, Y. Macrophage as cellular vehicles for delivery of nanoparticles. *J. Innov. Opt. Health Sci.* **2014**, *7*, 1450023. [CrossRef]
160. Xia, Y.; Rao, L.; Yao, H.; Wang, Z.; Ning, P.; Chen, X. Engineering Macrophages for Cancer Immunotherapy and Drug Delivery. *Adv. Mater.* **2020**, *32*, 2002054. [CrossRef]
161. Ibarra, L.E.; Beaugé, L.; Arias-Ramos, N.; Rivarola, V.A.; Chesta, C.A.; López-Larrubia, P.; Palacios, R.E. Trojan horse monocyte-mediated delivery of conjugated polymer nanoparticles for improved photodynamic therapy of glioblastoma. *Nanomedicine* **2020**, *15*, 1687–1707. [CrossRef]
162. Watson, D.C.; Bayik, D.; Srivatsan, A.; Bergamaschi, C.; Valentin, A.; Niu, G.; Bear, J.; Monninger, M.; Sun, M.; Morales-Kastresana, A.; et al. Efficient production and enhanced tumor delivery of engineered extracellular vesicles. *Biomaterials* **2016**, *105*, 195–205. [CrossRef]
163. Bhaskaran, M.; Devegowda, V.G.; Gupta, V.K.; Shivachar, A.; Bhosale, R.R.; Arunachalam, M.; Vaishnavi, T. Current Perspectives on Therapies, including Drug Delivery Systems, for Managing Glioblastoma Multiforme. *ACS Chem. Neurosci.* **2020**, *11*, 2962–2977. [CrossRef]
164. Ouyang, X.; Wang, X.; Kraatz, H.B.; Ahmadi, S.; Gao, J.; Lv, Y.; Sun, X.; Huang, Y. A Trojan horse biomimetic delivery strategy using mesenchymal stem cells for PDT/PTT therapy against lung melanoma metastasis. *Biomater. Sci.* **2020**, *8*, 1160–1170. [CrossRef]
165. Pang, L.; Zhu, Y.; Qin, J.; Zhao, W.; Wang, J. Primary M1 macrophages as multifunctional carrier combined with PLGA nanoparticle delivering anticancer drug for efficient glioma therapy. *Drug Deliv.* **2018**, *25*, 1922–1931. [CrossRef] [PubMed]
166. Habibi, N.; Brown, T.D.; Adu-Berchie, K.; Christau, S.; Raymond, J.E.; Mooney, D.J.; Mitragotri, S.; Lahann, J. Nanoparticle Properties Influence Transendothelial Migration of Monocytes. *Langmuir* **2022**, *38*, 5603–5616. [CrossRef] [PubMed]
167. Gardell, J.L.; Matsumoto, L.R.; Chinn, H.; Degolier, K.R.; Kreuser, S.A.; Prieskorn, B.; Balcaitis, S.; Davis, A.; Ellenbogen, R.G.; Crane, C.A. Human macrophages engineered to secrete a bispecific T cell engager support antigen-dependent T cell responses to glioblastoma. *J. Immunother. Cancer* **2020**, *8*, e001202. [CrossRef]
168. Madsen, S.J.; Hirschberg, H. Macrophages as delivery vehicles for anticancer agents. *Ther. Deliv.* **2019**, *10*, 189–201. [CrossRef]
169. Huang, W.C.; Chiang, W.H.; Cheng, Y.H.; Lin, W.C.; Yu, C.F.; Yen, C.Y.; Yeh, C.K.; Chern, C.S.; Chiang, C.S.; Chiu, H.C. Tumortropic monocyte-mediated delivery of echogenic polymer bubbles and therapeutic vesicles for chemotherapy of tumor hypoxia. *Biomaterials* **2015**, *71*, 71–83. [CrossRef]
170. Tripathi, C.; Tewari, B.N.; Kanchan, R.K.; Baghel, K.S.; Nautiyal, N.; Shrivastava, R.; Kaur, H.; Bramha Bhatt, M.L.; Bhadauria, S. Macrophages are recruited to hypoxic tumor areas and acquire a Pro-Angiogenic M2-Polarized phenotype via hypoxic cancer cell derived cytokines Oncostatin M and Eotaxin. *Oncotarget* **2014**, *5*, 5350–5368. [CrossRef] [PubMed]
171. Silva, V.L.; Al-Jamal, W.T. Exploiting the cancer niche: Tumor-associated macrophages and hypoxia as promising synergistic targets for nano-based therapy. *J. Control. Release* **2017**, *253*, 82–96. [CrossRef]
172. Bai, R.; Li, Y.; Jian, L.; Yang, Y.; Zhao, L.; Wei, M. The hypoxia-driven crosstalk between tumor and tumor-associated macrophages: Mechanisms and clinical treatment strategies. *Mol. Cancer* **2022**, *21*, 177. [CrossRef]
173. Mukhopadhyay, M. Macrophages enter CAR immunotherapy. *Nat. Methods* **2020**, *17*, 561. [CrossRef] [PubMed]
174. Pan, K.; Farrukh, H.; Chittepu, V.C.S.R.; Xu, H.; Pan, C.X.; Zhu, Z. CAR race to cancer immunotherapy: From CAR T, CAR NK to CAR macrophage therapy. *J. Exp. Clin. Cancer Res.* **2022**, *41*, 119. [CrossRef] [PubMed]
175. Gatto, L.; Di Nunno, V.; Franceschi, E.; Brandes, A.A. Chimeric antigen receptor macrophage for glioblastoma immunotherapy: The way forward. *Immunotherapy* **2021**, *13*, 879–883. [CrossRef]
176. Chen, C.; Jing, W.; Chen, Y.; Wang, G.; Abdalla, M.; Gao, L.; Han, M.; Shi, C.; Li, A.; Sun, P.; et al. Intracavity generation of glioma stem cell–specific CAR macrophages primes locoregional immunity for postoperative glioblastoma therapy. *Sci. Transl. Med.* **2022**, *14*, eabn1128. [CrossRef] [PubMed]

Disclaimer/Publisher's Note: The statements, opinions and data contained in all publications are solely those of the individual author(s) and contributor(s) and not of MDPI and/or the editor(s). MDPI and/or the editor(s) disclaim responsibility for any injury to people or property resulting from any ideas, methods, instructions or products referred to in the content.

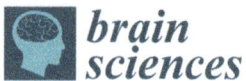

Review

An Update on Emergent Nano-Therapeutic Strategies against Pediatric Brain Tumors

Ammu V. V. V. Ravi Kiran [1], G. Kusuma Kumari [1], Praveen T. Krishnamurthy [1], Asha P. Johnson [2], Madhuchandra Kenchegowda [2], Riyaz Ali M. Osmani [2], Amr Selim Abu Lila [3], Afrasim Moin [3], H. V. Gangadharappa [2,*] and Syed Mohd Danish Rizvi [3,*]

[1] Department of Pharmacology, JSS College of Pharmacy, JSS Academy of Higher Education & Research, Rocklands, Ooty 643001, The Nilgiris, Tamil Nadu, India; devikiran006@gmail.com (A.V.V.V.R.K.); garikapatikusumakumari16@gmail.com (G.K.K.); praveentk@jssuni.edu.in (P.T.K.)

[2] Department of Pharmaceutics, JSS College of Pharmacy, JSS Academy of Higher Education & Research, Mysuru 570015, Karnataka, India; ashapjohnson19@gmail.com (A.P.J.); madhuchandra152@gmail.com (M.K.); riyazosmani@gmail.com (R.A.M.O.)

[3] Department of Pharmaceutics, College of Pharmacy, University of Ha'il, Ha'il 81442, Saudi Arabia; a.abulila@uoh.edu.sa (A.S.A.L.); a.moinuddin@uoh.edu.sa (A.M.)

* Correspondence: hvgangadharappa@jssuni.edu.in (H.V.G.); sm.danish@uoh.edu.sa (S.M.D.R.)

Abstract: Pediatric brain tumors are the major cause of pediatric cancer mortality. They comprise a diverse group of tumors with different developmental origins, genetic profiles, therapeutic options, and outcomes. Despite many technological advancements, the treatment of pediatric brain cancers has remained a challenge. Treatment options for pediatric brain cancers have been ineffective due to non-specificity, inability to cross the blood–brain barrier, and causing off-target side effects. In recent years, nanotechnological advancements in the medical field have proven to be effective in curing challenging cancers like brain tumors. Moreover, nanoparticles have emerged successfully, particularly in carrying larger payloads, as well as their stability, safety, and efficacy monitoring. In the present review, we will emphasize pediatric brain cancers, barriers to treating these cancers, and novel treatment options.

Keywords: brain tumors; childhood cancers; pediatrics; nanoparticles; liposomes

Citation: Ravi Kiran, A.V.V.V.; Kumari, G.K.; Krishnamurthy, P.T.; Johnson, A.P.; Kenchegowda, M.; Osmani, R.A.M.; Abu Lila, A.S.; Moin, A.; Gangadharappa, H.V.; Rizvi, S.M.D. An Update on Emergent Nano-Therapeutic Strategies against Pediatric Brain Tumors. Brain Sci. **2024**, 14, 185. https://doi.org/10.3390/brainsci14020185

Academic Editors: Luis Ibarra, Laura Natalia Milla Sanabria and Nuria Arias-Ramos

Received: 16 December 2023
Revised: 7 February 2024
Accepted: 13 February 2024
Published: 18 February 2024

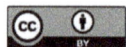

Copyright: © 2024 by the authors. Licensee MDPI, Basel, Switzerland. This article is an open access article distributed under the terms and conditions of the Creative Commons Attribution (CC BY) license (https://creativecommons.org/licenses/by/4.0/).

1. Introduction

Childhood/pediatric brain cancers are the second most common pediatric cancers, accounting for about one-fourth of all pediatric cancer cases [1]. The Industrial revolution and advancements in genetic screening and sequencing together ushered in new perspectives (both at the molecular and genetic levels) on these pediatric brain cancers. Mounting studies suggest that mutational burden is much lower in childhood brain cancers compared to adult brain cancers [1–3]. Furthermore, crucial targets in adult brain cancers cannot necessarily be exploited in childhood brain cancers due to their unique biology, which differs from adult cancers [1,4–6]. Over the past few decades, remarkable progress has been made in the treatment of childhood brain cancers, improving the patient survival rate by at least 5 years. Despite these improvements, many pediatric brain tumors are still incurable with high morbidity rates. Additionally, with the intensification of the therapy, the adverse effects of the chemo- and radiotherapies have become gradually apparent; for example, anthracyclines such as doxorubicin could cause cardiomyopathic problems [1,4].

In recent years, cancer nanomedicine has emerged as an important advancement in improving the therapeutic benefit [7,8]. Different nanoparticles, including organic, inorganic, or lipid-based nanoparticles, have been widely tested in delivering cancer theranostics. Further, these nanoparticles proved to be more advantageous than conventional methods due to their higher payload capacity, stability, and prolonged circulation time, thereby improving safety and efficacy [7,8]. In the present review, we will discuss the various pediatric brain cancers, barriers to treating these cancers, and novel treatment options. For selecting the recent relevant and informative research articles, a focused search using the keywords 'brain tumors', 'childhood cancers', 'pediatrics', 'nanoparticles', and 'nanotheranostics' was run using the databases such as Scopus, Web of Science, PubMed, ScienceDirect, Directory of Open Access Journals (DOAJ), etc. Articles showing more than 95% content and keyword match were included, and the rest were excluded.

2. Pediatric Brain Cancers: Targets and Mechanisms

Over the past few decades, cancer has been a long-lasting disease due to its heterogeneity [9,10]. In order to develop novel therapeutics, a thorough understanding of the underlying pathophysiological and molecular pathways is essential, especially in distinguishing childhood and adult cancers [11,12]. Unlike adult cancers, pediatric cancers are not triggered by lifestyle changes and are less inherited. Though the chance of risk development increases gradually with age, there are still a few exceptions. For instance, the occurrence of bone, brain, and blood cancers is greater in children than in adults. Further, the kinetic profile and therapeutic outcome differ in children than in adults (e.g., genitourinary pH, intestinal mobility, etc.) [11,13]. Additionally, pediatric tissues are immature and in the continuous growing phase, possessing greater metabolic rates and toxicity issues. Lastly, genetic variations in pediatric cancers, such as acute lymphocytic leukemia, Ewing sarcoma, etc., are greatly driven by fusion oncogenes due to chromosomal translocations. Unlike adult cancers, pediatric cancers possess a lower mutational rate, making their therapeutic targeting more challenging [13,14].

Considering the above-mentioned reasons, there is an imminent need to understand novel therapeutic targets and develop new therapeutic options. In this section, we will be discussing the various pediatric brain tumors and treatable options.

2.1. Medulloblastoma

Medulloblastoma (MB) is highly malignant and is the most common childhood brain cancer formed in the cerebellum [15]. MB is categorized into four molecular subgroups: Sonic hedgehog (SHH), WNT, group 3, and group 4 [15,16]. These subgroups are identified as powerful predictors of therapy outcomes. For instance, patients with WNT tumors have greater survival after therapy than group 3 tumors.

2.1.1. WNT Subgroup

WNT-associated MB is most common in children over the age of three, with a 5-year survival rate, and is seldom metastatic. WNT-MB has no focal somatic copy number aberrations (SCNAs) and typically has chromosome 6 monosomy. Initially, it was recognized that people with Turcot syndrome, a genetic disorder caused by mutations in the adenomatous polyposis coli (APC) gene, a repressor of WNT signaling, had a higher incidence of MB [16]. Later, it was discovered that a subgroup of sporadic MBs had WNT pathway mutations, notably in CTNNB1 (encoding β-catenin). β-catenin enhances WNT target gene transcription by interacting with a number of chromatin modifiers such as histone acetyltransferases, SMARCA4, and CREBBP. Furthermore, whole-genome sequencing (WGS) has revealed that CTNNB1 mutations commonly coincide with missense variations in the DEAD-box RNA helicase DDX3X [17,18]. WNT-MB tumors are thought to form in the dorsal brainstem from progenitor cells in the lower rhombic lip.

Despite WNT-MB's favorable prognosis, recent clinical trials have focused on lowering chemotherapy or radiation doses in the hopes of reducing off-target implications [16,17]. It is worth noting that WNT signaling has been proposed to play a role in WNT-MB's exceptional response to standard therapy. Further studies revealed that these tumors release soluble WNT antagonists, which may disrupt the blood–brain barrier and sensitize tumors to chemotherapy.

2.1.2. SHH Subgroup

Patients with SHH-activated MB were considered to have high-risk disease (survival rate of 50–75%), which is lower than WNT patients but higher than patients in group 3. SHH-MB, like WNT-MB, has a relatively even gender distribution. Unlike WNT-MB, most SHH-MB patients are newborns or adults; just a few youngsters have this tumor subtype. SHH-MB's genome contains substantially more SCNAs than WNT-MB's genome [13,17,18]. Initially, SHH signaling in MB was discovered in the context of Gorlin syndrome, a hereditary disorder embodied by basal cell carcinomas of the skin, craniofacial abnormalities, and an elevated prevalence of MB. Gorlin patients have germline mutations in PTCH1, a repressor of the SHH pathway. Germline mutations in the gene encoding Suppressor of Fused (SUFU) also predispose to SHH-MB [13,17]. Furthermore, spontaneous MBs in the SHH subgroup exhibit PTCH1 and SUFU loss-of-function mutations, Smoothened (SMO) and SHH activation mutations, GLI2, and MYCN amplifications. SHH pathway gene mutations are discovered in an age-dependent manner: All age groups have PTCH1 mutations; however, infants and adults are more likely to have SUFU mutations, infants are more likely to have SMO mutations, and children under the age of three are more likely to have MYCN and GLI2 amplifications. Mice with Gli2, Smo, Ptch1, and Sufu mutations are also susceptible to MB, indicating the function of these genes as tumorigenesis elicitors. A subset of SHH-MB patients, notably older adolescents and teenagers, have significant "chromothripsis" (chromosome shattering) [17]. Using WGS, Rausch et al. [19] discovered that these individuals typically had germline or somatic TP53 mutations, the former of which is related to Li-Fraumeni syndrome (LFS). Chromothripsis can cause SHH pathway gene amplification, such as GLI2 and MYCN, which increases SHH target gene expression and drives tumor development. For years, scientists have researched the genesis of SHH-MB tumors; however, most recent research indicates that these tumors are caused by granule neuron progenitors (GNPs). Small-molecule SHH pathway antagonists have made it possible to treat this subset of tumors in innovative ways. SMO inhibitors (SMOis), in particular GDC-0449 (vismodegib) and NVP-LDE225 (erismodegib), have been linked in clinical studies to strong (albeit frequently transitory) responses in MB patients [17]. SMO mutations may sometimes prevent long-term therapeutic benefits from occurring; in other circumstances, mutations in downstream components of the SHH pathway (for instance, MYCN or GLI2 amplifications) or in other pathways might render tumor cells resistant to these medications. The antifungal drug itraconazole and the cyclopamine derivative IPI-926 (saridegib) are two examples of second-site SMOis that have shown potential in preclinical research [20,21]. Arsenic trioxide, an inhibitor of downstream components of the SHH pathway, can accelerate GLI2 degradation [13].

2.1.3. Group 3 Subgroup

Group 3-MBs account for about ~20–25% with very little prognosis and occur more in pediatrics than adults. At the time of diagnosis, most group 3-MB patients have the highest metastasis. Most group 3-MB originate in the midline in the proximity of the fourth ventricle of the brainstem [13,17]. The possibility of higher metastasis is due to this location, which facilitates access to the cerebrospinal fluid. Contrastingly, no germline mutations are known for the formation of group 3-MB [18]. The prominence of these tumors is majorly due to the amplification of the MYC oncogene, which fuses with the plasmacytoma variant translocation 1 (PVT1), which stabilizes the MYC proteins. Group 3-MB exhibits orthodenticle homeobox 2 (OTX2) amplification, which upregulates MYC expression, thereby promoting tumor formation. Further, genomic instability in group 3-MB is associated with the loss or gain of chromosomes. One of the key events in group 3-MB that happens in chromosome 17 is the simultaneous loss of 17p and gain of 17q chromosomes [18].

In order to identify novel therapeutics for group 3-MB, a high-throughput screening has been generated. The same study has revealed that gemcitabine and pemetrexed suppressed the group 3-MB in both mouse and human models. Despite improvement in survival having been observed in in vivo models, the involvement of tumor microenvironment has enhanced drug resistance in tumors. Another potential undruggable target in group 3-MBs is the overexpressed MYC gene. Treatment options for MYC can be achieved by bromodomain protein inhibitors such as JQ1, which arrest the G1 phase of the cell cycle, causing apoptosis [18].

2.1.4. Group 4 Subgroup

Group 4-MBs account for more than one-third of all cases, with metastatic hallmark being the most common [13,18]. Unlike adult patients, infants and young adults with group 4-MBs have an intermediate survival rate. Similar to group 3-MBs, group 4-MBs originate adjacent to the fourth ventricle. Most of group-4 MBs possess chromosomal instability (esp. chromosome 17), causing the prevalence of SCNAs resulting from tetraploidization. Further, group 4-MBs possess < 10% mutations in KDM6A, ZMYM3, CTDNEP1, etc. An increase in SCNAs is reported to affect the NF-κB signaling, implying the potential therapeutic target [13]. Although the origin of group 4-MBs is unknown, gene signature has led to the glutamate-secreting neurons, suggesting from glutamatergic progenitors. Further studies revealed that the nuclear transitory zone (NTZ) is the main origin of group 4-MBs [22]. Due to the absence of a suitable animal model that mimics the group 4-MBs, proper therapeutic strategies against these tumors are limited. Few therapeutic options exist for treating group 4-MBs; for tumors that express MYCN and CDK6 amplification, bromodomain inhibitors and cyclin-dependent kinase (CDK) inhibitors along with MYC-destabilizing Aurora kinase A inhibitors may be preferred [23,24].

2.2. Gliomas/High-Grade Gliomas (HGGs)

Pediatric high-grade gliomas (HGGs) are the most common malignant brain tumors, majorly consisting of glioblastoma, astrocytoma, etc. [25]. World Health organization (WHO) has classified glioblastomas as grade IV due to their high proliferation, neovascularization, and necrosis [26,27]. Diffuse intrinsic pontine gliomas (DIPGs) are tumors that resemble gliomas histologically but possess diffusely metastatic growth inside the brainstem. Glioblastomas exhibit higher methylation of O6-methylguanine-DNA methyltransferase (MGMT), which results in impairment of DNA repair with the use of alkylating agents. To date, no therapeutic options have been available for improving survival for HGGs [26,27].

2.3. Neuroblastomas

Neuroblastomas are one of the major causes of death in pediatrics, accounting for about ~10–13% of all pediatric cancer cases [14,28]. Neuroblastomas originate from primordial neural crest cells, which form the adrenal medulla and sympathetic ganglia. Similar to glioblastomas, neuroblastomas also exhibit greater amplification of N-myc, which is associated with the expression of MRP and chromosome 1p deletion [28,29]. Overexpressed MRP on the neuroblastoma surface enhances the chemoresistance potential. Further, amplification of N-myc has downregulated the expression of CD44 receptors, which is a potential marker for aggressive tumor behavior. Additionally, low expression of Trk, a tyrosine kinase receptor, is associated with amplification of N-myc and even advanced stages of neuroblastomas. ALK amplification is another set of somatic mutations, accounting for ~14% of high-risk neuroblastomas [30]. Gain-of-function in ALK could drive the neuroblastoma but requires cooperation from MYCN amplification. Further, ALK upregulates the proto-oncogene RET and RET-driven sympathetic markers of the cholinergic lineage, which offer new therapeutic options, i.e., targeting both ALK and RET [30,31].

2.4. Ependymoma

Ependymoma (EPN) is one of the pediatric brain cancers which can occur in any part of the brain. The most popular originating location is the posterior fossa (cerebellum and brainstem), followed by supratentorial sites (cerebral hemispheres) and spinal cord [32,33].

The only option for treating ependymomas is surgery or radiation, as standard chemotherapy is ineffective. The molecular characteristics of EPNs are heterogeneous, mainly with dysregulation in growth factors such as epidermal growth factor receptor (EGFR), fibroblast growth factor receptor (FGFR), etc. EPNs originating from the posterior fossa (PF-EPN) are classified as PF-EPN-A and -B. PF-EPN-A is reported to be more deadly than PF-EPN-B [34]. Further, treatment with small molecule inhibitors, such as 3-deazaneplanocin A, causes degradation of PRC2 complex or with EZH2 (a GSK343 inhibitor), which competitively binds with S-adenosyl-L-methionine. EPNs originating from supratentorial (ST-EPNs) are reported to harbor fusion between RELA, NF-κB, and C11orf95 [35]. Further studies revealed that RELA fusion proteins alone could initiate the transformation of the neural stem cells [36]. Treatment options against ST-EPNs are mostly common chemotherapeutics such as temozolomide, vincristine, etc. [37] or HDAC inhibitors, including entinostat and vorinostat [38]. Ongoing research using preclinical models of ST-EPNs to evaluate potential druggable targets holds promise for developing treatment of tumors with RELA fusion proteins [32,34].

3. Nano-Based Approaches for Treating Pediatric Brain Cancers

Many research groups have emphasized utilizing nanotechnology to curb tumor progression, especially in pediatrics. In the present section, we will discuss nanotechnological advancements, especially for treating pediatric brain cancer. A schematic outline of diverse nanotherapeutic approached adopted for augmented pediatric brain cancer is depicted in Figure 1.

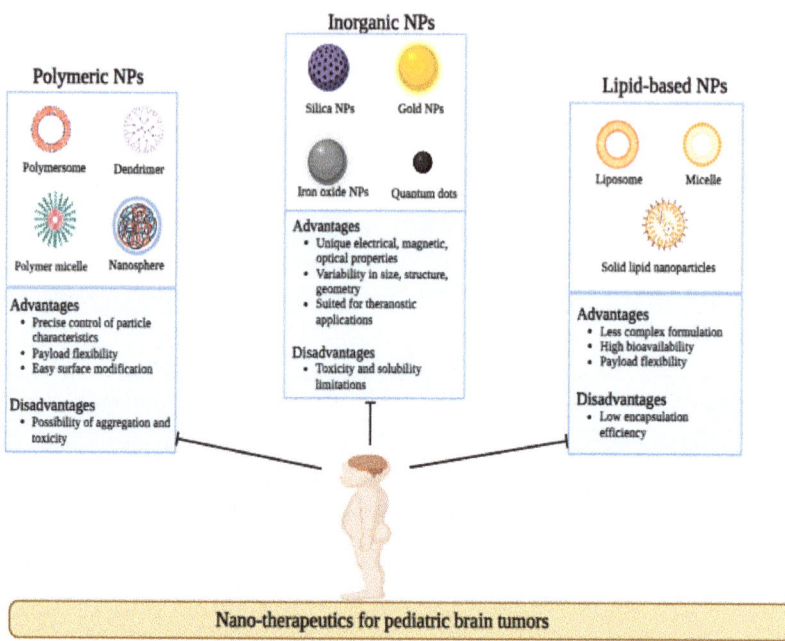

Figure 1. Schematic representation of nano-therapeutics for pediatric brain tumors.

3.1. Nanotechnology and Blood–Brain Barrier

Due to its highly selective nature, the blood-brain-barrier (BBB) has become the first crucial barrier for many brain therapeutics and diagnostic entities. To develop a novel target-specific, an in-depth understanding of the physiology of BBB and overcoming strategies for nanoparticles is essential [39–41].

3.2. Physiology of BBB and Overcoming Strategies

BBB comprises highly specialized cells, which act as a protective barrier around the brain, especially in maintaining brain homeostasis. The cellular architecture of BBB mainly consists of brain capillary endothelial cells (BCECs), astrocytes, and pericytes [42]. Tight junctions between BCECs restrict the cellular diffusion of aqueous moieties. Further, in intact condition, BBB restricts the entry of ~99% of small drug molecules. BBB offers many transport mechanisms internally, i.e., via the transcellular lipophilic pathway, carrier-mediated transport (CMT), or receptor-mediated transport (RMT) [42,43]. However, the delivery of small molecules can be compromised by a large number of efflux pumps (such as adenosine triphosphate binding cassette transporters including multi-drug resistant protein (MRP) and p-glycoprotein (p-gp)), evade the foreign material into the bloodstream. Further, biological compounds, including inflammatory mediators (e.g., bradykinin, prostaglandin, vascular endothelial growth factors (VEGF)), signal receptors to increase BBB permeability [43].

Currently, drug delivery systems that are used in clinics are especially focused on local delivery. However, local delivery has limitations, including high rates of infection and excessive cerebrospinal fluid requirement. A non-invasive with direct delivery of therapeutic agents to the brain is the "intranasal route", which is currently preferred but requires adjusting parameters such as dosage and positioning [42]. Transient opening of BBB can be achieved by biological (e.g., VEGF) or chemical stimuli (e.g., mannitol, oleic acid, cyclodextrins) but could have non-specific uptake, causing unwanted side effects. Therefore, an ideal approach to disrupting BBB is essential, one that would be controllable, reversible, specific, transient, and selective [43].

One of the best and most convenient approaches for drug delivery is intravenous administration with proper dosing. As discussed earlier, with the proper utilization of transporter proteins, specific receptors could be utilized for active targeting of nanoparticles-based drug deliveries. Further, disruption of BBB using either biological or chemical stimuli or nano-drug delivery systems, using either passive or active targeting, could achieve better BBB transport [41,42]. Moreover, most of the nano-drug delivery systems are lipophilic in nature, which is a crucial feature in bypassing the BBB.

Nanomedicines are small-sized nanocarriers that have been adopted to cure brain illnesses, including brain cancer and Alzheimer's disease (AD). Functionalized nanoparticles are considered the most useful applicable approach to delivering these recommended drugs to the affected part of the brain. Nanomedicines have a set of unique properties that enable them to deliver anticancer drugs at target sites in the brain. Nanomedicines have the advantages of reduced dimensions and increased biocompatibility that facilitate the easy transport of therapeutic substances into the brain. Small-size nanomedicines can easily interact with the proteins and molecules on the cell surface as well as inside the cell. NP-functionalized nanomedicines have central core structures that ensure the encapsulation or conjugation of drugs and provide protection and prolonged circulation in the blood (Figure 2). Nanomedicines are also specialized to target cells or even an intracellular compartment and thus can deliver the drug at a predetermined dosage directly to the pathological site. Nanomedicines can minimize the dose and frequency and then improve patient compliance. Regardless of some clinical issues, nanomedicines have potential advantages of favorability to the brain, greater stability, biocompatibility and biodegradability, protection from enzymatic degradation, increased half-life, improved bioavailability, and controlled release over other conventional ways of drug delivery to the brain to cure AD (Figure 2) [44].

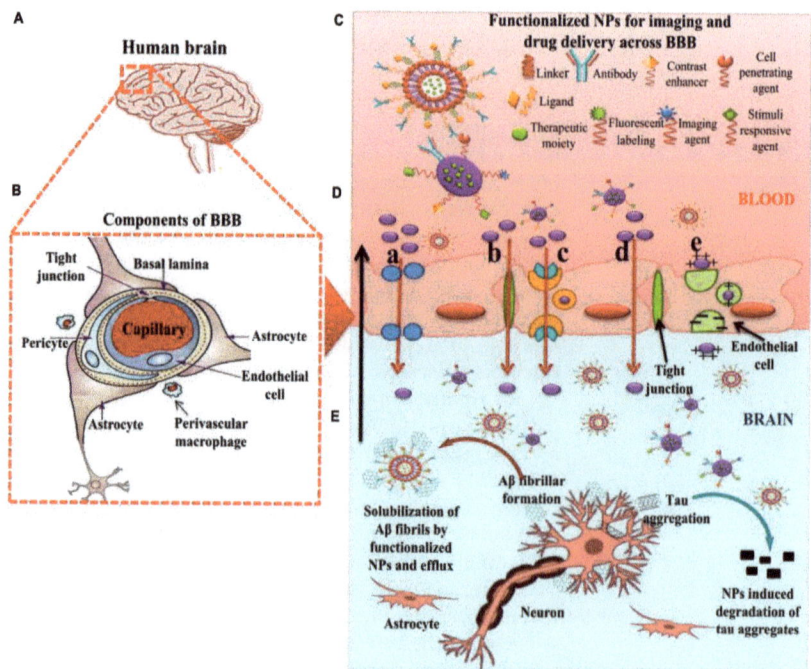

Figure 2. The role of nanoparticles in overcoming the BBB for efficient delivery of therapeutic moieties to treat AD. (**A**) Image of the human brain. (**B**) Components of the BBB. (**C**) Functionalized nanoparticles (NPs) for imaging and targeted drug delivery to the AD brain. (**D**) Different pathways of transport (a–e) across BBB are utilized by functionalized NPs. (a) Transport of NPs through cellular transport proteins; (b) transport of NPs through tight junctions; (c) transport of NPs via receptor-mediated transcytosis; (d) transport of NPs via transcellular pathway following diffusion, specifically adopted by gold NPs; and (e) transport of cationic NPs and liposomes via adsorption-mediated transcytosis. (**E**) Effect of functionalized NPs in treating AD via the degradation of tau aggregates and efflux of Aβ fibrils after getting solubilized by the NPs. AD: Alzheimer's disease; NPs: nanoparticles; BBB: blood–brain barrier. Adapted with permission from [44].

3.3. Nanoformulations Used for the Treatment of Medulloblastoma

Nanoparticle-based approaches are potential treatment options for pediatric medulloblastoma. NPs-based strategies mainly aim to improve the delivery of drugs by active or passive targeting and improve BBB crossing while reducing the side effects to surrounding healthy tissues.

Recently, herpes simplex virus type I thymidine kinase gene encoded plasmid loaded with poly (beta-amino ester) (PBAE) nanoparticles for gene therapy to medulloblastoma (MB) and atypical teratoid/rhabdoid tumors (AT/RT). The treatment with gene-encapsulated nanoparticles showed controlled apoptosis in transfected cells. In MB and AT/RT implanted mice, the gene therapy exhibited greater overall median survival [45]. An engineered biomimetic nanoparticle with dual targeting was designed to target the cancer stem-like cell population in sonic hedgehog medulloblastoma (SHH-MB). Treatment failure and poor outcomes are the significant struggles associated with the SHH-MB. High-density lipoprotein-mimetic nanoparticles (eHNPs) were used to cross BBB and load SHH inhibitors for the effective treatment of SHH-MB. Multi-component eHNPs were designed using microfluidic technology and are encapsulated with apolipoprotein A1, anti-CD15, and LDE225 (SHH inhibitor). eHNP-A1 improves the stability of the drug and has a therapeutic effect by SR-B1-mediated intracellular cholesterol depletion in tumor cells. These multifunctional nanoparticles exhibited promising effects in SHH-MB treatment and are applicable to other drugs that cannot cross BBB and have low bioavailability [46].

In a study, researchers developed a brain tumor model consisting of DAOY (MB cell lines) aggregates and cerebellum slices for evaluation of a poly(glycerol-adipate) (PGA) nanoparticle drug delivery system. PGA nanoparticles exhibited higher uptake than normal host cells. This novel tumor model suggests the effective evaluation of a drug delivery system between tumor cells and brain cells [47]. Kumar et al. [48] used Hedgehog inhibitor MDB5 and BRD4/PI3K dual inhibitor SF2523 to obtain the synergistic inhibition of medulloblastoma cell lines and to prevent resistance. They designed mPEG-b-PCC-g-DC copolymer-based NPs for effective loading of MDB5 and SF2523. NPs exhibit sustained release of loaded molecules. Targeted NPs were prepared by mixing COG-133-PEG-b-PBC and mPEG-b-PCC-g-DC copolymer and were found to be efficient in the reduction of tumors in orthotopic SHH-MB tumor-bearing NSG mice [48].

3.4. Nanoformulations Used for the Treatment of Glioma

Gliomas are the most common malignancy affecting the central nervous system. The primary treatment barrier for this disease is the difficulty of crossing the BBB by drug molecules. Nanoparticle-based approaches are familiar in overcoming these issues.

In a study, Temozolomide, an anti-glioma drug, was loaded on liposomes using proliposomes. The liposomes showed a slow release of temozolomide compared to the drug solution. The loading of temozolomide in liposomes improves the pharmacokinetic parameters compared to pure drug solution. Liposomes prolong the circulation time and improve the area under the curve (AUC). The biodistribution after IV injection revealed that the drug accumulation in the heart and lung is decreasing, and the concentration of the drug is increasing in the brain [49]. In another study, a targeted drug delivery platform was designed with PAMAM-PEG and transferrin for the encapsulation of temozolomide for the effective targeting of glioma stem cells. Glioma stem cells are responsible for the development of resistance. High cellular uptake and cytotoxicity were observed with transferrin-targeted temozolomide nanoparticles. The nanoparticle effectively crossed the BBB and delivered the drug specifically to the tumor. The PAMAM-PEG-trf nanoparticles induced potent cell apoptosis in drug-resistant glioma stem cells [50].

Gu et al. [51] designed MT1-AF7p peptide-decorated paclitaxel-loaded PEG-PLA nanoparticles for glioma management. MT1-AF7p peptide has high binding to membrane type-1 matrix metalloproteinase (MT1-MMP) overexpressed on glioma cells. To improve the penetration of nanoparticles to glioma cells, the nanoparticles were co-administered with Tumor-homing and penetrating peptide iRGD. In C6 glioma cells, the peptide-decorated NPs showed significant cellular uptake via energy-dependent macropinocytosis and lipid raft-mediated endocytosis compared to non-peptide NPs. The nanoparticle's extravasation across BBB and accumulation in glioma parenchyma was improved significantly in in vivo imaging and glioma distribution with MT1-AF7p functionalization and iRGD co-administration. Intracranial C6 glioma-bearing nude mice exhibited higher survival time with MT1-AF7p functionalization and iRGD co-administration (Figure 3) [51]. Bhunia et al. [52] have tailored a large amino acid transporter-1 (LAT1) conjugated nanometric liposomal carriers functionalized with amphiphile L-3,4-dihydroxyphenylalanine (L-DOPA) (Amphi-DOPA). Glioma-bearing mice showed higher uptake of NIR-dye labeled Amphi-DOPA to brain tissue. WP1066 labeled Amphi-DOPA enhanced the overall survivability of glioma-bearing C57BL/6J mice by 60% compared to the untreated group [52].

A red blood cell membrane-coated nanoparticle (RBCNP) with a neurotoxin-derived targeting ligand was designed for brain-targeted drug delivery. RBCNP can provide the biological function of natural cell membranes and desirable properties for drug delivery. The targeting moiety CDX peptide derived from candoxin has a high binding affinity to nicotinic acetylcholine receptors overexpressed on brain endothelial cells decorated on RBCNP. In vitro and in vivo results suggest that RBCNP-CDX has promising brain-targeting efficiency. In glioma mouse models, Dox-loaded RBCNP-CDX NPs showed superior therapeutic efficacy with less toxicity [53].

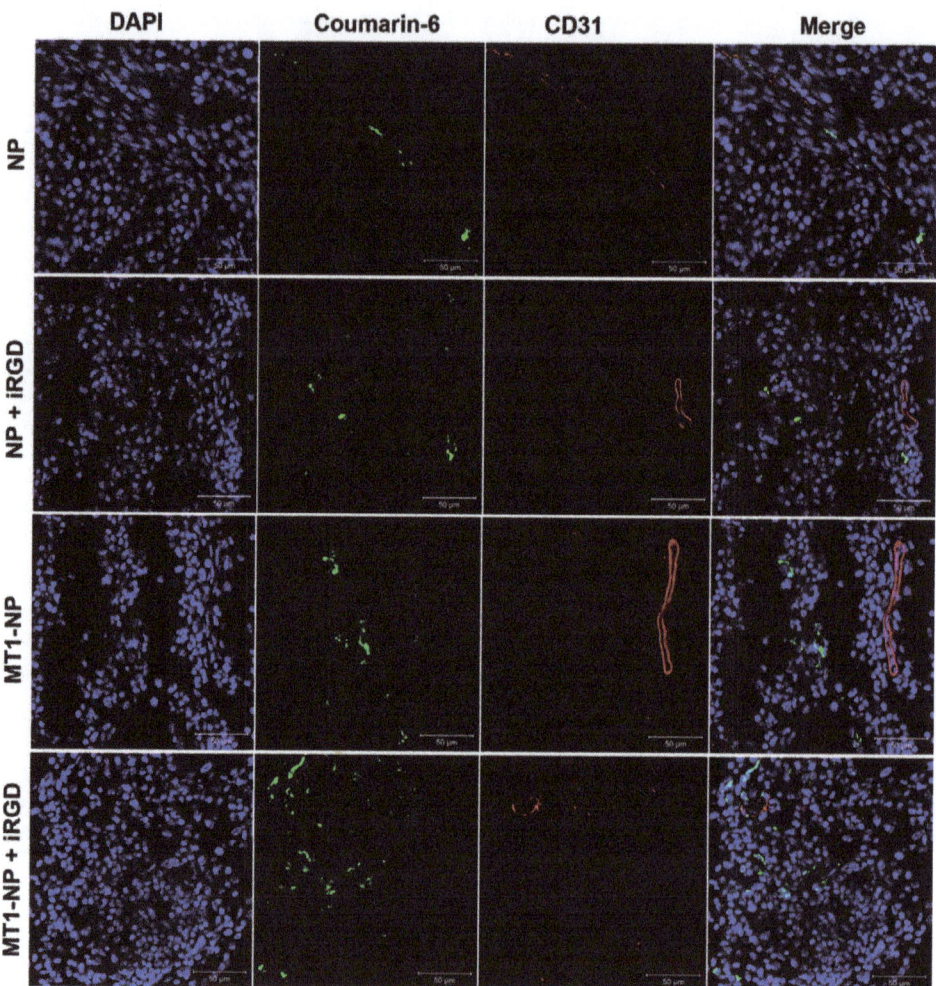

Figure 3. Observation of coumarin-6-labeled NP, NP co-administered with iRGD, MT1-NP, and MT1-NP co-administered with iRGD distribution in the brains of nude mice with intracranial C6 glioma, 3 h after intravenous administration. Analysis conducted on frozen sections using a confocal microscope revealed blood vessels marked with anti-CD31 (red), nuclei stained with DAPI (blue), and NPs depicted in green. Scale bars indicate 50 mm. Adapted with permission from reference [51].

AS1411 aptamer functionalized poly (L-γ-glutamyl-glutamine)-paclitaxel (PGG-PTX) nanoconjugates were designed to achieve active targeting and optimized solubilization of paclitaxel. The tumor uptake of the nanoconjugate was mediated through nucleolin receptors, over-expressed in glioblastoma cells and neovascular endothelial cells. The in vivo fluorescence imaging and biodistribution studies suggest that the AS1411-PGG-PTX has higher tumor accumulation than PGG-PTX. In glioma-bearing mice, this nanoconjugate exhibited prolonged median survival time and most tumor cell apoptosis compared to PGG-PTX [54]. A dual-targeted liposome was designed for the co-delivery of doxorubicin

(DOX) and vincristine (VCR) for glioma management. T7 (a ligand of transferrin receptors) and ^{D}A7R (ligand of VEGFR 2) peptides were used to target glioma. The dual targeting strategy exhibited higher cellular uptake when compared to the single targeting strategy. The dual targeting and dual drug delivery showed the most favorable anti-glioma effect in vivo [55].

Nanocarrier-based immunotherapy has emerged as a promising approach for the treatment of various cancers, including glioblastoma. Gliomas are highly invasive. They usually infiltrate the normal tissues and make surgical removal of the tissue difficult. Immunotherapy in glioma can target and eliminate the infiltrating glioma cells to the neighboring tissues. Gliomas usually lead to an immunosuppressive environment and prevent normal immune cell reactions against cancer cells. Hence, immunotherapy is the best strategy to overcome the challenges and activate the immune system against tumor formation. Gliomas are known for their molecular and cellular heterogeneity. Immunotherapy can target specific antigens expressed on tumor cells, including tumor-associated antigens and neoantigens, addressing the diversity of cancer cells within the tumor [56,57].

Immunotherapy coupled with nanocarrier-based drug delivery presents a revolutionary approach to treating glioblastoma. Overcoming the BBB, nanocarriers enabled targeted delivery of immunotherapeutic agents, and enhanced drug bioavailability while minimizing systemic side effects are the advantages of nanocarrier-based immunotherapy in gliomas. The personalized nature of nanocarrier systems, tailored to individual tumor characteristics, promises a more effective and precise treatment. By encapsulating immunomodulatory agents, these carriers boost the immune response within the tumor microenvironment. Additionally, the ability to administer combination therapies and mitigate systemic toxicity underscores the potential of this innovative strategy in overcoming the challenges posed by glioblastoma, offering hope for improved patient outcomes. Checkpoint inhibitors, cytokines, and antigenic peptides are major immunomodulatory agents that can be delivered using nanocarriers to modulate the immune system's response against glioblastoma [58,59].

Kuang et al. studied the effect of macrophage-directed immunotherapy with chemotherapy in orthotopic glioma. Doxorubicin and an immune checkpoint inhibitor (1-methyltryptophan, 1MT) were loaded on mesoporous silica nanoparticles modified with iRGD. The nanocarrier showed the ability to penetrate the BBB and accumulate drug molecules. The nanocarrier leads to the activation of cytotoxic CD8+ T lymphocytes and ions of CD4+ T cells in both GL261 cells cocultured with splenocytes in vitro and GL261-luc orthotopic tumors in vivo. The expression of antitumor cytokines was found to be upregulated, while protumor proteins were downregulated in the tumor tissues [60].

The Applications of Nanoparticles for medulloblastoma and glioma therapy are summarized in Table 1.

Table 1. Applications of Nanoparticles for medulloblastoma and glioma therapy.

Carriers [#]	Targeting Ligand [#]	Targeting Receptor/Area [#]	Therapeutic Molecule [#]	Cell Line and/or Animal Model Used [#]	Outcome/Key Findings [#]	Ref.
Poly (beta-amino ester) (PBAE) nanoparticles	-	-	Herpes simplex virus type I thymidine kinase	AT/RT implanted mice	Greater median overall survival in mice implanted with AT/RT	[45]
High-density lipoprotein-mimetic nanoparticles	apolipoprotein A1 anti-CD15	SR-B1 CD15 antigen	LDE225	SHH MB cells	SR-B1-mediated intracellular cholesterol depletion in SHH MB cells.	[46]
mPEG-b-PCC-g-DC copolymer-based NPs	ApoE-targeting peptide COG-133	ApoE receptor	MDB5 SF2523	SHH-MB tumor-bearing NSG mice	Reduction in tumors in orthotopic SHH-MB tumor-bearing NSG mice	[48]
Liposomes	-	-	Temozolomide	Mice	Preferential accumulation in the brain	[49]
PAMAM-PEG-nanoparticles	Transferrin	Transferrin-1 receptors	Temozolomide	nude mouse intracranial xenograft models.	Anticancer activity against O6-methylguanine-DNA-methyltransferase gene promoter methylation.	[50]

Table 1. Cont.

Carriers [#]	Targeting Ligand [#]	Targeting Receptor/Area [#]	Therapeutic Molecule [#]	Cell Line and/or Animal Model Used [#]	Outcome/Key Findings [#]	Ref.
PEG-PLA nanoparticles	MT1-AF7p peptide	Membrane type-1 matrix metalloproteinase	paclitaxel	C6 glioma-bearing nude mice	Enhanced survival time in intracranial C6 glioma-bearing nude mice	[51]
liposome	LAT 1	LAT-1 receptor	Amphi-DOPA	glioma-bearing C57BL/6J mice	Overall survivability increased by 60% in glioma-bearing C57BL/6J mice	[52]
RBC coated nanoparticle	CDX peptide	nAChRs	Doxorubicin	glioma bearing nude mice	High brain targeting, superior therapeutic activity with less toxicity	[53]
poly (L-γ-glutamyl-glutamine)-nanoconjugates	aptamer AS1411	Nucleolin	Paclitaxel	U87 MG cells and intracranial glioblastoma-bearing nude mice	Higher anti-glioma effect with enhanced median survival time	[54]
Liposome	T7 ^{D}A7R	Transferrin receptors, VEGFR 2 receptors	Doxorubicin and vincristine	HUVEC cells, C6 Cells, glioma-bearing mice	High anti-glioma effect in in vivo studies	[55]
Chitosan-coated PLGA nanoparticles	-	Brain	Carmustine	U87 MG cell line Albino Wistar rats	Enhanced cytotoxicity in cell lines and AUC in brain	[61]
PG-SPIONs	Folic acid	Folate receptors	Lomustine	U87 MG cell line	Enhanced cellular uptake	[62]
CGT nanoparticles	CGT	integrins αvβ3 and αvβ5	-	Rat glioblastoma model	UTMD with CGT therapy improved the CGT delivery, prolonged tumor retention, apoptosis, and median survival period	[63]
Human serum albumin nanoparticles	Folic acid	Folate receptors	Erlotinib	U87MG and C6 cells rat glioblastoma model	Improved apoptosis and tumor reduction compared to pure drug	[64]
Liposomes	-	-	Doxorubicin and erlotinib	U87 MG cell lines	Improved apoptosis	[65]
poly (butyl cyanoacrylate) (PBCA) NPs	mAb	-	Carboplatin.	Rat glioblastoma model	Longer survival time	[66]

[#] ApoE—Apolipoprotein E, AT—Atypical Teratoid, CGT—Cilengitide, DOPA—Dihydroxyphenylalanine, HUVEC—Human Umbilical Vein Endothelial Cells, LAT 1—Large Amino Acid Transporter1, mAb—Mono clonal antibody, nAChRs—Nicotinic Acetylcholine Receptors, NSG—NOD Scid Gamma, PAMAM—Polyamidoamine, PBAE—Poly (Beta-Amino Ester), PEG-PLA—Poly (Ethylene Glycol)—Poly (Lactic Acid), PG-SPIONS—polyglycerol coated superparamagnetic iron oxide nanoparticles, RT—Rhabdoid Tumors, SHH-MB—Sonic Hedgehog Medulloblastoma, SR-B1—Scavenger Receptor Class B Type 1, UTMD—ultrasound-targeted microbubble destruction, VEGFR—Vascular Endothelial Growth Factor Receptor.

3.5. Nanoformulations Used for the Treatment of Neuroblastoma

Neuroblastoma (NB) is a complex pediatric tumor that originates from the neural crest and is the most common extracranial solid tumor in children, accounting for 15% of pediatric tumor-related deaths and 8–10% of all childhood malignancies. Most of the malignant cells are found in the adrenal medulla, but they can manifest as localized or metastatic tumors in the paraspinal ganglia, thorax, pelvis, and neck [67]. There are now several alternative therapeutic options for localized NB at different stages. Since most children are inoperable at the time of diagnosis due to metastases, even though complete resection of the primary NB is expected to greatly improve overall survival, the primary treatments in most cases still involve radiotherapy, chemotherapy, immunotherapy, differentiation-inducing therapy, and autologous hematopoietic stem cell transplantation [68]. Nano-based methods for treating pediatric neuroblastoma are an emerging area of interest and possible treatment plans in the upcoming years.

Treatment for neuroblastoma, a cancer of the nerve tissue that affects young children, is still challenging. When it comes to targeted therapy, imaging, and drug distribution for neuroblastoma, nano-based methods have distinct benefits. Solid lipid NPs, polymer micelles, nanoliposomes, nanocapsules, nanospheres, and nanomedicines are the primary forms of nanoparticles (NPs) [40]. Graphene oxide nanoribbons were developed by Mari et al. [69] to investigate their effects on human neuroblastoma cells. In one of the cell lines, they discovered that these nanoribbons stimulated autophagy and increased the synthesis of reactive oxygen species (ROS) within the first 48 h of exposure. Both cell lines observed a brief increase in ROS generation and autophagy at low doses; however, neither cell growth inhibition nor cell death was brought about by these effects [69]. Li et al. [70] studied zinc oxide nanoparticles (ZnO NPs) that were produced using Clausena lansium Peel aqueous extracts and zinc nitrate. These developed ZnO NPs were found to affect the regulation of autophagy and apoptotic proteins in SH-SY5Y neuroblastoma cells, leading to DNA damage, ROS generation, decreased cell stability, and viability. The utilization of N-acetyl-L-cysteine (NAC) was shown to mitigate ROS effects and prevent apoptosis, suggesting that ZnO NPs have the potential to induce cell death in neuroblastoma cells through the production of intracellular ROS. Kalashnikova et al. [71] developed and tested nanoceria and dextran-nanoceria formulations loaded with curcumin for treating childhood neuroblastoma. The formulations effectively killed neuroblastoma cells, particularly in MYCN-amplified cases, without damaging the healthy cells. This nanoparticle-induced oxidative stress stabilized HIF-1α and triggered the caspase-dependent apoptosis. These results offer a promising alternative to traditional drug therapies for aggressive cancers. Mohammadniaei et al. [72] developed a promising cell differentiation therapy using silver-coated bismuth selenide nanoparticles. The developed nanoparticles can be functionalized with a unique RNA structure to inhibit micro-RNA-17 and release retinoic acid, facilitating the transformation of cancer cells into neurons. This innovative research reports on the hydrophobicity challenges and offers a new method for drug delivery and real-time monitoring of the differentiation process, potentially advancing diagnostic and therapeutic agents. Zhang et al. [73] have demonstrated that Nab-paclitaxel exerted significant cytotoxicity against various pediatric solid tumor cell lines in vitro, with dose-dependent effects studied. In vivo studies on rhabdomyosarcoma and neuroblastoma xenograft models showed antitumor activity and increased survival in the metastatic model. Nab-paclitaxel induced tumor cell-cycle arrest and apoptosis, and its higher tumor/plasma drug ratio favored its efficacy compared to paclitaxel, even in paclitaxel-resistant relapsed tumors [73]. The applications of nanoparticles for neuroblastoma therapy are summarized in Table 2.

Table 2. Applications of nanoparticles for neuroblastoma therapy.

Carriers/Moieties [#]	Therapeutic Molecule [#]	In Vitro/In Vivo Models [#]	Outcome/Key Findings [#]	Ref.
Silica-PAMAM dendrimer Hybrid	Anthocyanins	Neuro-2A brain neuroblastoma from mouse and Vero (African green monkey kidney) normal cell lines	The Hybrid nanoparticles (134.8 nm) with +19.78 mV zeta potential showed effective cytotoxicity against Neuroblastoma (Neuro 2A) cells, with 87.9% inhibition due to anthocyanin release. This system appears to be primarily therapeutic in its current application. The placebo nanoparticles were non-toxic to the cells.	[74]
Liposomes	Pyrazolo[3,4-d]pyrimidines	Sprague Dawley rats	Liposomal encapsulation effectively overcame the poor water solubility of pyrazolo[3,4-d]pyrimidines; this study focuses on the therapeutic approach and makes them more suitable for clinical drug development.	[75]
PLA- and PLGA-based nanoparticles	Doxorubicin	Neuroblastoma cell line UKF-NB-3	These kinds of nanoparticles can enhance in vivo drug activity through the EPR effect and overcome transporter-mediated drug resistance. The primary focus of the study is on delivering doxorubicin as a therapeutic agent against neuroblastoma cells.	[76]
PLGA (Poly(lactic-co-glycolic acid) nanoparticles	Paclitaxel (taxol)	Human neuroblastoma cells (SH-SY5Y)	Paclitaxel-loaded PLGA nanoparticles exhibited cytotoxicity with cell viability below 50% at concentrations > 10 nM and induced genotoxic effects, suggesting their potential as a biocompatible carrier for neuroblastoma treatment and the developed system was used for a therapeutic approach.	[77]
Cyclodextrin-Fibrin gels (FBGs)	Doxorubicin (Dox)	Mouse orthotopic NB model (SHSY5YLuc+ cells implanted into the left adrenal gland	Increase in the therapeutic index of Dox when locally administered via FBGs loaded with oCD-NH2/Dox for neuroblastoma treatment. Overall, the research presented in the article focuses on improving the therapeutic efficacy of Dox delivery for neuroblastoma treatment, with possibilities for exploring theranostic applications in the future.	[78]
Biomimetic Core-Shell NNs	Therapeutic miRNA	Human neuroblastoma CHLA-255 cells and CHLA-255-luc tumor-bearing nonobese diabetic/severe combined immunodeficient (NOD/SCID) mice	NN/NKEXO cocktail for targeted neuroblastoma therapy, efficient miRNA delivery, dual tumor growth inhibition, and potential clinical application. Prepared systems are primarily focused on a therapeutic approach.	[79]

Table 2. *Cont.*

Carriers/Moieties [#]	Therapeutic Molecule [#]	In Vitro/In Vivo Models [#]	Outcome/Key Findings [#]	Ref.
Soluplus or Chitosan Nanoparticles	Posidonia oceanica (POE)	SH-SY5Y human neuroblastoma cell line	NPs improved the aqueous solubility and stability of POE and enhanced its inhibitory effect on cancer cell migration, likely due to efficient encapsulation. Overall, the research presented in the article focuses on improving the therapeutic application of the nano-formulations.	[80]
Alginate-TiO2 TMZ Nanoparticles	Temozolomide (TMZ)	Human neuroblastoma cells SH-SY5Y	The developed system seems to focus primarily on a therapeutic approach, as these nanoparticles exhibit higher cytotoxicity against neuroblastoma cells, potentially impacting neuroblastoma treatment.	[81]
Solid lipid (Precirol®) and α_v integrins (ligand)	Etoposide and Cilengitide	HR-NB cell lines and MYCN-amplified cell lines	Combination therapy with cilengitide enhanced efficacy against high-risk neuroblastoma cells. This research offers theragnostic potential by targeting ECM-tumor cell interactions, inhibiting VN-integrin binding, modulating ECM stiffness, and employing nanoencapsulated chemotherapeutic agents to enhance the therapeutic index and overall effectiveness in high-risk neuroblastoma treatment.	[82]
Bacterial Membrane-coated Nanoparticle (BNP)	PC7A/CpG polyplex core with bacterial membrane	B78 melanoma tumors engrafted in syngeneic mice	BNP enhances immune recognition of tumor neoantigens post-radiation, improving dendritic cell uptake and cross-presentation, resulting in robust antitumor T-cell responses in mice with melanoma or neuroblastoma. The developed system seems to focus primarily on a therapeutic approach; therefore, the current application leans toward immunotherapy.	[83]
Synthetic High-Density Lipoprotein (HDL) Nanoparticles	4,19,27-tri acetyl withanolide A	Human NB cell lines SH-EP, SH-SY5Y, IMR32 and SK-N-As and tumor-bearing mice	Treatment reduced sphere formation, invasion, migration, and cancer stem cell markers in neuroblastoma cells. However, the targeting of SR-B1 and its potential for influencing CSC functions also suggest the potential for theranostic applications, where the nanoparticles could be used for both diagnosis and treatment.	[84]
Core-Shell MOF of Zinc	Titanocene Dichloride (TC) loaded Lactoferrin (Lf)	Neuroblastoma-IMR-32 cells and Wistar rats	ZIF-8 framework loaded with Lf-TC and 5-Fluorouracil exhibited potential for Neuroblastoma therapy, confirmed through in vitro cell studies and in vivo safety assessments in Wistar rats. The Lf-TC and 5FU-loaded ZIF-8 framework serves as nanoplatforms for tumor phototherapy, with the potential for transformation into a theranostic platform through additional imaging moiety modifications.	[85]
Graphene Quantum Dots (GQDs)	Anti-GD2 Antibody	NIH3T3 mouse fibroblast cell line and BE(2)-M17 human neuroblastoma cell line and nude mice	This study focuses on the theranostics potential of anti-GD2/GQDs and demonstrates the potential use of Anti-GD2/GQDs for targeting and imaging of neuroblastomas in vivo.	[86]
Nanocarriers coated-cationic liposomes functionalized with antibodies against GD2 receptor	miR-34a and let-7b	NB tumor cells, orthotopic xenografts, pseudometastatic models, athymic mice	Promising therapeutic efficacy of miR-34a and let-7b combined replacement, Support for clinical application as adjuvant therapy for high-risk NB patients.	[87]

[#] NKEXOs: Natural killer cell-derived exosomes, NNs: core–shell nanoparticles, TiO_2: Titanium dioxide, NB: Neuroblastoma, ECM: Extracellular matrix, CSC: Cancer Stem Cell, ZIF-8: Zeolitic Imidazolate Framework.

3.6. Nanoformulations Used for the Treatment of Retinoblastoma

Retinoblastoma is a disease in which malignant (cancer) cells form in the tissues of the retina. Retinoblastoma can expand to other parts of the body, such as the brain and spine [88]. Pediatric retinoblastoma (RB) is an uncommon and occasionally inherited malignancy. Because of alterations in the tumor-suppressor genes and the lack of a targeted, efficient, and cost-effective therapy, retinoblastoma is an uncommon form of cancer that is difficult to diagnose and treat. As such, there is a critical need for innovative treatments to address these issues [89]. External beam radiation, episcleral plaque radiation, cryotherapy, enucleation, and photocoagulation were conventional therapies for children with RB [90]. Ocular malignancies present unique problems, and improved penetration of the retinal pigment epithelium by monotherapies is required [91].

Several nano-applications have been investigated recently to overcome these obstacles. The application of nanotechnologies in the detection and management of cancers and eye conditions has grown rapidly in recent years [92–94]. Among the most useful nanotechnology-based ocular delivery methods include nanoliposomes, polymeric nanoparticles (PNPs), nanocapsules, nanocages, nano-micelles, nano-dendrimers, and nanohydrogels, which offer several benefits over standard diagnostics and treatments [95–97]. Moradi et al. [98] assess the combined effects of gold nanoparticles (Au-NPs) and ultrasonic hyperthermia on Y79 cells. Cells were exposed to ultrasonic irradiation with or without 60 nm Au-NPs, and their viability was measured 48 h later. Results showed that hyperthermia alone reduced cell viability after 4 min, while in the presence of Au-NPs, this effect was observed after 4.5 min. Higher Au-NP concentrations increased cytotoxicity. This research concludes that the use of Au-NPs enhances the sensitivity of cells to hyperthermia induced by ultrasound [98]. A multifunctional nanoparticle system has been developed for the diagnosis and treatment of retinoblastoma. The nanoparticles, consisting of magnetic hollow mesoporous gold nanocages (AuNCs) loaded with muramyl dipeptide (MDP) and perfluoropentane (PFP), enable advanced imaging (photoacoustic, ultrasound, and magnetic resonance) for diagnosis and enhance low-intensity focused ultrasound (LIFU) therapy. These nanoparticles, when combined with LIFU, effectively target and treat RB tumors, leading to tumor cell death, while MDP activates dendritic cells (DCs) for improved immune response. The multifunctional nanoparticles offer potential for multimodal imaging-guided LIFU therapy and show promise for RB treatment with high safety [99]. Silver nanoparticles (AgNPs) are increasingly used in medical and commercial products due to their potent antibacterial properties. Rajanahalli et al. [100] have investigated the impact of AgNPs on mouse embryonic stem cells (mESCs). They revealed that AgNPs with different surface coatings altered cell morphology, induced cell cycle arrest at G1 and S phases, and reduced pluripotency marker Oct4A while promoting the expression of stress-related isoforms. The findings suggested that AgNPs' toxicity is linked to excessive reactive oxygen species (ROS) production, with polysaccharide coating mitigating this effect [100]. Qu et al. [98,101] developed EpCAM-conjugated mesoporous silica nanoparticles (EpCMSN) to effectively deliver carboplatin (CRB) for the treatment of retinoblastoma (RB), a rare eye tumor. EpCMSN demonstrated enhanced cellular uptake and superior anticancer effects compared to free CRB, with a significantly lower IC_{50} value of 1.38 µg/mL. The specific receptor-mediated internalization of EpCMSN, targeting EpCAM receptors, suggests a promising approach for targeted treatment of RB and other ocular malignancies [101]. Photothermal therapy, with its minimal invasiveness and high specificity, addresses issues associated with traditional drug treatment for tumors. However, its limited tissue penetration hinders clinical application. Using a nano-platform comprising liposomes and indocyanine green (ICG) introduced a novel strategy for treating retinoblastoma by enhancing ICG stability and enabling imaging-guided photothermal therapy, making use of the eye's transparency to infrared light. In this study, ICG-loaded liposome nanoparticles (ILP) were developed, offering targeted tumor treatment and improved imaging capabilities, holding promise for image-guided tumor phototherapy. Figure 4 depicts the fluorescence and photoacoustic imaging capabilities of ILP [102]. Cerium-doped titania nanoparticles (Ce-doped TiO_2) were studied by Kartha et al. [103] using a cost-effective sol-gel method, and their enhanced photodynamic anticancer effects were evaluated on Y79 retinoblastoma cells. The study investigated the structural and optical properties of pure and Ce-doped TiO_2, revealing cerium's presence through X-ray diffraction and Raman spectra. Additionally, microscopy analysis showed that both TiO_2 variants exhibited spherical shapes. The findings indicated that cerium doping in TiO_2 enhances its photodynamic anticancer activity [103]. The applications of nanoparticles for retinoblastoma therapy are discussed in Table 3.

Table 3. Applications of nanoparticles for retinoblastoma therapy.

Carriers/Moieties [#]	Therapeutic Molecule [#]	In Vitro/In Vivo Models [#]	Outcome/Key Findings [#]	Ref.
AuNP-PEI-EpCAM Antibody (EpAb)	EpCAM-specific siRNA	Y79 retinoblastoma cells	Novel nanocarrier successfully delivered EpCAM-specific siRNA to retinoblastoma (RB) cells, leading to significant gene knockdown. The nanoparticles were well-tolerated by cells, and their conjugation with the EpCAM antibody enhanced internalization and therapeutic efficacy for RB. Gold nanoparticles also hold the potential for imaging in diagnosis.	[104]
Galactose-Chitosan Anchored Etoposide PLGA NPs (GC-ENP)	Etoposide (ETP)	Y-79 retinoblastoma cells	GC-ENP, with high entrapment efficiency and galactose targeting, demonstrates increased uptake in retinoblastoma cells (Y-79) and enhanced cytotoxicity, making it a promising drug delivery system for retinoblastoma treatment and enhancing the therapeutic application of the developed system.	[105]

Table 3. Cont.

Carriers/Moieties [#]	Therapeutic Molecule [#]	In Vitro/In Vivo Models [#]	Outcome/Key Findings [#]	Ref.
PLGA Nanoparticles	Melphalan	Y79 cells	Surface modification improves efficacy in retinoblastoma cells, particularly with MPG-NPs. Prepared systems are primarily focused on a therapeutic approach, and this system enhances cell association, but some NPs remain on the cell surface rather than internalizing.	[106]
Nanospheres (NSs) of PGZ	Pioglitazone (PGZ)	Y-79 cell line and male pigs	The Polymeric nanoparticles effectively encapsulated PGZ, showing optimal characteristics with sustained drug release, good ocular tolerance, and significant in vivo anti-inflammatory potential, offering a promising approach for ocular inflammation treatment and suggesting a purely therapeutic approach.	[107]
CMD-TCs-NPs		Y79 retinoblastoma cells and Wistar albino rats	CMD-TCs-NPs show smaller size, positive zeta potential, and higher affinity for retinoblastoma tumors in rat eyes when administered intravitreally, while CMD-TMC-NPs remained in the vitreous and did not reach the retina. These findings suggest CMD-TCs-NPs' potential for more effective drug delivery in retinoblastoma treatment.	[108]
Thiolated Chitosan Nanoparticles (TPH-TCs-NPs)	Topotecan (TPH)	Human retinoblastoma cells (Y79), xenograft-rat-model of retinoblastoma	TPH-TCs-NPs enhanced drug loading, improved control over drug release, and increased treatment efficacy for retinoblastoma. Thiolated chitosan demonstrates improved interaction with cell membranes, leading to higher cellular uptake of the drug. Therefore, this study primarily focuses on the therapeutic approach.	[109]
siRNA-loaded switchable LNP	Survivin siRNA	Y79 retinoblastoma cells and primary human RB cells.	Sequential siRNA survivin followed by chemotherapy sensitizes cancer cells to carboplatin and melphalan, showing promise in treating retinoblastoma (RB) without affecting healthy cells. The study suggests careful drug screening to find synergy with survivin for future in vivo testing.	[110]
Lipid Nanoparticles (LNP)	Melphalan and miR-181a	Y79 retinoblastoma cells and Sprague Dawley rats	Co-delivery of melphalan and miR-181a using 171 nm switchable LNP with high encapsulation efficiencies enhanced therapeutic efficiency, reducing the expression of anti-proliferative and anti-apoptotic genes while increasing pro-apoptotic gene expression.	[111]
Lactoferrin nanoparticles (Lf-Nps)	Carboplatin (CPT) and Etoposide (ETP)	Retinoblastoma (Rb) Y79 cells	The Nanoformulations of Lf-CPT and Lf-ETP enhance drug uptake, intracellular retention, and cytotoxicity, particularly in Rb Y79 CSCs, offering the potential for improved targeted therapy and therapeutic efficacy and better clinical outcomes by overcoming chemoresistance in cancer stem cells (CSCs).	[112]
Apo-nano-carbo and Lacto-nano-carbo nanoparticles	Carboplatin	Human retinoblastoma cell line Y79	These nanoparticles demonstrated pH-dependent drug release and receptor-mediated endocytosis for targeted delivery, resulting in greater intracellular uptake and anti-proliferative activity (IC$_{50}$ = 4.31 µg ml^{-1} and 4.16 µg ml^{-1}, respectively) compared to soluble carboplatin (IC50 = 13.498 µg ml^{-1}).	[113]
Polymethylmethacrylate nanoparticles	Carboplatin	Sprague Dawley rats	Intra-vitreal carboplatin concentrations were significantly higher with novel carboplatin-loaded polymethylmethacrylate nanoparticles (NPC) compared to the commercially available carboplatin (CAC), indicating enhanced trans-scleral permeability for potential use in treating advanced retinoblastoma. Therefore, this study primarily focuses on the therapeutic approach.	[114]
Folic Acid-Conjugated Polymeric Micelles	Curcumin-Difluorinated (CDF)	Retinoblastoma cell lines (Y-79 and WERI-RB1)	The Folic acid-conjugated micelles loaded with CDF increased CDF solubility and showed significant anticancer activity on retinoblastoma cell lines (Y-79 and WERI-RB). This formulation holds promise as an alternative approach to retinoblastoma therapies; therefore, the study focuses on the therapeutic potential of the developed system.	[115]
EpCAM antibody-functionalized PLGA NPs.	Paclitaxel	Y79 retinoblastoma cells	EpCAM antibody-functionalized biodegradable NPs show potential for tumor-selective drug delivery and overcoming drug resistance in retinoblastoma treatment. Therefore, this study primarily focuses on the therapeutic approach.	[116]
Hybrid Lipid Polymer Nanoparticles	Beta-lapachone (β-Lap)	Retinoblastoma cells	This study focuses on a combined chemo- and photodynamic therapy (PDT) approach, aiming to synergistically treat retinoblastoma with both β-Lap and m-THPC encapsulated in LNPs.	[117]
Mesoporous silica nanoparticles	anti-MRC2 and/or anti-CD209	Human retinoblastoma cancer cells (Y-79 and WERI-Rb1)	Identifies elevated expression of two receptors, MRC2 and CD209, in retinoblastoma, leading to the creation of mesoporous silica nanoparticles (MSN) equipped with anti-MRC2 and/or anti-CD209 antibodies for targeted PDT and imaging.	[118]

[#] AuNP-PEI-EpCAM Antibody: Gold nanoparticles-polyethyleneimine-Epithelial cell adhesion molecule monoclonal antibody conjugated, CMD-TCs-NPs thiolated and methylated chitosan-carboxymethyl dextran nanoparticles, siLNP: siRNA-loaded switchable lipid nanoparticles, Apo-nano-carbo: carboplatin loaded apotranferrin and Lacto-nano-carbo: lactoferrin loaded nanoparticles, PLGA NPs: Poly(lactic-co-glycolic acid) nanoparticles, PDT: Photodynamic therapy.

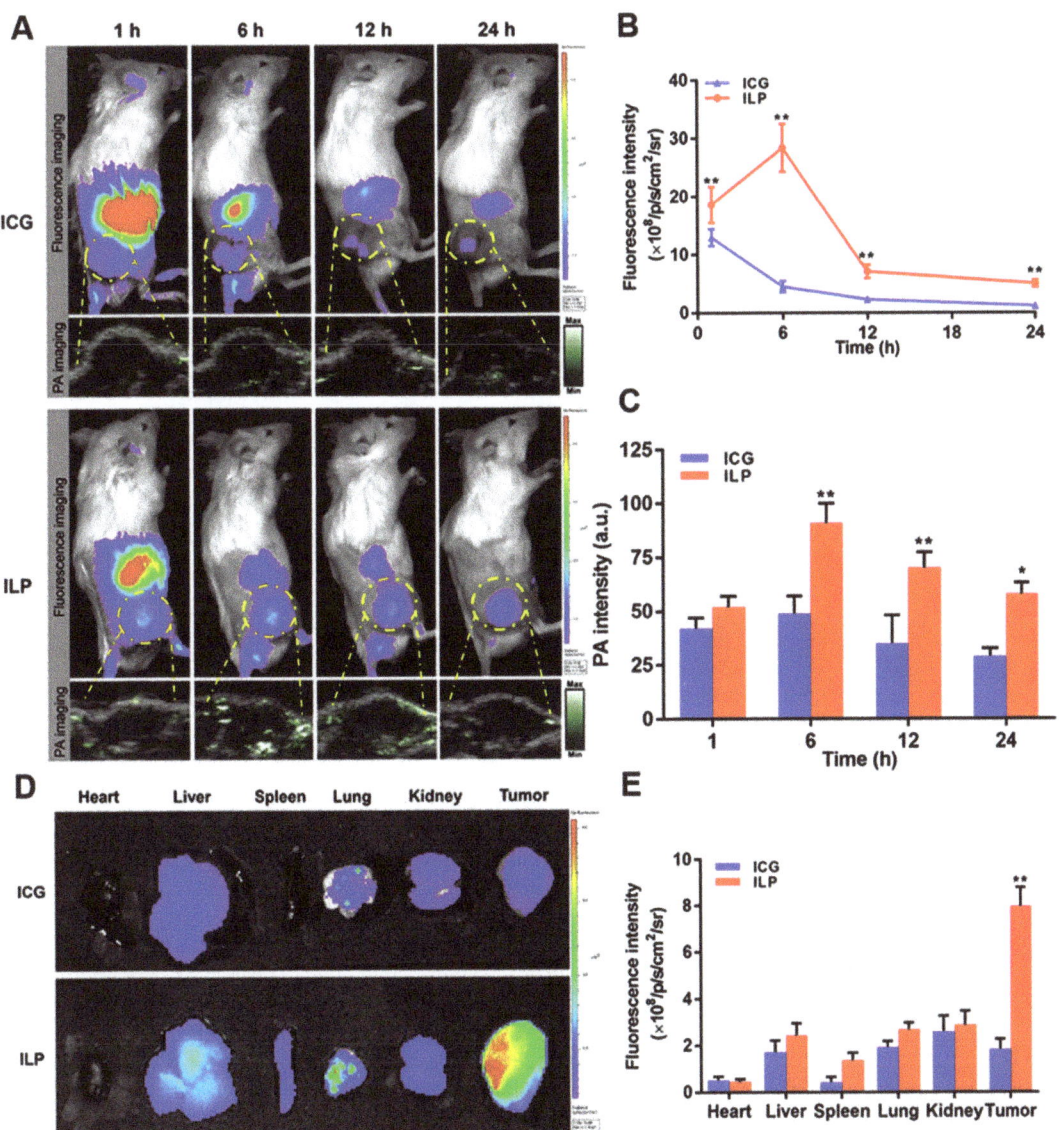

Figure 4. Assessing the fluorescence and photoacoustic imaging capabilities of ILP. (**A**) In vivo, observe the fluorescence and photoacoustic images of ICG and ILP at various time intervals. (**B**,**C**) Analyze the fluorescent intensity (**B**) and photoacoustic intensity (**C**) of tumor tissue quantitatively. (**D**) Examine ex vivo fluorescence images of ICG and ILP at 6 h. (**E**) Quantify the fluorescent intensity of different tissues at the 6 h mark. Herein $p < 0.05$ is flagged with one star (*) and $p < 0.01$ is flagged with two stars (**). Adapted with permission from reference [102].

4. Clinical Trials

Pediatric brain tumors are some of the most devastating childhood diseases, with high mortality rates and significant long-term morbidity for survivors. Conventional treatment options like surgery, radiation, and chemotherapy often have severe side effects and limited efficacy. As mentioned in Table 4 (retrieved from https://clinicaltrials.gov/, accessed on 15 February 2024), emerging nanotherapeutic strategies offer a promising avenue for improving the treatment of pediatric brain tumors by overcoming these limitations. Nanoparticles, with their unique size and properties, can be designed to target tumor cells more effectively, deliver drugs with greater precision, and reduce systemic toxicity. Here is a brief overview of some ongoing clinical studies exploring nano-therapeutic strategies against pediatric brain tumors.

Table 4. Clinical trials using nano-therapeutics in pediatric brain tumors.

Carriers/Nanoparticles [#]	Condition [#]	Therapeutic Agent [#]	Phase [#]	Status [#]	NCT Code
Liposomes	Glioblastoma	C225-ILs-dox	Phase 1	Completed	NCT03603379
Gold Nanoparticle	Recurrent Glioblastoma	NU-0129 IV	Early Phase 1	Completed	NCT03020017
Ultra-small iron oxide particle	Brain Neoplasms	Combidex as MRI contrast agent	Phase 2	Terminated	NCT00659334
Small iron particles	Childhood Brain Neoplasm	DSC-MRI with ferumoxytol	Early Phase 1	Completed	NCT00978562
Nanoparticle Formulation MTX110	Diffuse Intrinsic Pontine Glioma	Panobinostat	Phase 1 Phase 2	Completed	NCT03566199
Liposomes	Brain tumor	Doxorubicin	Phase 1	Completed	NCT00019630
Liposomes	Brain and Central Nervous System Tumors	Cytarabine	Phase 1	Unknown status	NCT00003073
MTX110 and gadolinium	Diffuse Intrinsic Pontine Glioma	Infusate	Phase 1	Completed	NCT04264143
Liposomes	Neuroblastoma	Doxorubicin	Phase 1	Terminated	NCT02536183
Liposome	Neuroblastoma	Doxorubicin	Phase 1	Withdrawn	NCT02557854
Liposome	Neuroblastoma	Irinotecan Sucrosofate	Phase 1	Recruiting	NCT02013336

[#] C225-ILs-dox: Doxorubicin-loaded Anti-EGFR-immunoliposomes.

5. Conclusions

Pediatric brain tumors are considered the most frequent type of pediatric cancer, and they pose a tremendous therapeutic challenge owing to their tendency to infiltrate and disseminate to surrounding tissues, restricting the use of surgery as a feasible monotherapeutic strategy. Furthermore, the difficulty in delivering medications to the brain tumor site in effective therapeutic concentrations while evading the blood–brain barrier (BBB) represents another challenge for cancer conquering. Consequently, nanomedicines have emerged as a promising therapeutic approach to circumvent the hurdles encountered with conventional therapy, along with improving the bioavailability of drug payloads. Nanotechnology-based delivery systems can effectively cross the BBB, and when decorated with receptors that are overexpressed both by BBB-building cells and cancer cells, they can discriminate cancer cells from surrounding healthy ones, thus directing the therapeutic agents towards malignant cells. However, various challenges must be carefully considered, including biocompatibility issues and clearance modulation. Nonetheless, various strategies have been implemented in recent years to overcome these drawbacks, and, along with the growing body of knowledge in the molecular genetics of brain tumors, the scientific community is unquestionably close to a major breakthrough in the development of efficient, safe, and low-cost nanosystems capable of imaging and treating brain cancers without inflicting remarkable damage to healthy tissue.

Author Contributions: Conceptualization, A.V.V.V.R.K., H.V.G. and S.M.D.R.; validation, A.P.J., M.K. and R.A.M.O.; formal analysis, G.K.K., A.S.A.L., A.M. and S.M.D.R.; resources, P.T.K., H.V.G. and A.M.; data curation, A.P.J., M.K. and R.A.M.O.; writing—original draft preparation, A.V.V.V.R.K., G.K.K., P.T.K. and A.P.J.; writing—review and editing, P.T.K., M.K., R.A.M.O., A.S.A.L., and A.M.; visualization, A.V.V.V.R.K., G.K.K. and A.S.A.L.; supervision, H.V.G. and S.M.D.R. All authors have read and agreed to the published version of the manuscript.

Funding: This research received no external funding.

Institutional Review Board Statement: Not applicable.

Informed Consent Statement: Not applicable.

Data Availability Statement: Data are contained within the article.

Conflicts of Interest: The authors declare no conflicts of interest.

References

1. Mueller, S.; Chang, S. Pediatric brain tumors: Current treatment strategies and future therapeutic approaches. *Neurotherapeutics* **2009**, *6*, 570–586. [CrossRef] [PubMed]
2. Moin, A.; Rizvi, S.M.D.; Hussain, T.; Gowda, D.V.; Subaiea, G.M.; Elsayed, M.M.A.; Ansari, M.; Alanazi, A.S.; Yadav, H. Current Status of Brain Tumor in the Kingdom of Saudi Arabia and Application of Nanobiotechnology for Its Treatment: A Comprehensive Review. *Life* **2021**, *11*, 421. [CrossRef] [PubMed]
3. Abedalthagafi, M.; Mobark, N.; Al-Rashed, M.; AlHarbi, M. Epigenomics and immunotherapeutic advances in pediatric brain tumors. *NPJ Precis. Oncol.* **2021**, *5*, 34. [CrossRef] [PubMed]
4. Udaka, Y.T.; Packer, R.J. Pediatric Brain Tumors. *Neurol. Clin.* **2018**, *36*, 533–556. [CrossRef] [PubMed]
5. Yang, S.; Wallach, M.; Krishna, A.; Kurmasheva, R.; Sridhar, S. Recent Developments in Nanomedicine for Pediatric Cancer. *J. Clin. Med.* **2021**, *10*, 1437. [CrossRef] [PubMed]
6. Pui, C.H.; Gajjar, A.J.; Kane, J.R.; Qaddoumi, I.A.; Pappo, A.S. Challenging issues in pediatric oncology. *Nat. Rev. Clin. Oncol.* **2011**, *8*, 540–549. [CrossRef] [PubMed]
7. Surendiran, A.; Sandhiya, S.; Pradhan, S.C.; Adithan, C. Novel applications of nanotechnology in medicine. *Indian J. Med. Res.* **2009**, *130*, 689–701. [PubMed]
8. Emerich, D.F.; Thanos, C.G. Nanotechnology and medicine. *Expert Opin. Biol. Ther.* **2003**, *3*, 655–663. [CrossRef]
9. Ando, H.; Kobayashi, S.; Abu Lila, A.S.; Eldin, N.E.; Kato, C.; Shimizu, T.; Ukawa, M.; Kawazoe, K.; Ishida, T. Advanced therapeutic approach for the treatment of malignant pleural mesothelioma via the intrapleural administration of liposomal pemetrexed. *J. Control. Release* **2015**, *220*, 29–36. [CrossRef]
10. Abu Lila, A.S.; Ishida, T.; Kiwada, H. Recent advances in tumor vasculature targeting using liposomal drug delivery systems. *Expert Opin. Drug Deliv.* **2009**, *6*, 1297–1309. [CrossRef]
11. Knudson, A.G., Jr. Genetics and the etiology of childhood cancer. *Pediatr. Res.* **1976**, *10*, 513–517. [CrossRef] [PubMed]
12. Castaneda, M.; den Hollander, P.; Kuburich, N.A.; Rosen, J.M.; Mani, S.A. Mechanisms of cancer metastasis. *Semin. Cancer Biol.* **2022**, *87*, 17–31. [CrossRef] [PubMed]
13. Liu, K.-W.; Pajtler, K.W.; Worst, B.C.; Pfister, S.M.; Wechsler-Reya, R.J. Molecular mechanisms and therapeutic targets in pediatric brain tumors. *Sci. Signal.* **2017**, *10*, eaaf7593. [CrossRef] [PubMed]
14. Kim, S.; Chung, D.H. Pediatric solid malignancies: Neuroblastoma and Wilms' tumor. *Surg. Clin. N. Am.* **2006**, *86*, 469–487. [CrossRef] [PubMed]
15. Dhall, G. Medulloblastoma. *J. Child. Neurol.* **2009**, *24*, 1418–1430. [CrossRef] [PubMed]
16. Millard, N.E.; De Braganca, K.C. Medulloblastoma. *J. Child. Neurol.* **2016**, *31*, 1341–1353. [CrossRef] [PubMed]
17. Packer, R.J.; Cogen, P.; Vezina, G.; Rorke, L.B. Medulloblastoma: Clinical and biologic aspects. *Neuro-Oncology* **1999**, *1*, 232–250. [CrossRef] [PubMed]
18. Kijima, N.; Kanemura, Y. Molecular Classification of Medulloblastoma. *Neurol. Med. Chir.* **2016**, *56*, 687–697. [CrossRef]
19. Rausch, T.; Jones, D.T.; Zapatka, M.; Stütz, A.M.; Zichner, T.; Weischenfeldt, J.; Jäger, N.; Remke, M.; Shih, D.; Northcott, P.A.; et al. Genome sequencing of pediatric medulloblastoma links catastrophic DNA rearrangements with TP53 mutations. *Cell* **2012**, *148*, 59–71. [CrossRef]
20. Lee, M.J.; Hatton, B.A.; Villavicencio, E.H.; Khanna, P.C.; Friedman, S.D.; Ditzler, S.; Pullar, B.; Robison, K.; White, K.F.; Tunkey, C.; et al. Hedgehog pathway inhibitor saridegib (IPI-926) increases lifespan in a mouse medulloblastoma model. *Proc. Natl. Acad. Sci. USA* **2012**, *109*, 7859–7864. [CrossRef]
21. Kim, J.; Tang, J.Y.; Gong, R.; Lee, J.J.; Clemons, K.V.; Chong, C.R.; Chang, K.S.; Fereshteh, M.; Gardner, D.; Reya, T.; et al. Itraconazole, a commonly used antifungal that inhibits Hedgehog pathway activity and cancer growth. *Cancer Cell* **2010**, *17*, 388–399. [CrossRef]
22. Roussel, M.F.; Stripay, J.L. Modeling pediatric medulloblastoma. *Brain Pathol.* **2020**, *30*, 703–712. [CrossRef] [PubMed]
23. Bolin, S.; Borgenvik, A.; Persson, C.U.; Sundström, A.; Qi, J.; Bradner, J.E.; Weiss, W.A.; Cho, Y.-J.; Weishaupt, H.; Swartling, F.J. Combined BET bromodomain and CDK2 inhibition in MYC-driven medulloblastoma. *Oncogene* **2018**, *37*, 2850–2862. [CrossRef]
24. Borgenvik, A.; Čančer, M.; Hutter, S.; Swartling, F.J. Targeting MYCN in Molecularly Defined Malignant Brain Tumors. *Front. Oncol.* **2020**, *10*, 626751. [CrossRef]
25. Hussain, T.; Paranthaman, S.; Rizvi, S.M.D.; Moin, A.; Gowda, D.V.; Subaiea, G.M.; Ansari, M.; Alanazi, A.S. Fabrication and Characterization of Paclitaxel and Resveratrol Loaded Soluplus Polymeric Nanoparticles for Improved BBB Penetration for Glioma Management. *Polymers* **2021**, *13*, 3210. [CrossRef] [PubMed]
26. MacDonald, T.J.; Aguilera, D.; Kramm, C.M. Treatment of high-grade glioma in children and adolescents. *Neuro-Oncology* **2011**, *13*, 1049–1058. [CrossRef]
27. Minturn, J.E.; Fisher, M.J. Gliomas in children. *Curr. Treat. Options Neurol.* **2013**, *15*, 316–327. [CrossRef] [PubMed]
28. Maris, J.M. Recent advances in neuroblastoma. *N. Engl. J. Med.* **2010**, *362*, 2202–2211. [CrossRef] [PubMed]

29. Mei, H.; Wang, Y.; Lin, Z.; Tong, Q. The mTOR signaling pathway in pediatric neuroblastoma. *Pediatr. Hematol. Oncol.* **2013**, *30*, 605–615. [CrossRef]
30. Louis, C.U.; Shohet, J.M. Neuroblastoma: Molecular pathogenesis and therapy. *Annu. Rev. Med.* **2015**, *66*, 49–63. [CrossRef]
31. Mora, J. Dinutuximab for the treatment of pediatric patients with high-risk neuroblastoma. *Expert Rev. Clin. Pharmacol.* **2016**, *9*, 647–653. [CrossRef] [PubMed]
32. Vitanza, N.A.; Partap, S. Pediatric Ependymoma. *J. Child. Neurol.* **2016**, *31*, 1354–1366. [CrossRef] [PubMed]
33. Kilday, J.P.; Rahman, R.; Dyer, S.; Ridley, L.; Lowe, J.; Coyle, B.; Grundy, R. Pediatric ependymoma: Biological perspectives. *Mol. Cancer Res.* **2009**, *7*, 765–786. [CrossRef] [PubMed]
34. Merchant, T.E.; Fouladi, M. Ependymoma: New therapeutic approaches including radiation and chemotherapy. *J. Neurooncol.* **2005**, *75*, 287–299. [CrossRef] [PubMed]
35. Thorp, N.; Gandola, L. Management of Ependymoma in Children, Adolescents and Young Adults. *Clin. Oncol. R Coll. Radiol.* **2019**, *31*, 162–170. [CrossRef] [PubMed]
36. Arabzade, A.; Zhao, Y.; Varadharajan, S.; Chen, H.C.; Jessa, S.; Rivas, B.; Stuckert, A.J.; Solis, M.; Kardian, A.; Tlais, D.; et al. ZFTA-RELA Dictates Oncogenic Transcriptional Programs to Drive Aggressive Supratentorial Ependymoma. *Cancer Discov.* **2021**, *11*, 2200–2215. [CrossRef] [PubMed]
37. Rudà, R.; Bosa, C.; Magistrello, M.; Franchino, F.; Pellerino, A.; Fiano, V.; Trevisan, M.; Cassoni, P.; Soffietti, R. Temozolomide as salvage treatment for recurrent intracranial ependymomas of the adult: A retrospective study. *Neuro-Oncology* **2016**, *18*, 261–268. [CrossRef]
38. Antonelli, R.; Jiménez, C.; Riley, M.; Servidei, T.; Riccardi, R.; Soriano, A.; Roma, J.; Martínez-Saez, E.; Martini, M.; Ruggiero, A.; et al. CN133, a Novel Brain-Penetrating Histone Deacetylase Inhibitor, Hampers Tumor Growth in Patient-Derived Pediatric Posterior Fossa Ependymoma Models. *Cancers* **2020**, *12*, 1922. [CrossRef]
39. Nehra, M.; Uthappa, U.T.; Kumar, V.; Kumar, R.; Dixit, C.; Dilbaghi, N.; Mishra, Y.K.; Kumar, S.; Kaushik, A. Nanobiotechnology-assisted therapies to manage brain cancer in personalized manner. *J. Control. Release* **2021**, *338*, 224–243. [CrossRef]
40. Aleassa, E.M.; Xing, M.; Keijzer, R. Nanomedicine as an innovative therapeutic strategy for pediatric cancer. *Pediatr. Surg. Int.* **2015**, *31*, 611–616. [CrossRef]
41. Rodríguez-Nogales, C.; González-Fernández, Y.; Aldaz, A.; Couvreur, P.; Blanco-Prieto, M.J. Nanomedicines for Pediatric Cancers. *ACS Nano* **2018**, *12*, 7482–7496. [CrossRef]
42. Pandit, R.; Chen, L.; Götz, J. The blood-brain barrier: Physiology and strategies for drug delivery. *Adv. Drug Deliv. Rev.* **2020**, *165-166*, 1–14. [CrossRef] [PubMed]
43. Tang, W.; Fan, W.; Lau, J.; Deng, L.; Shen, Z.; Chen, X. Emerging blood–brain-barrier-crossing nanotechnology for brain cancer theranostics. *Chem. Soc. Rev.* **2019**, *48*, 2967–3014. [CrossRef] [PubMed]
44. Khan, N.H.; Mir, M.; Ngowi, E.E.; Zafar, U.; Khakwani, M.M.A.K.; Khattak, S.; Zhai, Y.K.; Jiang, E.S.; Zheng, M.; Duan, S.F.; et al. Nanomedicine: A Promising Way to Manage Alzheimer's Disease. *Front. Bioeng. Biotechnol.* **2021**, *9*, 630055. [CrossRef]
45. Choi, J.; Rui, Y.; Kim, J.; Gorelick, N.; Wilson, D.R.; Kozielski, K.; Mangraviti, A.; Sankey, E.; Brem, H.; Tyler, B.; et al. Nonviral polymeric nanoparticles for gene therapy in pediatric CNS malignancies. *Nanomedicine* **2020**, *23*, 102115. [CrossRef] [PubMed]
46. Kim, J.; Dey, A.; Malhotra, A.; Liu, J.; Ahn, S.I.; Sei, Y.J.; Kenney, A.M.; MacDonald, T.J.; Kim, Y. Engineered biomimetic nanoparticle for dual targeting of the cancer stem-like cell population in sonic hedgehog medulloblastoma. *Proc. Natl. Acad. Sci. USA* **2020**, *117*, 24205–24212. [CrossRef] [PubMed]
47. Meng, W.; Kallinteri, P.; Walker, D.A.; Parker, T.L.; Garnett, M.C. Evaluation of poly (glycerol-adipate) nanoparticle uptake in an in vitro 3-D brain tumor co-culture model. *Exp. Biol. Med.* **2007**, *232*, 1100–1108. [CrossRef] [PubMed]
48. Kumar, V.; Wang, Q.; Sethi, B.; Lin, F.; Coulter, D.W.; Dong, Y.; Mahato, R.I. Polymeric nanomedicine for overcoming resistance mechanisms in hedgehog and Myc-amplified medulloblastoma. *Biomaterials* **2021**, *278*, 121138. [CrossRef]
49. Gao, J.; Wang, Z.; Liu, H.; Wang, L.; Huang, G. Liposome encapsulated of temozolomide for the treatment of glioma tumor: Preparation, characterization and evaluation. *Drug Discov. Ther.* **2015**, *9*, 205–212. [CrossRef]
50. Sun, T.; Wu, H.; Li, Y.; Huang, Y.; Yao, L.; Chen, X.; Han, X.; Zhou, Y.; Du, Z. Targeting transferrin receptor delivery of temozolomide for a potential glioma stem cell-mediated therapy. *Oncotarget* **2017**, *8*, 74451–74465. [CrossRef]
51. Gu, G.; Gao, X.; Hu, Q.; Kang, T.; Liu, Z.; Jiang, M.; Miao, D.; Song, Q.; Yao, L.; Tu, Y.; et al. The influence of the penetrating peptide iRGD on the effect of paclitaxel-loaded MT1-AF7p-conjugated nanoparticles on glioma cells. *Biomaterials* **2013**, *34*, 5138–5148. [CrossRef]
52. Bhunia, S.; Vangala, V.; Bhattacharya, D.; Ravuri, H.G.; Kuncha, M.; Chakravarty, S.; Sistla, R.; Chaudhuri, A. Large Amino Acid Transporter 1 Selective Liposomes of l-DOPA Functionalized Amphiphile for Combating Glioblastoma. *Mol. Pharm.* **2017**, *14*, 3834–3847. [CrossRef] [PubMed]
53. Chai, Z.; Hu, X.; Wei, X.; Zhan, C.; Lu, L.; Jiang, K.; Su, B.; Ruan, H.; Ran, D.; Fang, R.H.; et al. A facile approach to functionalizing cell membrane-coated nanoparticles with neurotoxin-derived peptide for brain-targeted drug delivery. *J. Control. Release* **2017**, *264*, 102–111. [CrossRef] [PubMed]
54. Luo, Z.; Yan, Z.; Jin, K.; Pang, Q.; Jiang, T.; Lu, H.; Liu, X.; Pang, Z.; Yu, L.; Jiang, X. Precise glioblastoma targeting by AS1411 aptamer-functionalized poly (l-γ-glutamylglutamine)-paclitaxel nanoconjugates. *J. Colloid Interface Sci.* **2017**, *490*, 783–796. [CrossRef] [PubMed]

55. Zhang, Y.; Zhai, M.; Chen, Z.; Han, X.; Yu, F.; Li, Z.; Xie, X.; Han, C.; Yu, L.; Yang, Y.; et al. Dual-modified liposome codelivery of doxorubicin and vincristine improve targeting and therapeutic efficacy of glioma. *Drug Deliv.* **2017**, *24*, 1045–1055. [CrossRef] [PubMed]
56. Segura-Collar, B.; Hiller-Vallina, S.; de Dios, O.; Caamaño-Moreno, M.; Mondejar-Ruescas, L.; Sepulveda-Sanchez, J.M.; Gargini, R. Advanced Immunotherapies for Glioblastoma: Tumor Neoantigen Vaccines in Combination with Immunomodulators. *Acta Neuropathol. Commun.* **2023**, *11*, 79. [CrossRef] [PubMed]
57. Bovenberg, M.S.S.; Degeling, M.H.; Tannous, B.A. Cell-Based Immunotherapy Against Gliomas: From Bench to Bedside. *Mol. Ther.* **2013**, *21*, 1297–1305. [CrossRef] [PubMed]
58. Tang, L.; Zhang, M.; Liu, C. Advances in Nanotechnology-Based Immunotherapy for Glioblastoma. *Front. Immunol.* **2022**, *13*, 882257. [CrossRef] [PubMed]
59. Šamec, N.; Zottel, A.; Paska, A.V.; Jovčevska, I. Nanomedicine and Immunotherapy: A Step Further towards Precision Medicine for Glioblastoma. *Molecules* **2020**, *25*, 490. [CrossRef]
60. Kuang, J.; Song, W.; Yin, J.; Zeng, X.; Han, S.; Zhao, Y.P.; Tao, J.; Liu, C.J.; He, X.H.; Zhang, X.Z. IRGD Modified Chemo-Immunotherapeutic Nanoparticles for Enhanced Immunotherapy against Glioblastoma. *Adv. Funct. Mater.* **2018**, *28*, 1800025. [CrossRef]
61. Ahmad, S.; Khan, I.; Pandit, J.; Emad, N.A.; Bano, S.; Dar, K.I.; Rizvi, M.M.A.; Ansari, M.D.; Aqil, M.; Sultana, Y. Brain Targeted Delivery of Carmustine Using Chitosan Coated Nanoparticles via Nasal Route for Glioblastoma Treatment. *Int. J. Biol. Macromol.* **2022**, *221*, 435–445. [CrossRef]
62. Jafari, S.; Tavakoli, M.B.; Zarrabi, A. Lomustine Loaded Superparamagnetic Iron Oxide Nanoparticles Conjugated with Folic Acid for Treatment of Glioblastoma Multiforma (GBM). *Iran. J. Pharm. Res.* **2020**, *19*, 134. [CrossRef]
63. Zhao, Y.Z.; Lin, Q.; Wong, H.L.; Shen, X.T.; Yang, W.; Xu, H.L.; Mao, K.L.; Tian, F.R.; Yang, J.J.; Xu, J.; et al. Glioma-Targeted Therapy Using Cilengitide Nanoparticles Combined with UTMD Enhanced Delivery. *J. Control. Release* **2016**, *224*, 112–125. [CrossRef]
64. Kamali, M.; Webster, T.J.; Amani, A.; Hadjighassem, M.R.; Malekpour, M.R.; Tirgar, F.; Khosravani, M.; Adabi, M. Effect of Folate-Targeted Erlotinib Loaded Human Serum Albumin Nanoparticles on Tumor Size and Survival Rate in a Rat Model of Glioblastoma. *Life Sci.* **2023**, *313*, 121248. [CrossRef] [PubMed]
65. Lakkadwala, S.; Singh, J. Co-Delivery of Doxorubicin and Erlotinib through Liposomal Nanoparticles for Glioblastoma Tumor Regression Using an in Vitro Brain Tumor Model. *Colloids Surf. B Biointerfaces* **2019**, *173*, 27–35. [CrossRef] [PubMed]
66. Hassanzadeganroudsari, M.; Soltani, M.; Heydarinasab, A.; Apostolopoulos, V.; Akbarzadehkhiyavi, A.; Nurgali, K. Targeted Nano-Drug Delivery System for Glioblastoma Therapy: In Vitro and in Vivo Study. *J. Drug Deliv. Sci. Technol.* **2020**, *60*, 102039. [CrossRef]
67. Mobasheri, T.; Rayzan, E.; Shabani, M.; Hosseini, M.; Mahmoodi Chalbatani, G.; Rezaei, N. Neuroblastoma-targeted nanoparticles and novel nanotechnology-based treatment methods. *J. Cell Physiol.* **2021**, *236*, 1751–1775. [CrossRef] [PubMed]
68. Perkins, S.M.; Shinohara, E.T.; DeWees, T.; Frangoul, H. Outcome for children with metastatic solid tumors over the last four decades. *PLoS ONE* **2014**, *9*, e100396. [CrossRef]
69. Mari, E.; Mardente, S.; Morgante, E.; Tafani, M.; Lococo, E.; Fico, F.; Valentini, F.; Zicari, A. Graphene Oxide Nanoribbons Induce Autophagic Vacuoles in Neuroblastoma Cell Lines. *Int. J. Mol. Sci.* **2016**, *17*, 1995. [CrossRef] [PubMed]
70. Li, F.; Song, L.; Yang, X.; Huang, Z.; Mou, X.; Syed, A.; Bahkali, A.H.; Zheng, L. Anticancer and genotoxicity effect of (*Clausena lansium* (Lour.) Skeels) Peel ZnONPs on neuroblastoma (SH-SY5Y) cells through the modulation of autophagy mechanism. *J. Photochem. Photobiol. B* **2020**, *203*, 111748. [CrossRef]
71. Kalashnikova, I.; Mazar, J.; Neal, C.J.; Rosado, A.L.; Das, S.; Westmoreland, T.J.; Seal, S. Nanoparticle delivery of curcumin induces cellular hypoxia and ROS-mediated apoptosis via modulation of Bcl-2/Bax in human neuroblastoma. *Nanoscale* **2017**, *9*, 10375–10387. [CrossRef]
72. Mohammadniaei, M.; Yoon, J.; Choi, H.K.; Placide, V.; Bharate, B.G.; Lee, T.; Choi, J.-W. Multifunctional Nanobiohybrid Material Composed of Ag@Bi$_2$Se$_3$/RNA Three-Way Junction/miRNA/Retinoic Acid for Neuroblastoma Differentiation. *ACS Appl. Mater. Interfaces* **2019**, *11*, 8779–8788. [CrossRef]
73. Zhang, L.; Marrano, P.; Kumar, S.; Leadley, M.; Elias, E.; Thorner, P.; Baruchel, S. Nab-paclitaxel is an active drug in preclinical model of pediatric solid tumors. *Clin. Cancer Res.* **2013**, *19*, 5972–5983. [CrossRef] [PubMed]
74. Yesil-Celiktas, O.; Pala, C.; Cetin-Uyanikgil, E.O.; Sevimli-Gur, C. Synthesis of silica-PAMAM dendrimer nanoparticles as promising carriers in Neuro blastoma cells. *Anal. Biochem.* **2017**, *519*, 1–7. [CrossRef] [PubMed]
75. Vignaroli, G.; Calandro, P.; Zamperini, C.; Coniglio, F.; Iovenitti, G.; Tavanti, M.; Colecchia, D.; Dreassi, E.; Valoti, M.; Schenone, S.; et al. Improvement of pyrazolo[3,4-d]pyrimidines pharmacokinetic properties: Nanosystem approaches for drug delivery. *Sci. Rep.* **2016**, *6*, 21509. [CrossRef] [PubMed]
76. Pieper, S.; Onafuye, H.; Mulac, D.; Cinatl, J., Jr.; Wass, M.N.; Michaelis, M.; Langer, K. Incorporation of doxorubicin in different polymer nanoparticles and their anticancer activity. *Beilstein J. Nanotechnol.* **2019**, *10*, 2062–2072. [CrossRef]
77. Bacanlı, M.; Eşi, M.Ö.; Erdoğan, H.; Sarper, M.; Erdem, O.; Özkan, Y. Evaluation of cytotoxic and genotoxic effects of paclitaxel-loaded PLGA nanoparticles in neuroblastoma cells. *Food Chem. Toxicol.* **2021**, *154*, 112323. [CrossRef] [PubMed]

78. Viale, M.; Vecchio, G.; Monticone, M.; Bertone, V.; Giglio, V.; Maric, I.; Cilli, M.; Bocchini, V.; Profumo, A.; Ponzoni, M.; et al. Fibrin Gels Entrapment of a Poly-Cyclodextrin Nanocarrier as a Doxorubicin Delivery System in an Orthotopic Model of Neuroblastoma: Evaluation of In Vitro Activity and In Vivo Toxicity. *Pharm. Res.* **2019**, *36*, 115. [CrossRef]
79. Wang, G.; Hu, W.; Chen, H.; Shou, X.; Ye, T.; Xu, Y. Cocktail Strategy Based on NK Cell-Derived Exosomes and Their Biomimetic Nanoparticles for Dual Tumor Therapy. *Cancers* **2019**, *11*, 560. [CrossRef]
80. Piazzini, V.; Vasarri, M.; Degl'Innocenti, D.; Guastini, A.; Barletta, E.; Salvatici, M.C.; Bergonzi, M.C. Comparison of Chitosan Nanoparticles and Soluplus Micelles to Optimize the Bioactivity of Posidonia oceanica Extract on Human Neuroblastoma Cell Migration. *Pharmaceutics* **2019**, *11*, 655. [CrossRef]
81. Zhao, J.; Yao, L.; Nie, S.; Xu, Y. Low-viscosity sodium alginate combined with TiO2 nanoparticles for improving neuroblastoma treatment. *Int. J. Biol. Macromol.* **2021**, *167*, 921–933. [CrossRef] [PubMed]
82. Burgos-Panadero, R.; El Moukhtari, S.H.; Noguera, I.; Rodríguez-Nogales, C.; Martín-Vañó, S.; Vicente-Munuera, P.; Cañete, A.; Navarro, S.; Blanco-Prieto, M.J.; Noguera, R. Unraveling the extracellular matrix-tumor cell interactions to aid better targeted therapies for neuroblastoma. *Int. J. Pharm.* **2021**, *608*, 121058. [CrossRef]
83. Patel, R.B.; Ye, M.; Carlson, P.M.; Jaquish, A.; Zangl, L.; Ma, B.; Wang, Y.; Arthur, I.; Xie, R.; Brown, R.J.; et al. Development of an In Situ Cancer Vaccine via Combinational Radiation and Bacterial-Membrane-Coated Nanoparticles. *Adv. Mater.* **2019**, *31*, e1902626. [CrossRef] [PubMed]
84. Subramanian, C.; White, P.T.; Kuai, R.; Kalidindi, A.; Castle, V.P.; Moon, J.J.; Timmermann, B.N.; Schwendeman, A.; Cohen, M.S. Synthetic high-density lipoprotein nanoconjugate targets neuroblastoma stem cells, blocking migration and self-renewal. *Surgery* **2018**, *164*, 165–172. [CrossRef] [PubMed]
85. Kulkarni, S.; Pandey, A.; Nikam, A.N.; Nannuri, S.H.; George, S.D.; Fayaz, S.M.A.; Vincent, A.P.; Mutalik, S. ZIF-8 nano confined protein-titanocene complex core-shell MOFs for efficient therapy of Neuroblastoma: Optimization, molecular dynamics and toxicity studies. *Int. J. Biol. Macromol.* **2021**, *178*, 444–463. [CrossRef] [PubMed]
86. Lin, Y.S.; Chen, Y.; Tsai, Y.H.; Tseng, S.H.; Lin, K.S. In Vivo Imaging of Neuroblastomas Using GD2-Targeting Graphene Quantum Dots. *J. Pediatr. Surg.* **2021**, *56*, 1227–1232. [CrossRef] [PubMed]
87. Di Paolo, D.; Pastorino, F.; Brignole, C.; Corrias, M.V.; Emionite, L.; Cilli, M.; Tamma, R.; Priddy, L.; Amaro, A.; Ferrari, D.; et al. Combined Replenishment of MiR-34a and Let-7b by Targeted Nanoparticles Inhibits Tumor Growth in Neuroblastoma Preclinical Models. *Small* **2020**, *16*, 1906426. [CrossRef]
88. Dimaras, H.; Corson, T.W. Retinoblastoma, the visible CNS tumor: A review. *J. Neurosci. Res.* **2019**, *97*, 29–44. [CrossRef]
89. Fabian, I.D.; Onadim, Z.; Karaa, E.; Duncan, C.; Chowdhury, T.; Scheimberg, I.; Ohnuma, S.I.; Reddy, M.A.; Sagoo, M.S. The management of retinoblastoma. *Oncogene* **2018**, *37*, 1551–1560. [CrossRef]
90. Shields, C.L.; Shields, J.A.; De Potter, P.; Minelli, S.; Hernandez, C.; Brady, L.W.; Cater, J.R. Plaque radiotherapy in the management of retinoblastoma. Use as a primary and secondary treatment. *Ophthalmology* **1993**, *100*, 216–224. [CrossRef]
91. Bhavsar, D.; Subramanian, K.; Sethuraman, S.; Krishnan, U.M. Management of retinoblastoma: Opportunities and challenges. *Drug Deliv.* **2016**, *23*, 2488–2496. [CrossRef] [PubMed]
92. Wei, D.; Zhang, N.; Qu, S.; Wang, H.; Li, J. Advances in nanotechnology for the treatment of GBM. *Front. Neurosci.* **2023**, *17*, 1180943. [CrossRef] [PubMed]
93. Barzegar Behrooz, A.; Talaie, Z.; Syahir, A. Nanotechnology-Based Combinatorial Anti-Glioblastoma Therapies: Moving from Terminal to Treatable. *Pharmaceutics* **2022**, *14*, 1697. [CrossRef] [PubMed]
94. Gusmão, L.A.; Matsuo, F.S.; Barbosa, H.F.G.; Tedesco, A.C. Advances in nano-based materials for glioblastoma multiforme diagnosis: A mini-review. *Front. Nanotechnol.* **2022**, *4*, 836802. [CrossRef]
95. Barani, M.; Mukhtar, M.; Rahdar, A.; Sargazi, G.; Thysiadou, A.; Kyzas, G.Z. Progress in the Application of Nanoparticles and Graphene as Drug Carriers and on the Diagnosis of Brain Infections. *Molecules* **2021**, *26*, 186. [CrossRef] [PubMed]
96. Kenchegowda, M.; Rahamathulla, M.; Hani, U.; Begum, M.Y.; Guruswamy, S.; Osmani, R.A.M.; Gowrav, M.P.; Alshehri, S.; Ghoneim, M.M.; Alshlowi, A.; et al. Smart Nanocarriers as an Emerging Platform for Cancer Therapy: A Review. *Molecules* **2021**, *27*, 146. [CrossRef] [PubMed]
97. Bilal, M.; Barani, M.; Sabir, F.; Rahdar, A.; Kyzas, G.Z. Nanomaterials for the treatment and diagnosis of Alzheimer's disease: An overview. *NanoImpact* **2020**, *20*, 100251. [CrossRef]
98. Moradi, S.; Mokhtari-Dizaji, M.; Ghassemi, F.; Sheibani, S.; Amoli, F.A. The effect of ultrasound hyperthermia with gold nanoparticles on retinoblastoma Y79 cells. *Gold. Bull.* **2020**, *53*, 111–120. [CrossRef]
99. Wang, W.; Yang, Q.; Li, M.; Zou, H.; Wang, Z.; Ran, H.; Zheng, Y.; Jian, J.; Zhou, Y.; Luo, Y.; et al. Multifunctional Nanoparticles for Multimodal Imaging-Guided Low-Intensity Focused Ultrasound/Immunosynergistic Retinoblastoma Therapy. *ACS Appl. Mater. Interfaces* **2020**, *12*, 5642–5657. [CrossRef]
100. Rajanahalli, P.; Stucke, C.J.; Hong, Y. The effects of silver nanoparticles on mouse embryonic stem cell self-renewal and proliferation. *Toxicol. Rep.* **2015**, *2*, 758–764. [CrossRef]
101. Qu, W.; Meng, B.; Yu, Y.; Wang, S. EpCAM antibody-conjugated mesoporous silica nanoparticles to enhance the anticancer efficacy of carboplatin in retinoblastoma. *Mater. Sci. Eng. C Mater. Biol. Appl.* **2017**, *76*, 646–651. [CrossRef] [PubMed]
102. Liu, Y.; Han, Y.; Chen, S.; Liu, J.; Wang, D.; Huang, Y. Liposome-based multifunctional nanoplatform as effective therapeutics for the treatment of retinoblastoma. *Acta Pharm. Sin. B* **2022**, *12*, 2731–2739. [CrossRef]

103. Kartha, B.; Thanikachalam, K.; Vijayakumar, N.; Alharbi, N.S.; Kadaikunnan, S.; Khaled, J.M.; Gopinath, K.; Govindarajan, M. Synthesis and characterization of Ce-doped TiO2 nanoparticles and their enhanced anticancer activity in Y79 retinoblastoma cancer cells. *Green Process. Synth.* **2022**, *11*, 143–149. [CrossRef]
104. Mitra, M.; Kandalam, M.; Rangasamy, J.; Shankar, B.; Maheswari, U.K.; Swaminathan, S.; Krishnakumar, S. Novel epithelial cell adhesion molecule antibody conjugated polyethyleneimine-capped gold nanoparticles for enhanced and targeted small interfering RNA delivery to retinoblastoma cells. *Mol. Vis.* **2013**, *19*, 1029–1038.
105. Godse, R.; Rathod, M.; De, A.; Shinde, U. Intravitreal galactose conjugated polymeric nanoparticles of etoposide for retinoblastoma. *J. Drug Deliv. Sci. Technol.* **2021**, *61*, 102259. [CrossRef]
106. Sims, L.B.; Tyo, K.M.; Stocke, S.; Mahmoud, M.Y.; Ramasubramanian, A.; Steinbach-Rankins, J.M. Surface-Modified Melphalan Nanoparticles for Intravitreal Chemotherapy of Retinoblastoma. *Invest. Ophthalmol. Vis. Sci.* **2019**, *60*, 1696–1705. [CrossRef] [PubMed]
107. Silva-Abreu, M.; Calpena, A.C.; Espina, M.; Silva, A.M.; Gimeno, A.; Egea, M.A.; García, M.L. Optimization, Biopharmaceutical Profile and Therapeutic Efficacy of Pioglitazone-loaded PLGA-PEG Nanospheres as a Novel Strategy for Ocular Inflammatory Disorders. *Pharm. Res.* **2018**, *35*, 11. [CrossRef]
108. Delrish, E.; Ghassemi, F.; Jabbarvand, M.; Lashay, A.; Atyabi, F.; Soleimani, M.; Dinarvand, R. Biodistribution of Cy5-labeled Thiolated and Methylated Chitosan-Carboxymethyl Dextran Nanoparticles in an Animal Model of Retinoblastoma. *J. Ophthalmic Vis. Res.* **2022**, *17*, 58–68. [CrossRef]
109. Delrish, E.; Jabbarvand, M.; Ghassemi, F.; Amoli, F.A.; Atyabi, F.; Lashay, A.; Soleimani, M.; Aghajanpour, L.; Dinarvand, R. Efficacy of topotecan nanoparticles for intravitreal chemotherapy of retinoblastoma. *Exp. Eye Res.* **2021**, *204*, 108423. [CrossRef]
110. Passos Gibson, V.; Derbali, R.M.; Phan, H.T.; Tahiri, H.; Allen, C.; Hardy, P.; Chain, J.L. Survivin silencing improved the cytotoxicity of carboplatin and melphalan in Y79 and primary retinoblastoma cells. *Int. J. Pharm.* **2020**, *589*, 119824. [CrossRef]
111. Tabatabaei, S.N.; Derbali, R.M.; Yang, C.; Superstein, R.; Hamel, P.; Chain, J.L.; Hardy, P. Co-delivery of miR-181a and melphalan by lipid nanoparticles for treatment of seeded retinoblastoma. *J. Control. Release* **2019**, *298*, 177–185. [CrossRef] [PubMed]
112. Narayana, R.V.L.; Jana, P.; Tomar, N.; Prabhu, V.; Nair, R.M.; Manukonda, R.; Kaliki, S.; Coupland, S.E.; Alexander, J.; Kalirai, H.; et al. Carboplatin- and Etoposide-Loaded Lactoferrin Protein Nanoparticles for Targeting Cancer Stem Cells in Retinoblastoma In Vitro. *Invest. Ophthalmol. Vis. Sci.* **2021**, *62*, 13. [CrossRef]
113. Ahmed, F.; Ali, M.J.; Kondapi, A.K. Carboplatin loaded protein nanoparticles exhibit improve anti-proliferative activity in retinoblastoma cells. *Int. J. Biol. Macromol.* **2014**, *70*, 572–582. [CrossRef] [PubMed]
114. Shome, D.; Kalita, D.; Jain, V.; Sarin, R.; Maru, G.B.; Bellare, J.R. Carboplatin loaded polymethylmethacrylate nano-particles in an adjunctive role in retinoblastoma: An animal trial. *Indian J. Ophthalmol.* **2014**, *62*, 585–589. [CrossRef] [PubMed]
115. Alsaab, H.; Alzhrani, R.M.; Kesharwani, P.; Sau, S.; Boddu, S.H.; Iyer, A.K. Folate Decorated Nanomicelles Loaded with a Potent Curcumin Analogue for Targeting Retinoblastoma. *Pharmaceutics* **2017**, *9*, 15. [CrossRef] [PubMed]
116. Mitra, M.; Misra, R.; Harilal, A.; Sahoo, S.K.; Krishnakumar, S. Enhanced in Vitro Antiproliferative Effects of EpCAM Antibody-Functionalized Paclitaxel-Loaded PLGA Nanoparticles in Retinoblastoma Cells. *Mol. Vis.* **2011**, *17*, 2724. [PubMed]
117. N'Diaye, M.; Vergnaud-Gauduchon, J.; Nicolas, V.; Faure, V.; Denis, S.; Abreu, S.; Chaminade, P.; Rosilio, V. Hybrid Lipid Polymer Nanoparticles for Combined Chemo- And Photodynamic Therapy. *Mol. Pharm.* **2019**, *16*, 4045–4058. [CrossRef]
118. Gallud, A.; Warther, D.; Maynadier, M.; Sefta, M.; Poyer, F.; Thomas, C.D.; Rouxel, C.; Mongin, O.; Blanchard-Desce, M.; Morère, A.; et al. Identification of MRC2 and CD209 Receptors as Targets for Photodynamic Therapy of Retinoblastoma Using Mesoporous Silica Nanoparticles. *RSC Adv.* **2015**, *5*, 75167–75172. [CrossRef]

Disclaimer/Publisher's Note: The statements, opinions and data contained in all publications are solely those of the individual author(s) and contributor(s) and not of MDPI and/or the editor(s). MDPI and/or the editor(s) disclaim responsibility for any injury to people or property resulting from any ideas, methods, instructions or products referred to in the content.

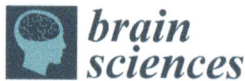

Article

Integrative Magnetic Resonance Imaging and Metabolomic Characterization of a Glioblastoma Rat Model

Nuria Arias-Ramos, Cecilia Vieira, Rocío Pérez-Carro and Pilar López-Larrubia *

Instituto de Investigaciones Biomédicas Sols-Morreale, Consejo Superior de Investigaciones Científicas-Universidad Autónoma de Madrid (CSIC-UAM), 28029 Madrid, Spain; narias@iib.uam.es (N.A.-R.)
* Correspondence: plopez@iib.uam.es

Abstract: Glioblastoma (GBM) stands as the most prevalent and lethal malignant brain tumor, characterized by its highly infiltrative nature. This study aimed to identify additional MRI and metabolomic biomarkers of GBM and its impact on healthy tissue using an advanced-stage C6 glioma rat model. Wistar rats underwent a stereotactic injection of C6 cells (GBM group, n = 10) or cell medium (sham group, n = 4). A multiparametric MRI, including anatomical T_2W and T_1W images, relaxometry maps (T_2, T_2^*, and T_1), the magnetization transfer ratio (MTR), and diffusion tensor imaging (DTI), was performed. Additionally, ex vivo magnetic resonance spectroscopy (MRS) HRMAS spectra were acquired. The MRI analysis revealed significant differences in the T_2 maps, T_1 maps, MTR, and mean diffusivity parameters between the GBM tumor and the rest of the studied regions, which were the contralateral areas of the GBM rats and both regions of the sham rats (the ipsilateral and contralateral). The ex vivo spectra revealed markers of neuronal loss, apoptosis, and higher glucose uptake by the tumor. Notably, the myo-inositol and phosphocholine levels were elevated in both the tumor and the contralateral regions of the GBM rats compared to the sham rats, suggesting the effects of the tumor on the healthy tissue. The MRI parameters related to inflammation, cellularity, and tissue integrity, along with MRS-detected metabolites, serve as potential biomarkers for the tumor evolution, treatment response, and impact on healthy tissue. These techniques can be potent tools for evaluating new drugs and treatment targets.

Keywords: glioblastoma; magnetic resonance imaging; magnetic resonance spectroscopy; HRMAS; preclinical models

1. Introduction

Brain cancer is a life-threatening neurological disorder in which malignant cells grow, proliferate, and invade the cerebral structures of the host, seriously hampering an adequate brain function [1]. Glioblastoma (GBM) stands as the most common primary malignant brain tumor, accounting for approximately 50% of all primary malignant tumors. It is classified as a grade IV tumor by the World Health Organization (WHO) [2], the most aggressive subtype. It has an incidence of 3.26 cases/100,000 inhabitants per year in the United States, with a very poor prognosis: a 5-year survival rate of less than 7%, despite a therapeutic approach that includes surgical resection, immunotherapy, chemotherapy, and radiotherapy [3]. The infiltrative nature of this type of tumor, which makes its complete resection virtually impossible, implies an inevitable impact on the surrounding brain tissue and, ultimately, on the healthy brain tissue and its microenvironment [4]. Furthermore, the presence of the blood–brain barrier (BBB), which can hinder the delivery of drugs to the tumor [5], highlights the critical importance of researching new drug delivery methods and enhancing our tumor targeting capabilities. The current research and advancements in theranostic approaches and nanomedicine can significantly contribute to addressing this challenge [6–8].

Magnetic resonance imaging (MRI) stands out as one of the most powerful techniques for accurately studying and monitoring the progression of brain tumors and their effects on healthy tissue, as well as their response to treatment. Its main advantage lies in the fact it provides a wealth of information ranging from high-contrast, high-resolution anatomical images to metabolomic information with details on cell density, vascular supply, and hypoxia [9], among others.

Despite improvements, accurately assessing the tumor progression and the response to treatments using imaging techniques remains challenging. Traditionally, post-treatment tumor changes are evaluated based on anatomical post-contrast T_1-weighted MRI images, where a decrease in the contrast-enhanced areas is interpreted as a reduced tumor burden. However, the interpretation of the image is not always straightforward due to post-surgical changes in the brain anatomy and radiation-induced necrotic areas. Additionally, the phenomenon of 'pseudo-progression' may raise doubts when interpreting the images [10]. Multiparametric MRI techniques offer a valuable alternative, allowing for a comprehensive assessment of the characteristics of the tumor and the healthy tissue. Diffusion tensor imaging (DTI) provides information on the tissue microstructure [11] and magnetic transfer (MT) imaging offers insights into cellularity [12], while the T_2, T_2^*, and T_1 mapping provide data on inflammation and vasogenic oedema [13], hemorrhage/neoangiogenesis and oxygen levels [14], and interstitial water content and BBB disruption [15], respectively. As a result, these approaches provide data that serve as imaging biomarkers of the disease progression following the therapeutic interventions that target the pathological features of the tumor. Indeed, multiparametric MRI has been utilized by other researchers in both clinical and preclinical studies for various purposes, including investigating the evolution of the development of the tumor [16], distinguishing between primary GBM tumors and metastases [17], and monitoring treatments for this disease [18,19].

On the other hand, metabolomics plays a key role in understanding the behavior of tumors and their microenvironment. The metabolites detected and identified by in vivo magnetic resonance spectroscopy (MRS), such as choline (Cho), lactate (Lac), lipids, N-acetylaspartic acid (NAA), and myo-inositol (mI), are well-studied biomarkers of the characteristics and disease progression of GBM [20]. Additionally, ex vivo High-Resolution Magic Angle Spinning (HRMAS) provides metabolomic information of a wider range of metabolites from unprocessed small tissue samples or biopsies [21,22].

Given the significant challenges posed by glioblastoma (GBM) and the increasing recognition of the importance of multiparametric MRI in understanding its pathophysiology, we aimed to characterize an advanced-stage GBM tumor model using in vivo multiparametric MRI evaluations and ex vivo metabolomic HRMAS MRS studies. Building upon prior studies utilizing multiparametric MRI in GBM research, our approach sought to provide a comprehensive assessment of the progression of a tumor and its microenvironment. By investigating both the tumor and the contralateral regions potentially affected by the tumor, along with the equivalent regions in sham animals, we aimed to discern the parameters that serve as biomarkers to monitor the disease progression. Furthermore, we aimed to explore the potential of our methodology in preclinical and clinical research, particularly in validating new drugs, including theranostic nanodrugs.

2. Materials and Methods
2.1. Animal Models

All experimental procedures complied with the national (R.D.53/2013) and European Community guidelines (2010/62/UE) for the care and management of experimental animals and were approved by the Ethics Committee of the Community of Madrid (PROEX 047/18; approved 2 November 2015). Male Wistar albino rats (*Rattus novergicus*) with a body weight (b.w.) of 230 ± 20 g were used. The animals were housed in cages in a light-controlled (12 h cycle of light and darkness) and temperature-controlled (22 ± 2 °C) room with access to water and food ad libitum in the IIBM animal facility (Reg. No. ES280790000188) and cared for by specialized personnel.

2.2. Cell Line Culture

An authenticated C6 glioma cell line obtained from the American Type Culture Collection (ATCC number: CCL-107) (Manassas, VA, USA) was used. The cells were cultured in Dulbecco's Modified Eagle Medium (DMEM), supplemented with 10% fetal bovine serum (FBS) (Gibco®, Thermo Fisher Scientific, Inc., Waltham, MA, USA) and antibiotics (10% of amphotericin B, 100 UI/mL of penicillin, 0.03 mg/mL of gentamicin, and 0.1 mg/mL of streptomycin), and were kept in an incubator at 37 °C and 5% of CO_2.

2.3. Surgical Procedure

The male Wistar rats (n = 14) were submitted to a surgical procedure using stereotaxic equipment (Model 900LS Small Animal Stereotaxic Instrument, Kopf Instruments®, Tujunga, CA, USA). Briefly, the animals were injected subcutaneously with the analgesic meloxicam (0.5 mg/kg b.w.) 30 min before the surgery. Then, the animals were anesthetized by an intraperitoneal injection of ketamine hydrochloride (75 mg/kg b.w.) and medetomidine hydrochloride (0.5 mg/kg b.w.) and placed in the stereotaxic device. Through a small burr hole, the tumor cells (10^5/10 µL of culture medium per animal, ten GBM rats) or the culture medium alone (10 µL, four sham rats) were injected on the right caudate–putamen, based on coordinates using the bregma as a reference: 0.35 mm from it on the right lateral and 0.55 mm from it on the ventral side. Once finished, the skull hole was sealed and the skin sutured. After the surgery, atipamezol hydrochloride (5 mg/kg b.w.) was administered subcutaneously to fasten the anesthesia recovery, and meloxicam (0.5 mg/kg b.w.) was used for analgesia and administrated during the following two days.

2.4. Magnetic Resonance Imaging

The MRI studies were carried out on a 7 T superconductor horizontal animal MR system (Bruker Medical GmbH, Ettlingen, Germany) equipped with a ^{1}H 38 mm bird cage resonator and a gradient insert of 90 mm in diameter (360 mT/m maximum strength). All data were acquired running Paravision 5.1 software (Bruker Medical GmbH®, Ettlingen, Germany) operating on a Linux platform.

The animals were anesthetized with 3–4% isoflurane in 100% O_2 in an induction box, followed by the administration of 1.5–2% isoflurane through a mask during the MRI acquisitions. The rats were placed in an animal holder with a heated blanket, which maintained their body temperature at ~37 °C. The temperature and respiratory rate of the animals were monitored by a monitoring and gating system (SA Instruments, Inc., Stony Brook, NY, USA). The GBM-bearing rats were placed in the MRI system with a tail catheter to allow the intravenous (i.v) administration of the contrast agent (CA).

Magnetic Resonance Imaging Studies

The tumor development in the GBM-bearing rats was followed up with T_2-weighted (T_2W) anatomical MRI weekly after the surgery. Multiparametric MRI studies were conducted between 2 and 3 weeks post-surgery, when the tumor reached a volume ≥ 100 mm^3, including T_2W and T_1-weighted (T_1W) images after the i.v. administration of the CA and parametric MRI acquisitions: relaxometry (T_2, T_2*, and T_1 maps), MT images, and DTI. The sham rats underwent the same multiparametric MRI studies.

- Anatomical MRI

The T_2W images were acquired with a rapid acquisition relaxation-enhanced (RARE) sequence with the following acquisition parameters: a repetition time (TR) = 3000 ms, an echo time (TE) = 60 ms, the number of experiments (NEX) = 3, the total acquisition time (TAT) of 3 min and 36 s, and a RARE factor = 8, with 10 slices in an axial orientation with a slice thickness (ST) = 1.5 mm—covering the whole brain—a field of view (FOV) = 35×35 mm^2, and a matrix = 256×256 pixels, corresponding to an in-plane resolution of 136.7×136.7 µm^2. The T_1W images were acquired after the i.v. administration of 0.3 M of Gd-diethylenetriaminepentaacetic acid (Magnevist®, Bayer, Whippany, NJ, USA) at a dose of 0.3 mmol/kg b.w. as the CA with the TR = 300 ms, TE = 10.5 ms, NEX = 3, and TAT = 2 min and 52 s. The same geometric parameters were used as in the T$_2$W images.

- Parametric MRI

The MRI studies to generate the parametric images were performed in an axial orientation using five slices (with an ST = 1.5 mm) placed at the central part of the tumor in the GBM-bearing rats and in an equivalent position in the sham rats, with a FOV of 35 × 35 mm^2 and a matrix = 128 × 128, corresponding to an in-plane resolution of 273.4 × 273.4 μm^2/pixel.

The T$_2$ maps were acquired using a multi-slice multi-echo (MSME) sequence with a TR = 5000 ms, employing 75 echoes; TE = 12–900 ms; NEX = 1; and TAT = 10 min and 40 s. The fitting curve for the calculation of T$_2$ is described in Equation (1):

$$S = S_0 \cdot e^{-TE/T_2} \quad (1)$$

where S is the value of the MRI signal at a given TE and S$_0$ is the value of the MR signal when TE = ∞.

The T$_2$* maps were acquired using a multi-gradient echo (MGE) sequence with a TR = 543.3 ms, emplying 20 echoes; TE = 2.73–83.86 ms; flip angle = 30°; NEX = 4; and TAT = 5 min and 37 s. The fitting curve for the calculation of T$_2$* is the one described in Equation (1), substituting T$_2$ for T$_2$*.

The T$_1$ maps were acquired employing a saturation–recovery sequence with eight values of TR = 125–6000 ms, TE = 12 ms, NEX = 1, and TAT = 24 min and 55 s. The fitting curve for the calculation of T$_1$ is described in Equation (2):

$$S = S_0 \cdot \left(1 - e^{-TR/T_1}\right) \quad (2)$$

where S is the value of the MR signal at a given TR and S$_0$ is the value of the MRI signal when TR = ∞.

The magnetization transfer ratio (MTR) maps were generated by acquiring two set of images, one applying an MT pulse (MT ON) and the other without applying it (MT OFF), with a TR = 2500 ms, TE = 10 ms, NEX = 1, and TAT = 5 min and 20 s. The MT ONs comprised a train of radiofrequency pulses (N = 50) of bandwidth = 550 Hz, length = 5 ms, power = 5.5 μT, and offset = 1500 Hz. The MT effect was calculated as an MT ratio according to Equation (3):

$$\%MTR = \frac{S_0 - S_{MT}}{S_0} * 100 \quad (3)$$

where S$_{MT}$ is the signal intensity of a pixel in the MT ON image and S$_0$ the signal of the same pixel in the MT OFF.

The DTI studies were performed using a Stejskal–Tanner sequence with a single-shot echo-planar readout, where the TR = 3000 ms, TE = 39.3 ms, NEX = 4, diffusion gradient separation (Δ) = 20 ms, and diffusion gradient duration (δ) = 4 ms, with one basal image and two b factors of 300 and 1400 s/mm^2 applied in seven directions and a TAT = 3 min. The mean diffusivity (MD) and fractional anisotropy (FA) parameters were calculated according to Equations (4) and (5), where the corresponding eigenvalues (λ1, λ2, and λ3) were obtained by solving the tensor:

$$MD = \frac{\lambda 1 + \lambda 2 + \lambda 2}{3} \quad (4)$$

$$FA = \frac{\sqrt{(\lambda 1 - MD)^2 + (\lambda 2 - MD)^2 + (\lambda 3 - MD)^2}}{2\left(\lambda 1^2 + \lambda 2^2 + \lambda 3^2\right)} \quad (5)$$

2.5. MRI Processing

The tumor volume development in the GBM-bearing rats was followed by using the T_2W anatomical images and manually selecting the tumor areas employing the software ImageJ (National Institutes of Health, Bethesda, MD, USA, http://rsbweb.nih.gov/ij/) and then calculated using Equation (6), where the TA (tumor area) represents the area of the tumor in each slice in mm^2:

$$\text{Tumor volume} \left(\text{mm}^3\right) = [\text{TAslice1} + \text{TAslice2} + (\ldots) + \text{TAslice10}] \times \text{ST} \quad (6)$$

Color-based maps were generated pixelwise from the images by fitting the signal to the appropriate equation using home-made software developed in MatLab version R2010b (The MathWorks, Nattick, MA, USA). Two regions of interest (ROIs) were manually selected and quantified using the Image J: tumoral area and the healthy contralateral region in all tumor-containing slices in the GBM-bearing rats and in the equivalent areas in the sham group (the ipsilateral and contralateral areas). Then, the mean value of each ROI, considering all selected slices for each rat, was used for the statistical analysis.

2.6. Ex Vivo Magnetic Resonance Spectroscopy

Immediately following the multiparametric MRI study, the rats were sacrificed using a high-power (5 kw) focused microwave (TMW-6402 C, Muromachi Kikai Co., Ltd., Tokyo, Japan), which causes an arrest of the cerebral metabolism. Then, the brains were removed from the skull and the tumor and the contralateral regions were resected from the GBM-bearing rats and the equivalent areas from the sham animals. The samples were immediately frozen in liquid nitrogen and stored at $-80\,°C$.

The HRMAS spectra were acquired in a 11.7 T Bruker AVANCE WB spectrometer (Bruker Medical GmbH, Ettlingen, Germany) operating at 500.13 MHz at a ^1H frequency, equipped with a triple nuclei HRMAS probe and using the Topspin 2.1 software. Briefly, a sample (10–15 mg) was placed on a zirconium oxide rotor (4 mm o.d.) and suspended in 50 µL of D_2O. The spectra were acquired in a probe cooled to 4 °C and spun at 5 kHz using a Carr–Purcell–Meiboom–Gill sequence with the following parameters: a water saturation pulse of 2 s, a relaxation delay of 5 s, 32 k data points, and 128 scans. Two spectra per sample were acquired, one with a total TE of 36 ms and another of 144 ms. Then, the detectable metabolites were quantified using the LCModel package (Linear Combination of Model Spectra, http://s-provencher.com/lcmodel.shtml), a prior knowledge spectral fit software. This program fits the sample spectra as a linear combination of the model spectra contained in a home-designed database of brain metabolites and taking into account the contributions for lipids and macromolecules, yielding values for the metabolite concentration and estimated standard deviation (SD) [23]. Only metabolites with an SD smaller than 20% were included in the final analysis of the data. The metabolite concentrations are presented normalized to the total creatine (PCr + Cr) content.

2.7. Statistical Analysis

The statistical analysis and data representation were performed using GraphPad Prism Software, version 9 (GraphPad Software, La Jolla, CA, USA). The Shapiro–Wilk test was used to assess the normality of the data. A two-way ANOVA followed by Tukey's post hoc for multiple comparison was used for the comparison among the different groups (the GBM rats vs. the sham rats). To compare the regions within the same group (tumor/ipsilateral vs. contralateral), a paired t-test with a Holm–Sidak correction was performed. The data are represented by boxplots, where the horizontal bar represents the median, the '+' symbol shows the mean, and the lower and upper limits of the box indicate the first and third quartile, respectively. The upper and lower whiskers extend to the most extreme data points 1.5× the interquartile range from the nearest box border (the quartile). A p-value < 0.05 was considered statistically significant.

3. Results

3.1. MRI Studies

The multiparametric MRI studies were conducted in the GBM rats between 16 and 21 days after the surgery, once the tumors had reached a volume of ≥ 100 mm^3, while the sham rats underwent the studies 21 days after surgery. The tumors were observed in the GBM animals as hyperintense areas on both the T$_2$WI (weighted images) and in the T$_1$WI after the administration of the CA (Figure 1). In addition, a higher uptake of the CA could be observed in the proliferative tumor periphery region than in the central core area due to the presence of necrosis. The scars resulting from the intracranial surgery were visible as hypointense areas on the T$_2$WI from the sham rats.

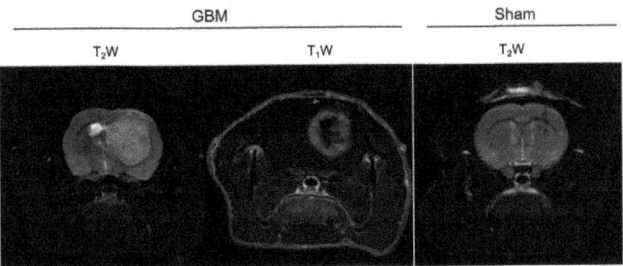

Figure 1. Anatomical images of a representative slice from the GBM and sham animals. The surgical scar is observed as a hypointense area in the T$_2$W image of the sham rat, while the tumor is detected as an hyperintense area in the T$_2$W and T$_1$W images after the CA administration in the GBM rat.

3.1.1. Relaxometry

The relaxation times, including the T$_2$, T$_2$*, and T$_1$ values from the assessed regions (the tumor/ipsilateral and contralateral areas), were quantified from the corresponding parametric maps (Figure 2). The mean relaxation values for each group are presented in Table 1.

Table 1. MRI parameters (mean ± SEM) measured in the different regions of the studied groups.

	GBM		Sham	
MRI Parameter	Tumor	Contralateral	Ipsilateral	Contralateral
T$_2$ (ms)	66.52 ± 2.43	51.26 ± 0.56	49.64 ± 0.35	49.91 ± 0.21
T$_2$* (ms)	22.75 ± 1.30	21.85 ± 1.54	22.59 ± 3.23	21.81 ± 2.69
T$_1$ (ms)	2574 ± 37	2090 ± 45	1937 ± 17	1942 ± 38
MTR (%)	15.15 ± 1.46	30.56 ± 1.99	30.03 ± 0.95	29.79 ± 1.10
MD (μm^2/s)	1064 ± 52	816 ± 30	815 ± 9	836 ± 16
FA	0.255 ± 0.045	0.284 ± 0.035	0.232 ± 0.012	0.231 ± 0.013

SEM: standard error of mean, MTR: magnetization transfer ratio, MD: mean diffusivity, and FA: fractional anisotropy.

The results obtained on the T$_2$ maps of this GBM model are depicted in Figure 2A. Higher T$_2$ values were observed in the tumor compared to the contralateral areas in the GBM rats ($p < 0.001$) and compared to the ipsilateral and contralateral regions of the sham rats ($p < 0.001$). Similar T$_2$ values were observed in the ipsilateral and contralateral regions of the sham rats.

No statistically significant differences in the T$_2$* values were found between the regions in the GBM or sham animals, nor among the groups (Figure 2B).

Regarding the T$_1$ values, similar results were obtained as for the T$_2$ values. The tumor regions of the GBM rats showed higher T$_1$ values than the corresponding contralateral areas ($p < 0.001$), and they were also higher than the ipsilateral and contralateral regions of the sham rats ($p < 0.001$). No statistically significant differences in the T$_1$ values were observed between the ipsilateral and contralateral regions of the sham rats (Figure 2C).

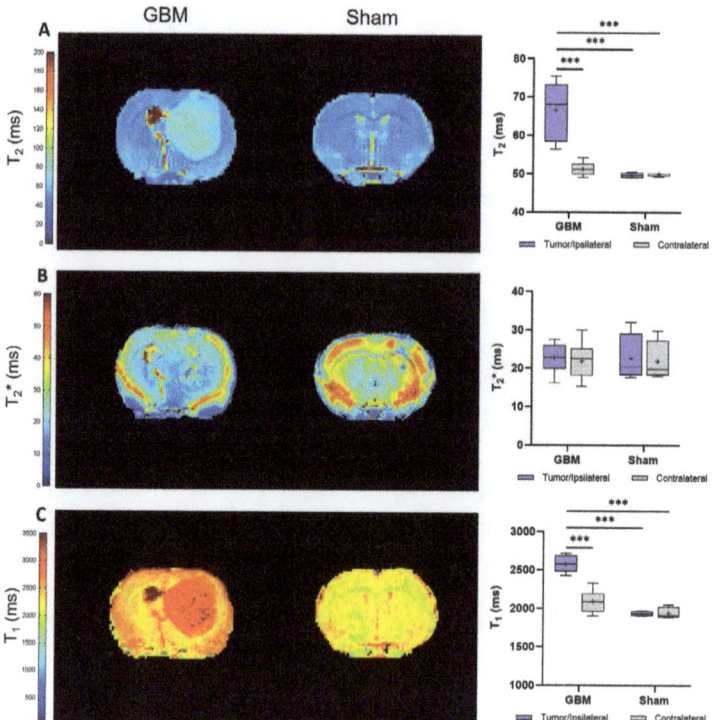

Figure 2. Parametric maps generated from the relaxometry images of a representative slice from the GBM and sham rats and a quantification of the studied regions: the tumor and contralateral areas in the GBM rats, as well as the ipsilateral and contralateral regions in the sham rats. (**A**). Parametric maps and quantification of the T_2 values. (**B**). Parametric maps and quantification of the T_2^* values. (**C**). Parametric maps and quantification of the T_1 values. *** $p < 0.001$.

3.1.2. Magnetization Transfer Images

The calculated MTR values showed trends that were consistent with the T_2 and T_1 analyses. However, notably, lower MTR values were detected in the tumor than in the contralateral areas ($p < 0.01$) of the GBM rats, as well as in comparison to both regions studied in the sham rats ($p < 0.001$), where no significant differences were detected between regions in this group (Figure 3). The mean MTR values from each group are presented in Table 1.

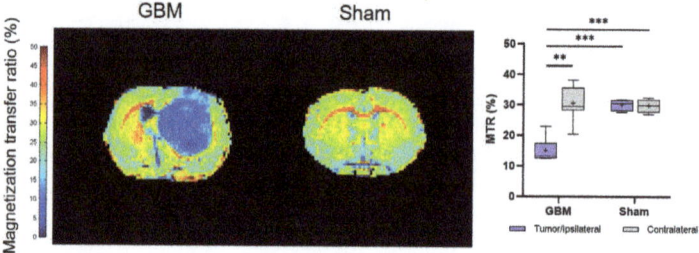

Figure 3. Parametric maps generated from the MT images of a representative slice from the GBM and sham rats and a quantification of the studied regions: the tumor and contralateral areas in the GBM rats, as well as the ipsilateral and contralateral regions in the sham rats. ** $p < 0.01$ and *** $p < 0.001$.

3.1.3. Diffusion Tensor Imaging

The DTI studies provide information about the restriction of the water molecule movement in the tissues and, therefore, about the tissues' microstructural organization through the mean diffusivity (MD) and fractional anisotropy (FA) parameters, respectively. The same trend observed in the T_2 and T_1 analyses was observed, with the tumor regions showing higher MD values than the respective contralateral area of the GBM rats ($p < 0.01$) and, also, when compared to the ipsilateral ($p < 0.01$) and contralateral areas ($p < 0.05$) of the sham rats, with no significant differences between the regions in this last group (Figure 4A). Regarding the FA, no statistically significant differences were detected either within or among the groups. However, a greater degree of data dispersion is evident in the boxplot representation of the tumor and contralateral areas of the GBM rats compared to the regions of the sham rats (Figure 4B). The mean MD and FA values from each group are presented in Table 1.

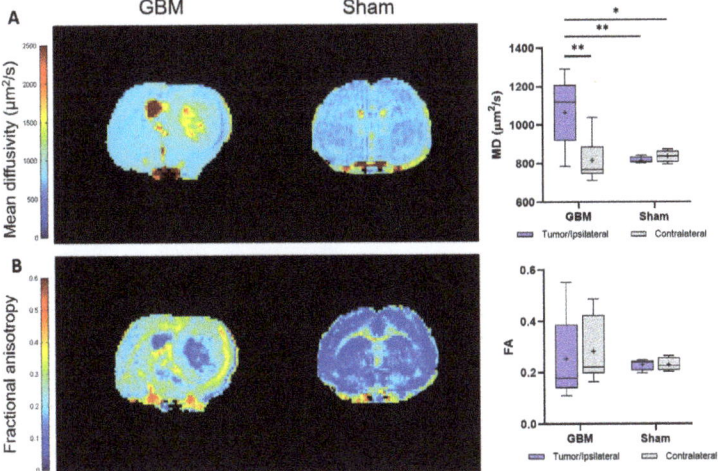

Figure 4. Parametric maps generated from the DTI images of a representative slice from the GBM and sham rats and a quantification of the studied regions: the tumor and contralateral areas in the GBM rats, as well as the ipsilateral and contralateral regions in the sham rats. (**A**). Parametric maps and quantification of MD values. (**B**). Parametric maps and quantification of FA values. * $p < 0.05$ and ** $p < 0.01$.

3.2. Metabolomic Studies: Ex Vivo Spectra

The metabolomic information was obtained from the ^{1}H HR-MAS spectra acquired from the regions of the animals across the different groups. Figure 5 shows the metabolites in which statistically significant differences were observed in the spectra acquired with a TE of 36 ms. The mean metabolite concentration data are presented in Table 2.

Higher concentrations were found in the tumor of the GBM rats when compared to the contralateral regions or when compared to the sham rats in alanine (Ala), lactate (Lac), choline + glycerophosphocholine + phosphocholine (Cho + GPC + PCh), and taurine (Tau). Similar concentrations were found when the contralateral area from the GBM rats and both regions of the sham rats were compared. The Ala and Lac exhibited statistically significant differences in the three comparisons: between the tumor and the contralateral regions in the GBM rats ($p < 0.001$), between the tumor and the sham rats ($p < 0.01$), and ($p < 0.05$) for the ipsilateral and contralateral regions in the sham animals (Figure 5A). For the Lac, all three comparisons showed significance ($p < 0.05$) (Figure 5B). A similar trend was observed for the Cho + GPC + PCh, when comparing the tumor region of the GBM rats to the ipsilateral area ($p < 0.001$) and the contralateral area ($p < 0.01$) of the sham rats. However, although there was a lower concentration in the contralateral area of the GBM rats, this difference was not statistically significant (Figure 5C). A comparable pattern to the Cho + GPC + PCh was found in the Tau, with statistically significant differences observed only between the GBM tumor and the sham ipsilateral region ($p < 0.01$) (Figure 5D).

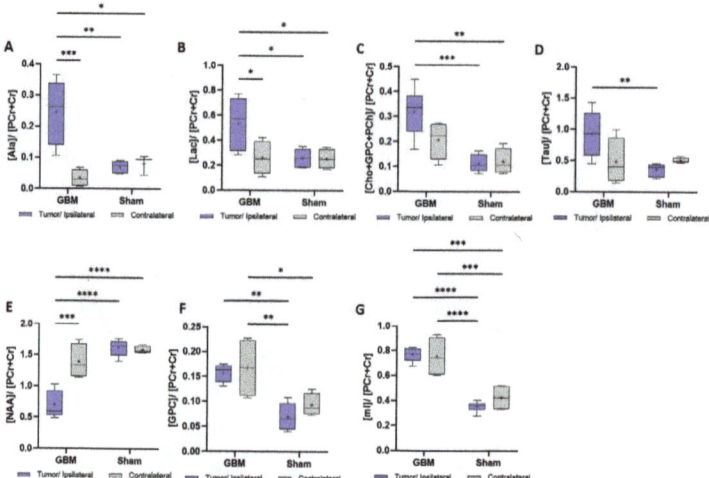

Figure 5. Metabolic data obtained from the ^{1}H HRMAS spectra with a TE = 36 ms from the tumor and contralateral regions of the GBM rats and the ipsilateral and contralateral regions of the sham rats. The metabolic concentrations are expressed relative to the phosphocreatine + creatine (PCr + Cr). (**A**). Ala: alanine. (**B**). Lac: lactate. (**C**). Cho + GPC + PCh: choline + glycerophosphocholine + phosphocholine. (**D**). Tau: taurine. (**E**). NAA: N-acetylaspartic acid. (**F**). GPC: glycerophosphocholine. (**G**). mI: myo-inositol. * $p < 0.05$, ** $p < 0.01$, *** $p < 0.001$, and **** $p < 0.0001$.

Table 2. Metabolite concentrations (mean ± SEM) obtained from the ex vivo ^{1}H HRMAS (TE = 36 ms) spectra from the different regions of the studied groups. The metabolic concentrations are expressed relative to the phosphocreatine + creatine (PCr + Cr).

	GBM		Sham	
[Metabolite]/[PCr + Cr]	Tumor	Contralateral	Ipsilateral	Contralateral
Ala	0.25 ± 0.04	0.03 ± 0.01	0.07 ± 0.01	0.08 ± 0.02
Lac	0.53 ± 0.10	0.26 ± 0.07	0.26 ± 0.03	0.26 ± 0.04
Cho + GPC + PCh	0.32 ± 0.04	0.21 ± 0.04	0.11 ± 0.01	0.12 ± 0.03
Tau	0.93 ± 0.15	0.48 ± 0.19	0.36 ± 0.04	0.51 ± 0.02
NAA	0.70 ± 0.10	1.39 ± 0.14	1.59 ± 0.06	1.59 ± 0.03
GPC	0.16 ± 0.01	0.17 ± 0.03	0.07 ± 0.01	0.09 ± 0.01
mI	0.77 ± 0.03	0.75 ± 0.08	0.35 ± 0.02	0.43 ± 0.05

SEM: standard error of mean; TE: echo time; PCr + Cr: phosphocreatine + creatine; Ala: alanine; Lac: lactate; Cho + GPC + PCh: choline + glycerophosphocholine + phosphocholine; Tau: taurine; NAA: N-acetylaspartic acid; GPC: glycerophosphocholine; and mI: myo-inositol.

In the case of the N-acetylaspartic acid (NAA), lower concentrations were found in the GBM tumor than in the contralateral region of the GBM rats ($p < 0.001$) and for the ipsilateral ($p < 0.0001$) and contralateral ($p < 0.0001$) sham regions (Figure 5E). In the case of the glycerophosphocholine (GPC) and myo-inositol (mI), a higher metabolite concentration was found in both the tumor and contralateral areas of the GBM rats compared to the ipsilateral and the contralateral regions of the sham rats. In the GPC, statistically significant differences were found between the tumor of the GBM rats and the ipsilateral area ($p < 0.01$) of the sham rats and, also, between the contralateral area of the GBM rats and the ipsilateral ($p < 0.01$) and contralateral areas ($p < 0.05$) of the sham rats (Figure 5F). Regarding the mI, statistically significant differences were found between the GBM tumor and the ipsilateral ($p < 0.0001$) and contralateral areas ($p < 0.0001$) of the sham rats and between the contralateral regions of the GBM rats and the ipsilateral ($p < 0.0001$) and contralateral areas of the sham rats ($p < 0.0001$) (Figure 5G).

The same trend was observed in the metabolite analysis obtained from the spectra acquired with a TE of 144 ms, shown in Figure S1 of the Supplementary Material.

4. Discussion

Despite advances in recent decades, GBM remains a fatal cancer with a dismal prognosis. This aggressive brain tumor presents formidable challenges in diagnosis and treatment. Efforts to improve patient outcomes hinge on the identification of precise diagnostic markers and the development of targeted therapies. The validation of these treatments is crucial for effective management. Advanced imaging modalities such as MRI and the utilization of animal models play pivotal roles in this endeavor, offering valuable insights into the tumor biology and aiding in the development and validation of novel therapeutic approaches. Furthermore, multiparametric MRI facilitates the non-invasive and quantitative assessment of multiple tissue characteristics, complementing the qualitative insights obtained from anatomical T_2W and T_1W images, which may also be very useful for validating theranostic approaches [8,24,25].

The aim of this study was to identify the biomarkers of GBM using in vivo MRI and ex vivo metabolomic analysis via HRMAS MRS, with the potential to enhance accurate diagnosis and an early therapy validation. Additionally, these methodologies can be applied to investigate preclinical models of GBM and to identify therapeutic targets, thereby aiding in the development of novel drugs against GBM. Moreover, beyond analyzing the tumor region, considering the infiltrative nature of GBM, our objective was to examine the apparently healthy tissue areas to ascertain potential tumor infiltration into the normal brain tissue.

Overall, we failed to detect significant signs of tumor invasion in the apparently healthy contralateral region. The most pronounced differences were observed between the tumor region of the GBM rats and the rest of the studied regions: the contralateral hemisphere of the GBM rats and the ipsilateral and contralateral regions of the sham rats. Although we were not able to detect any tumor invasion, the disparities observed within the tumor region can potentially serve as biomarkers for the detection and evolution of tumors and the therapy response. The T_2 and T_1 mapping showed statistically significant higher values in the tumor regions of the GBM rats. This observed increase in the T_1 and T_2 values can be attributed to several underlying factors. GBM typically exhibits high cellularity, increased tissue water content, and alterations in the tissue microstructure, all of which contribute to changes in the relaxation times. The higher cell density and water content in the tumor result in prolonged T_1 and T_2 values compared to healthy tissue. Additionally, the presence of vasogenic edema, necrotic regions, and altered vascularization within the GBM microenvironment further influences these MRI parameters, leading to an overall increase in the T_1 and T_2 values. Furthermore, the disruption of the BBB in the tumor contributes to the increase in the T_2 values.

T_2 represents the time it takes for the transverse component of the magnetization in the MRI signal to decay, and it is correlated with, among other aspects, the content of free-water in the tissue. It is indicative of the presence of vasogenic edema, a common feature in human GBM and peritumoral areas [13]. Elevated mean T_2 values in GBM compared to normal contralateral tissues have been reported in both human and preclinical models. This can be attributed to the presence of gliosis, necrosis, and irregular vasculature within the tumor [13,26–28]. Moreover, decreased T_2 values induced in the tumor and peritumoral edema have been recognized as indicators of therapy response in GBM patients undergoing antiangiogenic treatment [29,30] and radiotherapy [31]. T_1 is the longitudinal relaxation time, corresponding to the time it takes for the longitudinal component of the magnetization to recover due to the exchange of energy between the water spins and the environment. This parameter, utilized to identify anatomical changes and BBB disruption through the extravasation of the CA, is also associated with the response of the tumor to therapy [32–34] and tumor infiltration [35]. While T_1 values have not typically been viewed as potential biomarkers without the use of contrast agents, previous studies indicate that quantitative T_1 values measured prior to injection can predict the potential of extravasation, thereby making T_1 a potential biomarker for BBB disruption without administrating a CA [15]. In our study, we found higher T_1 values in the tumor area than in the contralateral brain tissue and the sham rats, consistent with the existence of tumor infiltration [35], necrosis, and increased permeability of the vessels due to the BBB alteration [36,37]. This has also been observed in other preclinical models, such as neuroblastoma [38]. While perfusion evaluations were not included in our MRI protocol for this study, the data we obtained suggest that it would be beneficial to include them in future investigations.

In contrast, the obtained T_2^* values were similar among the regions. T_2^* refers to the transfer relaxation time in the presence of inhomogeneities in the magnetic field, as a result of variations in the local magnetic susceptibility. It has been reported that tumors induce the loss of brain homogeneity due to increased cellularity, aberrant microvasculature, blood accumulation from micro-hemorrhages, and edematous or necrotic areas, resulting in decreased T_2^* values in seminal pathological tissues [14]. However, this effect was not detected in our study, which warrants further investigation in future experiments.

Regarding the MTR, it is linked to the distinct distribution of water molecules between two different compartments: a free water pool (comprising water molecules with $T_2 > 10$ ms) and a pool of water molecules (those with $T_2 < 1$ ms) bound to macromolecules [39]. In normal physiological conditions, each type of tissue has its unique distribution of both water compartments, which may be altered in pathological situations [12]. We observed that the GBM tumor values were significantly lower than those in the contralateral hemisphere and the regions of the sham animals, consistent with prior studies using the C6 model, particularly when examining the tumor core [40]. This finding suggests the presence of necrotic areas, especially in the advanced tumor stages, as observed in our study. Furthermore, MT imaging has been identified as a biomarker of the response to therapy in human GBM, effectively distinguishing between responders and non-responder patients [41]. Interestingly, the same authors found no significant differences in this parameter between the contralateral areas of the GBM patients and healthy subjects [42], contrary to what occurs in our study.

The diffusion phenomenon is associated with the random Brownian motion of water molecules. In this study, we focused on analyzing two DTI parameters: MD and FA. The MD is influenced by various factors, including tissue organization, cell size and integrity, permeability barriers, and viscosity. Consistent with the T_2 and T_1 results, we observed higher MD values in the tumor region of the GBM rats compared to the other regions studied. In brain cancer, two significant factors affect the MD in opposite directions: vasogenic edema and necrosis increase the free water content, thereby elevating the MD values, while hypercellularity and cytotoxic edema decrease them [43]. Hence, our results suggest that vasogenic edema and/or necrosis in this tumor outweigh the impact of the increased cell density or cytotoxic edema, which is consistent with the results obtained from this preclinical model at an advanced stage [40,44]. The MD is associated with clinical outcomes in high-grade gliomas, serving as an indicator of changes from basal levels to post-therapeutic stages [45,46]. It is worth noting that, regarding tumor infiltration, there are some discrepancies with this parameter [47]. Furthermore, a preclinical study conducted in this C6 model, employing both fed and fasted rats, reported differences in the MD in the apparently healthy brain tissue between fasted GBM rats and fasted control rats [48].

The FA, on the other hand, reflects the degree of anisotropy in the translational movement of the water molecules and is highly dependent on the tissue composition.

Structural changes should be reflected on the FA indexes and the presence of a tumor can displace normal structures and disrupt fiber tracts, thereby altering the existing preferential directionality of the water motion, reducing the FA values. It also serves as an indicator of tumor invasion [49] and has been reported to be related to therapy response [46]. In this study, we did not observe differences in the FA between the tumor area and the contralateral hemisphere or the sham regions. However, the presence of a higher data dispersion in the two studied regions of the GBM rats compared with the sham rats could be reflecting the tumor heterogeneity among animals, which also affects the microstructure of the contralateral healthy brain regions. Nevertheless, some studies have reported not only similar but even higher FA levels in the tumor in this C6 GBM model. One possible explanation is that the tumor grows in a ring-like structure, thus elevating the FA values [40,44]. Differences in the FA were also detected in several apparently healthy brain tissue areas between the GBM and control rats in both fed and fasted states [48].

In this study, we conducted an analysis of metabolomic data using magnetic resonance spectroscopy. While in vivo ^{1}H MRS provides insights into tumor evolution, grading, and treatment response [50,51], a broader range of metabolites can be obtained ex vivo from biopsies using ^{1}H HRMAS in both humans and preclinical models such as C6GBM [21–23,52].

We observed significant differences among the studied regions in several metabolites or groups of metabolites. In four of these metabolites, higher concentrations were found in the tumor region of the GBM rats compared to either the contralateral region of the GBM rats or the regions examined in the sham animals These four metabolites are recognized as GBM markers: Ala, a glucogenic amino acid which is converted to pyruvate for rapidly proliferating tumor cells [53]; Lac, a marker of anerobic metabolism visualized in necrotic tissues with anerobic metabolism in high-grade tumors [51]; Cho + GPC + PCh, a marker of increased cell turnover which can be detected within tumors [51]; and Tau, which correlates with the presence of apoptosis [54]. However, it is worth noting that, in the latter two cases, Cho + GPC + PCh and Tau, although higher values of these metabolites were detected in the GBM tumor, no significant differences were recorded between the tumor and the contralateral region of the GBM rats. The choline (Cho) levels typically exhibit higher concentrations in the center of a solid mass, decreasing towards the periphery. Studies have indicated a correlation between the tumor grade and Cho levels in astrocytomas, with higher grade tumors often showing elevated Cho concentrations. However, this association may not be present in high-grade gliomas characterized by extensive necrosis, which tend to result in a low choline peak. In such cases, increased lactate and lipid concentrations typically suppress the peaks of other metabolites, including Cho [55,56].

As anticipated, we observed a lower detection of NAA in the GBM tumor region compared to both the contralateral region of the GBM rats and the regions studied in the sham animals. NAA serves as a neuronal marker whose reduction is typically detected in pathologies such as brain cancer, which involve neural loss [51].

Regarding GPC and mI, we observed increased levels of these metabolites in the two studied regions of the GBM rats, suggesting that the apparently healthy brain tissue may be affected by the presence of the tumor, potentially indicating tumor infiltration, a phenomenon we were not able to detect via MRI. Additionally, lower metabolite detection was observed in the ipsilateral and contralateral regions of the sham animals. GPC is the most abundant phospholipid in mammalian cell membranes [57], and increased levels of GPC are considered a marker of low grade gliomas [58,59]. It is also a potential marker of the prognosis and response to treatment in GBM, when related to the PCh content [58,60,61]. Similar levels of this metabolite have been reported in C6 tumors and their contralateral areas [22], but, in this article, the tumor data were not compared with healthy or sham animals. Based on these inconsistencies, further research is needed concerning GPC in this C6 GBM model.

Finally, mI is a precursor of phosphatidylinositol, and elevated levels of mI are typically observed in well-differentiated low-grade gliomas compared to high-grade gliomas [62]. Additionally, mI is considered a marker of GBM therapy response [63]. However, contrary to our observations in this study, it has been described that the mI levels in a GBM tumor are lower than in tissue with a normal appearance [62,64]. Interestingly, other authors have reported findings similar to what we detected in this study: a non-significant increase of mI in the tissue with a normal appearance of the contralateral hemisphere in patients with untreated glioblastoma, suggesting the detection of tumor cell infiltration [63,65].

Previous studies have conducted multiparametric MRI investigations, both clinically and preclinically, to explore GBM invasion. These investigations typically involve diffusion-weighted and DTI images, perfusion-weighted imaging (PWI), FLAIR images, and contrast-enhanced T1WI, suggesting the combined use of these acquisitions as invasion biomarkers [66–70]. While our study expands on these approaches by incorporating additional imaging modalities, such as T_2, T_2^*, and T_1 parametric maps, along with magnetization transfer studies and the metabolomic assessment, future research should strive to further delineate tumor invasion in this model. Specifically, integrating specific perfusion techniques to assess the permeability of the blood–brain barrier could deepen our understanding. Furthermore, the integration of the multiparametric MRI findings with the metabolomic data obtained through HRMAS MRS offers a comprehensive approach for assessing the GBM pathophysiology. Our results suggest that the combination of imaging biomarkers, such as relaxation, diffusion, and MT mapping with metabolite concentrations, can provide valuable insights into the characteristics and behavior of tumors. By incorporating these findings into diagnostic algorithms or predictive models, clinicians may enhance diagnostic accuracy and improve the patient management strategies for GBM.

In summary, while our research offers valuable insights into the use of multiparametric MRI in characterizing GBM, we acknowledge the need for continued refinement and validation of the imaging parameters, as well as the importance of developing customized examination protocols to address the diverse research and clinical needs.

5. Conclusions

Despite considerable advancements, GBM remains a highly fatal cancer with a bleak prognosis. The exploration of novel therapies that target GBM is imperative given its high mortality and aggressive nature. The inherent invasiveness and the tumor behavior of GBM pose significant challenges to its treatment. This underscores the importance of investigating new treatments with animal models that might play a pivotal role, such as the one employed in this study. Moreover, the pursuit of imaging biomarkers using techniques like multiparametric MRI emerges as a critical strategy in overcoming the challenge of accurately assessing and monitoring aggressive brain tumors with a non-invasive approach.

In this work, our findings highlight the utility of multiparametric MRI in assessing various tissue characteristics, complementing the qualitative insights derived from conventional imaging techniques. Notably, our exploration of the metabolomic data revealed significant differences among the studied regions, pointing towards there being distinctive metabolic signatures in GBM. Our study revealed notable differences in the MRI parameters between the GBM tumor region and other studied areas, including the contralateral hemisphere of the GBM animals and the ipsilateral and contralateral regions from the sham animals. Despite our inability to detect tumor invasion in the contralateral area of the GBM rats, this characteristic was discernible through an ex vivo HRMAS spectroscopy. Further investigations are warranted to enhance the imaging techniques to accurately identify tumor invasion. Moving forward, the integration of multiparametric MRI and metabolomic data into diagnostic algorithms or predictive models holds promise for enhancing diagnostic accuracy and improving the patient management strategies for GBM.

Supplementary Materials: The following supporting information can be downloaded at https://www.mdpi.com/article/10.3390/brainsci14050409/s1. Figure S1: metabolic data obtained by the ^{1}H HRMAS with a TE = 144 ms from the tumor and contralateral regions of the GBM rats and the ipsilateral and contralateral regions of the sham rats; and Table S1: the metabolite concentrations (mean ± SEM) obtained from the ex vivo ^{1}H HRMAS (TE = 144 ms) spectra from the different regions of the studied groups.

Author Contributions: Conceptualization, N.A.-R. and P.L.-L.; experimental acquisition and data processing, R.P.-C. and C.V.; formal analysis, N.A.-R.; data curation, N.A.-R.; writing—original draft preparation, R.P.-C., C.V. and N.A.-R.; writing—review and editing, N.A.-R. and P.L.-L.; supervision, N.A.-R. and P.L.-L.; and funding acquisition, P.L.-L. All authors have read and agreed to the published version of the manuscript.

Funding: This work was supported in part by grant PID2021-122528OB-I00 (MICINN/AEI/FEDER, UE) awarded to P.L.-L.

Institutional Review Board Statement: All experimental procedures were approved by the Ethics Committee of the Community of Madrid (PROEX 047/18; approved 2 November 2015) and follow the national (R.D.53/2013) and European Community guidelines (2010/62/UE) for the care and management of experimental animals.

Informed Consent Statement: Not applicable.

Data Availability Statement: The data presented in this study are available on request from the corresponding author due to the need for a formal data sharing agreement.

Acknowledgments: The authors are indebted to the staff of the Biomedical NMR Facility Sebastián Cerdán for their continuous technical support.

Conflicts of Interest: The authors declare no conflicts of interest.

References

1. Lauko, A.; Lo, A.; Ahluwalia, M.S.; Lathia, J.D. Cancer Cell Heterogeneity & Plasticity in Glioblastoma and Brain Tumors. *Semin. Cancer Biol.* **2022**, *82*, 162–175. [PubMed]
2. Louis, D.N.; Perry, A.; Wesseling, P.; Brat, D.J.; Cree, I.A.; Figarella-Branger, D.; Hawkins, C.; Ng, H.K.; Pfister, S.M.; Reifenberger, G.; et al. The 2021 WHO Classification of Tumors of the Central Nervous System: A Summary. *Neuro. Oncol.* **2021**, *23*, 1231–1251. [CrossRef] [PubMed]
3. Ostrom, Q.T.; Price, M.; Neff, C.; Cioffi, G.; Waite, K.A.; Kruchko, C.; Barnholtz-Sloan, J.S. CBTRUS Statistical Report: Primary Brain and Other Central Nervous System Tumors Diagnosed in the United States in 2015–2019. *Neuro. Oncol.* **2022**, *24*, V1–V95. [CrossRef] [PubMed]
4. de Gooijer, M.C.; Guillén Navarro, M.; Bernards, R.; Wurdinger, T.; van Tellingen, O. An Experimenter's Guide to Glioblastoma Invasion Pathways. *Trends Mol. Med.* **2018**, *24*, 763–780. [CrossRef] [PubMed]
5. Mo, F.; Pellerino, A.; Soffietti, R.; Rudà, R. Blood-Brain Barrier in Brain Tumors: Biology and Clinical Relevance. *Int. J. Mol. Sci.* **2021**, *22*, 12654. [CrossRef] [PubMed]
6. Haumann, R.; Videira, J.C.; Kaspers, G.J.L.; van Vuurden, D.G.; Hulleman, E. Overview of Current Drug Delivery Methods Across the Blood–Brain Barrier for the Treatment of Primary Brain Tumors. *CNS Drugs* **2020**, *34*, 1121–1131. [CrossRef] [PubMed]
7. Arias-Ramos, N.; Ibarra, L.E.; Serrano-Torres, M.; Yagüe, B.; Caverzán, M.D.; Chesta, C.A.; Palacios, R.E.; López-Larrubia, P. Iron Oxide Incorporated Conjugated Polymer Nanoparticles for Simultaneous Use in Magnetic Resonance and Fluorescent Imaging of Brain Tumors. *Pharmaceutics* **2021**, *13*, 1258. [CrossRef] [PubMed]
8. Suárez-García, S.; Arias-Ramos, N.; Frias, C.; Candiota, A.P.; Arús, C.; Lorenzo, J.; Ruiz-Molina, D.; Novio, F. Dual T1/T2 Nanoscale Coordination Polymers as Novel Contrast Agents for MRI: A Preclinical Study for Brain Tumor. *ACS Appl. Mater. Interfaces* **2018**, *10*, 38819–38832. [CrossRef] [PubMed]
9. McMillan, K.M.; Rogers, B.P.; Field, A.S.; Laird, A.R.; Fine, J.P.; Meyerand, M.E. Physiologic Characterisation of Glioblastoma Multiforme Using MRI-Based Hypoxia Mapping, Chemical Shift Imaging, Perfusion and Diffusion Maps. *J. Clin. Neurosci.* **2006**, *13*, 811–817. [CrossRef]
10. Abbasi, A.W.; Westerlaan, H.E.; Holtman, G.A.; Aden, K.M.; van Laar, P.J.; van der Hoorn, A. Incidence of Tumour Progression and Pseudoprogression in High-Grade Gliomas: A Systematic Review and Meta-Analysis. *Clin. Neuroradiol.* **2018**, *28*, 401–411. [CrossRef]
11. Huisman, T.A.G.M. Diffusion-Weighted and Diffusion Tensor Imaging of the Brain, Made Easy. *Cancer Imaging* **2010**, *10*, S163. [CrossRef]
12. Pui, M.H. Magnetization Transfer Analysis of Brain Tumor, Infection, and Infarction. *J. Magn. Reson. Imaging* **2000**, *12*, 395–399. [CrossRef]
13. Oh, J.; Cha, S.; Aiken, A.H.; Han, E.T.; Crane, J.C.; Stainsby, J.A.; Wright, G.A.; Dillon, W.P.; Nelson, S.J. Quantitative Apparent Diffusion Coefficients and T2 Relaxation Times in Characterizing Contrast Enhancing Brain Tumors and Regions of Peritumoral Edema. *J. Magn. Reson. Imaging* **2005**, *21*, 701–708. [CrossRef] [PubMed]
14. Chavhan, G.B.; Babyn, P.S.; Thomas, B.; Shroff, M.M.; Mark Haacke, E. Principles, Techniques, and Applications of T2*-Based MR Imaging and Its Special Applications. *Radiographics* **2009**, *29*, 1433–1449. [CrossRef] [PubMed]

15. Hattingen, E.; Müller, A.; Jurcoane, A.; Mädler, B.; Ditter, P.; Schild, H.; Herrlinger, U.; Glas, M.; Kebir, S. Value of Quantitative Magnetic Resonance Imaging T1-Relaxometry in Predicting Contrast-Enhancement in Glioblastoma Patients. *Oncotarget* 2017, *8*, 53542–53551. [CrossRef]
16. Le, T.N.T.; Lim, H.; Hamilton, A.M.; Parkins, K.M.; Chen, Y.; Scholl, T.J.; Ronald, J.A. Characterization of an Orthotopic Rat Model of Glioblastoma Using Multiparametric Magnetic Resonance Imaging and Bioluminescence Imaging. *Tomography* 2018, *4*, 55–65. [CrossRef] [PubMed]
17. Neska-Matuszewska, M.; Bladowska, J.; Sąsiadek, M.; Zimny, A. Differentiation of Glioblastoma Multiforme, Metastases and Primary Central Nervous System Lymphomas Using Multiparametric Perfusion and Diffusion MR Imaging of a Tumor Core and a Peritumoral Zone—Searching for a Practical Approach. *PLoS ONE* 2018, *13*, e0191341. [CrossRef] [PubMed]
18. Garteiser, P.; Doblas, S.; Watanabe, Y.; Saunders, D.; Hoyle, J.; Lerner, M.; He, T.; Floyd, R.A.; Towner, R.A. Multiparametric Assessment of the Anti-Glioma Properties of OKN007 by Magnetic Resonance Imaging. *J. Magn. Reson. Imaging* 2010, *31*, 796–806. [CrossRef] [PubMed]
19. Brekke, C.; Williams, S.C.; Price, J.; Thorsen, F.; Modo, M. Cellular Multiparametric MRI of Neural Stem Cell Therapy in a Rat Glioma Model. *Neuroimage* 2007, *37*, 769–782. [CrossRef]
20. Padelli, F.; Mazzi, F.; Erbetta, A.; Chiapparini, L.; Doniselli, F.M.; Palermo, S.; Aquino, D.; Bruzzone, M.G.; Cuccarini, V. In Vivo Brain MR Spectroscopy in Gliomas: Clinical and Pre-Clinical Chances. *Clin. Transl. Imaging* 2022, *10*, 495–515. [CrossRef]
21. Wright, A.J.; Fellows, G.A.; Griffiths, J.R.; Wilson, M.; Bell, B.A.; Howe, F.A. Ex-Vivo HRMAS of Adult Brain Tumours: Metabolite Quantification and Assignment of Tumour Biomarkers. *Mol. Cancer* 2010, *9*, 66. [CrossRef] [PubMed]
22. Coquery, N.; Stupar, V.; Farion, R.; Maunoir-Regimbal, S.; Barbier, E.L.; Rémy, C.; Fauvelle, F. The Three Glioma Rat Models C6, F98 and RG2 Exhibit Different Metabolic Profiles: In Vivo 1H MRS and Ex Vivo 1H HRMAS Combined with Multivariate Statistics. *Metabolomics* 2015, *11*, 1834–1847. [CrossRef]
23. Righi, V.; Garciá-Martín, M.L.; Mucci, A.; Schenetti, L.; Tugnoli, V.; Lopez-Larrubia, P.; Cerdán, S. Spatially Resolved Bioenergetic and Genetic Reprogramming Through the Brain of Rats Bearing Implanted C6 Gliomas As Detected by Multinuclear High-Resolution Magic Angle Spinning and Genomic Analysis. *J. Proteome Res.* 2018, *17*, 2953–2962. [CrossRef] [PubMed]
24. Israel, L.L.; Galstyan, A.; Holler, E.; Ljubimova, J.Y. Magnetic Iron Oxide Nanoparticles for Imaging, Targeting and Treatment of Primary and Metastatic Tumors of the Brain. *J. Control. Release* 2020, *320*, 45. [CrossRef] [PubMed]
25. Arias-Ramos, N.; Ferrer-Font, L.; Lope-Piedrafita, S.; Mocioiu, V.; Julià-Sapé, M.; Pumarola, M.; Arús, C.; Candiota, A.P. Metabolomics of Therapy Response in Preclinical Glioblastoma: A Multi-Slice MRSI-Based Volumetric Analysis for Noninvasive Assessment of Temozolomide Treatment. *Metabolites* 2017, *7*, 20. [CrossRef]
26. Dortch, R.D.; Yankeelov, T.E.; Yue, Z.; Quarles, C.C.; Gore, J.C.; Does, M.D. Evidence of Multiexponential T2 in Rat Glioblastoma. *NMR Biomed.* 2009, *22*, 609–618. [CrossRef] [PubMed]
27. Eis, M.; Els, T.; Hoehn-Berlage, M. High Resolution Quantitative Relaxation and Diffusion MRI of Three Different Experimental Brain Tumors in Rat. *Magn. Reson. Med.* 1995, *34*, 835–844. [CrossRef] [PubMed]
28. Blasiak, B.; Tomanek, B.; Abulrob, A.; Iqbal, U.; Stanimirovic, D.; Albaghdadi, H.; Foniok, T.; Lun, X.; Forsyth, P.; Sutherland, G.R. Detection of T2 Changes in an Early Mouse Brain Tumor. *Magn. Reson. Imaging* 2010, *28*, 784–789. [CrossRef] [PubMed]
29. Hattingen, E.; Jurcoane, A.; Daneshvar, K.; Pilatus, U.; Mittelbronn, M.; Steinbach, J.P.; Bähr, O. Quantitative T2 Mapping of Recurrent Glioblastoma under Bevacizumab Improves Monitoring for Non-Enhancing Tumor Progression and Predicts Overall Survival. *Neuro. Oncol.* 2013, *15*, 1395–1404. [CrossRef]
30. Lescher, S.; Jurcoane, A.; Veit, A.; Bähr, O.; Deichmann, R.; Hattingen, E. Quantitative T1 and T2 Mapping in Recurrent Glioblastomas under Bevacizumab: Earlier Detection of Tumor Progression Compared to Conventional MRI. *Neuroradiology* 2015, *57*, 11–20. [CrossRef]
31. Tomaszewski, M.R.; Dominguez-Viqueira, W.; Ortiz, A.; Shi, Y.; Costello, J.R.; Enderling, H.; Rosenberg, S.A.; Gillies, R.J. Heterogeneity Analysis of MRI T2 Maps for Measurement of Early Tumor Response to Radiotherapy. *NMR Biomed.* 2021, *34*, e4454. [CrossRef] [PubMed]
32. Kong, Z.; Yan, C.; Zhu, R.; Wang, J.; Wang, Y.; Wang, Y.; Wang, R.; Feng, F.; Ma, W. Imaging Biomarkers Guided Anti-Angiogenic Therapy for Malignant Gliomas. *NeuroImage Clin.* 2018, *20*, 51–60. [CrossRef] [PubMed]
33. Jain, R. Measurements of Tumor Vascular Leakiness Using DCE in Brain Tumors: Clinical Applications. *NMR Biomed.* 2013, *26*, 1042–1049. [CrossRef] [PubMed]
34. Herrmann, K.; Erokwu, B.O.; Johansen, M.L.; Basilion, J.P.; Gulani, V.; Griswold, M.A.; Flask, C.A.; Brady-Kalnay, S.M. Dynamic Quantitative T1 Mapping in Orthotopic Brain Tumor Xenografts. *Transl. Oncol.* 2016, *9*, 147–154. [CrossRef] [PubMed]
35. Nöth, U.; Tichy, J.; Tritt, S.; Bähr, O.; Deichmann, R.; Hattingen, E. Quantitative T1 Mapping Indicates Tumor Infiltration beyond the Enhancing Part of Glioblastomas. *NMR Biomed.* 2020, *33*, e4242. [CrossRef] [PubMed]
36. Araki, T.; Inouye, T.; Suzuki, H.; Machida, T.; Iio, M. Magnetic Resonance Imaging of Brain Tumors: Measurement of T1. Work in Progress. *Radiology* 1984, *150*, 95–98. [CrossRef] [PubMed]
37. Englund, E.; Brun, A.; Larsson, E.M.; Györffy-Wagner, Z.; Persson, B. Tumours of the Central Nervous System: Proton Magnetic Resonance Relaxation Times T1 and T2 and Histopathologic Correlates. *Acta Radiologica. Diagn.* 1986, *27*, 653–659. [CrossRef] [PubMed]

38. Zormpas-Petridis, K.; Poon, E.; Clarke, M.; Jerome, N.P.; Boult, J.K.R.; Blackledge, M.D.; Carceller, F.; Koers, A.; Barone, G.; Pearson, A.D.J.; et al. Noninvasive MRI Native T1 Mapping Detects Response to MYCN-Targeted Therapies in the Th- MYCN Model of Neuroblastoma. *Cancer Res.* **2020**, *80*, 3424–3435. [CrossRef] [PubMed]
39. Henkelman, R.M.; Stanisz, G.J.; Graham, S.J. Magnetization Transfer in MRI: A Review. *NMR Biomed.* **2001**, *14*, 57–64. [CrossRef]
40. Pérez-Carro, R.; Cauli, O.; López-Larrubia, P. Multiparametric Magnetic Resonance in the Assessment of the Gender Differences in a High-Grade Glioma Rat Model. *EJNMMI Res.* **2014**, *4*, 44. [CrossRef]
41. Mehrabian, H.; Myrehaug, S.; Soliman, H.; Sahgal, A.; Stanisz, G.J. Quantitative Magnetization Transfer in Monitoring Glioblastoma (GBM) Response to Therapy. *Sci. Rep.* **2018**, *8*, 2475. [CrossRef] [PubMed]
42. Mehrabian, H.; Lam, W.W.; Myrehaug, S.; Sahgal, A.; Stanisz, G.J. Glioblastoma (GBM) Effects on Quantitative MRI of Contralateral Normal Appearing White Matter. *J. Neurooncol.* **2018**, *139*, 97–106. [CrossRef] [PubMed]
43. Maier, S.E.; Sun, Y.; Mulkern, R.V. Diffusion Imaging of Brain Tumors. *NMR Biomed.* **2010**, *23*, 849–864. [CrossRef] [PubMed]
44. Lope-Piedrafita, S.; Garcia-Martin, M.L.; Galons, J.P.; Gillies, R.J.; Trouard, T.P. Longitudinal Diffusion Tensor Imaging in a Rat Brain Glioma Model. *NMR Biomed.* **2008**, *21*, 799–808. [CrossRef] [PubMed]
45. Chen, L.; Liu, M.; Bao, J.; Xia, Y.; Zhang, J.; Zhang, L.; Huang, X.; Wang, J. The Correlation between Apparent Diffusion Coefficient and Tumor Cellularity in Patients: A Meta-Analysis. *PLoS ONE* **2013**, *8*, e79008. [CrossRef] [PubMed]
46. Mousa, M.I.; Youssef, A.; Hamed, M.R.; Mousa, W.B.; Al Ajerami, Y.; Akhdar, H.; Eisa, M.H.; Ibnaouf, K.H.; Sulieman, A. Mapping High-Grade Glioma Response to Chemoradiotherapy: Insights from Fractional Anisotropy and Mean Diffusivity. *J. Radiat. Res. Appl. Sci.* **2023**, *16*, 100706. [CrossRef]
47. Kinoshita, M.; Goto, T.; Okita, Y.; Kagawa, N.; Kishima, H.; Hashimoto, N.; Yoshimine, T. Diffusion Tensor-Based Tumor Infiltration Index Cannot Discriminate Vasogenic Edema from Tumor-Infiltrated Edema. *J. Neurooncol.* **2010**, *96*, 409–415. [CrossRef] [PubMed]
48. Guadilla, I.; González, S.; Cerdán, S.; Lizarbe, B.; López-Larrubia, P. Magnetic Resonance Imaging to Assess the Brain Response to Fasting in Glioblastoma-Bearing Rats as a Model of Cancer Anorexia. *Cancer Imaging* **2023**, *23*, 36. [CrossRef]
49. Price, S.J.; Gillard, J.H. Imaging Biomarkers of Brain Tumour Margin and Tumour Invasion. *Br. J. Radiol.* **2011**, *84*, S159–S167. [CrossRef]
50. Wei, L.; Hong, S.; Yoon, Y.; Hwang, S.N.; Park, J.C.; Zhang, Z.; Olson, J.J.; Hu, X.P.; Shim, H. Early Prediction of Response to Vorinostat in an Orthotopic Rat Glioma Model. *NMR Biomed.* **2012**, *25*, 1104–1111. [CrossRef]
51. Weinberg, B.D.; Kuruva, M.; Shim, H.; Mullins, M.E. Clinical Applications of Magnetic Resonance Spectroscopy in Brain Tumors: From Diagnosis to Treatment. *Radiol. Clin. N. Am.* **2021**, *59*, 349–362. [CrossRef] [PubMed]
52. Cheng, L.L.; Anthony, D.C.; Comite, A.R.; Black, P.M.; Tzika, A.A.; Gonzalez, R.G. Quantification of Microheterogeneity in Glioblastoma Multiforme with Ex Vivo High-Resolution Magic-Angle Spinning (HRMAS) Proton Magnetic Resonance Spectroscopy. *Neuro. Oncol.* **2000**, *2*, 87–95. [CrossRef]
53. Firdous, S.; Abid, R.; Nawaz, Z.; Bukhari, F.; Anwer, A.; Cheng, L.L.; Sadaf, S. Dysregulated Alanine as a Potential Predictive Marker of Glioma—An Insight from Untargeted Hrmas-Nmr and Machine Learning Data. *Metabolites* **2021**, *11*, 507. [CrossRef] [PubMed]
54. Opstad, K.S.; Bell, B.A.; Griffiths, J.R.; Howe, F.A. Taurine: A Potential Marker of Apoptosis in Gliomas. *Br. J. Cancer* **2009**, *100*, 789–794. [CrossRef]
55. Horská, A.; Barker, P.B. Imaging of Brain Tumors: MR Spectroscopy and Metabolic Imaging. *Neuroimaging Clin. N. Am.* **2010**, *20*, 293–310. [CrossRef]
56. Farche, M.K.; Fachinetti, N.O.; da Silva, L.R.P.; Matos, L.A.; Appenzeller, S.; Cendes, F.; Reis, F. Revisiting the Use of Proton Magnetic Resonance Spectroscopy in Distinguishing between Primary and Secondary Malignant Tumors of the Central Nervous System. *Neuroradiol. J.* **2022**, *35*, 619–626. [CrossRef]
57. Sonkar, K.; Ayyappan, V.; Tressler, C.M.; Adelaja, O.; Cai, R.; Cheng, M.; Glunde, K. Focus on the Glycerophosphocholine Pathway in Choline Phospholipid Metabolism of Cancer. *NMR Biomed.* **2019**, *32*, e4112. [CrossRef] [PubMed]
58. Righi, V.; Roda, J.M.; Paz, J.; Mucci, A.; Tugnoli, V.; Rodriguez-Tarduchy, G.; Barrios, L.; Schenetti, L.; Cerdán, S.; García-Martín, M.L. 1H HR-MAS and Genomic Analysis of Human Tumor Biopsies Discriminate between High and Low Grade Astrocytomas. *NMR Biomed.* **2009**, *22*, 629–637. [CrossRef]
59. Gandía-González, M.L.; Cerdán, S.; Barrios, L.; López-Larrubia, P.; Feijoó, P.G.; Palpan, A.; Roda, J.M.; Solivera, J. Assessment of Overall Survival in Glioma Patients as Predicted by Metabolomic Criteria. *Front. Oncol.* **2019**, *9*, 454128. [CrossRef]
60. Kumar, M.; Arlauckas, S.P.; Saksena, S.; Verma, G.; Ittyerah, R.; Pickup, S.; Popov, A.V.; Delikatny, E.J.; Poptani, H. Magnetic Resonance Spectroscopy for Detection of Choline Kinase Inhibition in the Treatment of Brain Tumors. *Mol. Cancer Ther.* **2015**, *14*, 899–908. [CrossRef]
61. Hattingen, E.; Bähr, O.; Rieger, J.; Blasel, S.; Steinbach, J.; Pilatus, U. Phospholipid Metabolites in Recurrent Glioblastoma: In Vivo Markers Detect Different Tumor Phenotypes before and under Antiangiogenic Therapy. *PLoS ONE* **2013**, *8*, 56439. [CrossRef] [PubMed]
62. Castillo, M.; Smith, J.K.; Kwock, L. Correlation of Myo-Inositol Levels and Grading of Cerebral Astrocytomas. *AJNR Am. J. Neuroradiol.* **2000**, *21*, 1645.

63. Steidl, E.; Pilatus, U.; Hattingen, E.; Steinbach, J.P.; Zanella, F.; Ronellenfitsch, M.W.; Bahr, O. Myoinositol as a Biomarker in Recurrent Glioblastoma Treated with Bevacizumab: A 1H-Magnetic Resonance Spectroscopy Study. *PLoS ONE* **2016**, *11*, e0168113. [CrossRef]
64. Candiota, A.P.; Majós, C.; Julià-Sapé, M.; Cabañas, M.; Acebes, J.J.; Moreno-Torres, A.; Griffiths, J.R.; Arús, C. Non-Invasive Grading of Astrocytic Tumours from the Relative Contents of Myo-Inositol and Glycine Measured by in Vivo MRS. *JBR-BTR* **2011**, *94*, 319–329. [CrossRef]
65. Kallenberg, K.; Bock, H.C.; Helms, G.; Jung, K.; Wrede, A.; Buhk, J.H.; Giese, A.; Frahm, J.; Strik, H.; Dechent, P.; et al. Untreated Glioblastoma Multiforme: Increased Myo-Inositol and Glutamine Levels in the Contralateral Cerebral Hemisphere at Proton MR Spectroscopy. *Radiology* **2009**, *253*, 805–812. [CrossRef]
66. Durst, C.R.; Raghavan, P.; Shaffrey, M.E.; Schiff, D.; Lopes, M.B.; Sheehan, J.P.; Tustison, N.J.; Patrie, J.T.; Xin, W.; Elias, W.J.; et al. Multimodal MR Imaging Model to Predict Tumor Infiltration in Patients with Gliomas. *Neuroradiology* **2014**, *56*, 107–115. [CrossRef] [PubMed]
67. Fathi Kazerooni, A.; Nabil, M.; Zeinali Zadeh, M.; Firouznia, K.; Azmoudeh-Ardalan, F.; Frangi, A.F.; Davatzikos, C.; Saligheh Rad, H. Characterization of Active and Infiltrative Tumorous Subregions from Normal Tissue in Brain Gliomas Using Multiparametric MRI. *J. Magn. Reson. Imaging* **2018**, *48*, 938–950. [CrossRef]
68. Oltra-Sastre, M.; Fuster-Garcia, E.; Juan-Albarracin, J.; Sáez, C.; Perez-Girbes, A.; Sanz-Requena, R.; Revert-Ventura, A.; Mocholi, A.; Urchueguia, J.; Hervas, A.; et al. Multi-Parametric MR Imaging Biomarkers Associated to Clinical Outcomes in Gliomas: A Systematic Review. *Curr. Med. Imaging Former. Curr. Med. Imaging Rev.* **2019**, *15*, 933–947. [CrossRef] [PubMed]
69. Hu, L.S.; Ning, S.; Eschbacher, J.M.; Gaw, N.; Dueck, A.C.; Smith, K.A.; Nakaji, P.; Plasencia, J.; Ranjbar, S.; Price, S.J.; et al. Multi-Parametric MRI and Texture Analysis to Visualize Spatial Histologic Heterogeneity and Tumor Extent in Glioblastoma. *PLoS ONE* **2015**, *10*, e0141506. [CrossRef]
70. Li, C.; Wang, S.; Yan, J.L.; Torheim, T.; Boonzaier, N.R.; Sinha, R.; Matys, T.; Markowetz, F.; Price, S.J. Characterizing Tumor Invasiveness of Glioblastoma Using Multiparametric Magnetic Resonance Imaging. *J. Neurosurg.* **2020**, *132*, 1465–1472. [CrossRef]

Disclaimer/Publisher's Note: The statements, opinions and data contained in all publications are solely those of the individual author(s) and contributor(s) and not of MDPI and/or the editor(s). MDPI and/or the editor(s) disclaim responsibility for any injury to people or property resulting from any ideas, methods, instructions or products referred to in the content.

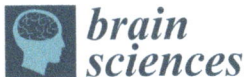

Article

Flavonoid Rutin Presented Anti-Glioblastoma Activity Related to the Modulation of Onco miRNA-125b Expression and STAT3 Signaling and Impact on Microglia Inflammatory Profile

Irlã Santos Lima [1], Érica Novaes Soares [1], Carolina Kymie Vasques Nonaka [2], Bruno Solano de Freitas Souza [2], Balbino Lino dos Santos [1,3,*] and Silvia Lima Costa [1,4,*]

1. Laboratory of Neurochemistry and Cellular Biology, Institute of Health Sciences, Federal University of Bahia, Salvador 40231-300, Brazil; irlalima@ufba.br (I.S.L.); ericanovaessoares@gmail.com (É.N.S.)
2. Center of Biotechnology and Cell Therapy, São Rafael Hospital, D'Or Institute for Research and Teaching (IDOR), Salvador 41253-190, Brazil; carolina.nonaka@hsr.com.br (C.K.V.N.); brunosolanosouza@gmail.com (B.S.d.F.S.)
3. College of Nursing, Federal University of Vale do São Francisco, Petrolina 56304-917, Brazil
4. National Institute of Translation Neuroscience (INNT), Rio de Janeiro 21941-902, Brazil
* Correspondence: balbino.lino@univasf.edu.br (B.L.d.S.); costasl@ufba.br (S.L.C.); Tel.: +55-71-32838919 (S.L.C.)

Abstract: Glioblastoma (GBM) is the most aggressive and treatment-resistant brain tumor. In the GBM microenvironment, interaction with microglia is associated with the dysregulation of cytokines, chemokines, and miRNAs, contributing to angiogenesis, proliferation, anti-apoptosis, and chemoresistance. The flavonoid rutin can inhibit glioma cell growth associated with microglial activation and production of pro-inflammatory mediators by mechanisms that are still poorly understood. The present study investigated the effect of rutin on viability, regulation of miRNA-125b, and the STAT3 expression in GBM cells, as well as the effects on the modulation of the inflammatory profile and STAT3 expression in microglia during indirect interaction with GBM cells. Human GL15-GBM cells and human C20 microglia were treated or not with rutin for 24 h. Rutin (30–50 µM) significantly reduced the viability of GL15 cells; however, it did not affect the viability of microglia. Rutin (30 µM) significantly reduced the expression of miRNA-125b in the cells and secretome and STAT3 expression. Microglia submitted to the conditioned medium from GBM cells treated with rutin showed reactive morphology associated with reduced expression of IL-6, TNF, and STAT3. These results reiterate the anti-glioma effects of the flavonoid, which may also modulate microglia towards a more responsive anti-tumor phenotype, constituting a promising molecule for adjuvant therapy to GBM.

Keywords: glioblastoma; miRNA-125b; STAT3; inflammatory cytokines; rutin

Citation: Lima, I.S.; Soares, É.N.; Nonaka, C.K.V.; Souza, B.S.d.F.; dos Santos, B.L.; Costa, S.L. Flavonoid Rutin Presented Anti-Glioblastoma Activity Related to the Modulation of Onco miRNA-125b Expression and STAT3 Signaling and Impact on Microglia Inflammatory Profile. *Brain Sci.* **2024**, *14*, 90. https://doi.org/10.3390/brainsci14010090

Academic Editors: Luis Exequiel Ibarra, Laura Natalia Milla Sanabria and Nuria Arias-Ramos

Received: 21 December 2023
Revised: 9 January 2024
Accepted: 13 January 2024
Published: 17 January 2024

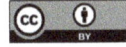

Copyright: © 2024 by the authors. Licensee MDPI, Basel, Switzerland. This article is an open access article distributed under the terms and conditions of the Creative Commons Attribution (CC BY) license (https://creativecommons.org/licenses/by/4.0/).

1. Introduction

Glioblastoma (GBM) is a highly aggressive brain tumor whose complete surgical resection is challenging due to its infiltrative nature [1]. Standard therapy involves surgery for tumor resection, followed by radiotherapy and chemotherapy, but the median survival is limited to about 15 months [2,3]. The tumor microenvironment (TME) emerges as a crucial factor in GBM progression, involving complex interactions between tumor cells and mesenchymal cells, glial cells, stem cells, fibroblasts, vascular cells, and tumor-associated macrophages (TAM) [3]. The activation of microglia, which is essential for the development of the central nervous system (CNS), plays an ambivalent role and may promote tumorigenesis or inflammatory response in the GBM [4]. This process acts as a vicious cycle, in which M2-type TAM cells are stimulated by the tumor itself, releasing factors like TNF and interleukins such as IL-6, IL-1b, and IL-10, which promote tumor proliferation and survival. An alternative to interrupting this cycle can be the inhibition of the anti-inflammatory phenotype of TAMs and far repolarization towards an inflammatory profile [5–7]. On the other hand, the activation of signaling pathways such as NFκB by TNF by microglia, astrocytes, or glioma cells themselves can induce an increase in IL6 expression, which can activate the JAK/STAT3 pathway and contribute to tumor proliferation, migration, and invasion. All these factors are associated with a poor prognosis [8–10]. Furthermore, several molecules that have epigenetic capacity have an impact on the regulation of TME plasticity. Several epigenetic modifications have been associated with the biological characteristics of this tumor, some playing essential roles as therapeutic targets [11]. In this context, there is evidence that miRNAs, which are small RNAs, do not have a protein-coding function. Nevertheless, they bind to mRNAs and play crucial roles in gene regulation [12,13]; miRNAs, such as miR125b, emerge as crucial components in oncogenic upregulation and are associated with the STAT3 signaling pathway [14,15]. Studies have pointed out that the modulation of miRNA expression by tumor cells associated with proliferation suppression can increase drug sensitivity and suppress metastasis and angiogenesis. Strategies to disrupt this mechanism include inhibition of miRNA-125b and repolarization of TAMs towards an inflammatory profile.

The flavonoid rutin, a glycone of quercetin, is widely distributed in plants [16] and has been associated with several beneficial pharmacological properties, including anti-inflammatory, neuroprotective, antiproliferative, anticarcinogenic, stress antioxidant, and anticancer effects [17]. According to transcriptome studies developed by bioinformatics tools, rutin can participate in the regulation of miRNAs [18]. In vitro and in vivo studies have demonstrated the impact of this natural agent on the regulation of different molecular mechanisms, such as Wnt/β-catenin, p53-independent pathway, PI3K/Akt, MAPK, p53, apoptosis and NF-κB, and JAK/STAT, which help mediate its anti-cancer impacts [19]. Furthermore, it was demonstrated that, combined with TMZ treatment, rutin increased the cytotoxicity and inhibition of cytoprotective autophagy of GBM cells [20]. Rutin also significantly reduced the expression of inflammatory mediators such as IL-6, TNF-α, IL-1β, and NO in microglial cells from BV-2 rats after stimulation with LPS [21]. In studies developed by our group, the properties of rutin were initially characterized at concentrations of 1 to 100 μM, which induced cytotoxicity and inhibited the proliferation of human GBM cells associated with the modulation of the ERK/MAPK signaling pathway [22]. Rutin was also able to inhibit GBM cell migration associated with the reduction of expression of extracellular components and matrix-associated metalloproteinases [22]. Subsequently, we demonstrated that rutin can modulate the inflammatory profile of isolated rat microglia [23] and, more recently, we have shown that this flavonoid and its aglycone quercetin exhibit anti-glioma effects associated with the property of modulating the inflammatory profile of microglia. In the study developed by Amorim et al. (2020) [24], it was also demonstrated that the rutin flavonoid can reduce the proliferation of tumor cells, as well as induce the chemotaxis of microglia to the tumor microenvironment in monocultures of cells of the C6 lineage, stimulate the upregulation of tumor necrosis factor (TNF) expression, and reduce the expression of cytokines and chemokines such as IL-10, MCI, and growth factors (IGF, GDNF). The antitumor effect of this molecule can also be observed in an indirect coculture model (via glioma conditioning medium), inducing microglial regulation to a pro-inflammatory profile by increasing the expression levels of cytokines such as IL-1β, IL-6, and IL-18.

In this context, in the present study, we analyzed the anti-glioma effects of rutin on viability, miRNA-125b expression, and STAT3 expression in human GBM cells, as well as its immunomodulatory property during indirect interaction (via secretome) with human microglia, relating inflammatory mediators and modulating STAT3 signaling. The results herein presented reiterate the anti-glioma potential of the flavonoid and reveal its property in modulating the expression of the onco miRNA-125b, which may be implicated in the modulation of the inflammatory profile of microglia towards a more responsive antitumor phenotype. Therefore, this work can contribute to a better understanding of miRNAs, target mechanisms, and immunological response associated with rutin treatment, offering valuable insights to guide more effective strategies, consolidating the basis for the successful application of rutin in adjuvant therapies in the treatment of GBM.

2. Results

2.1. Rutin Selectively Reduces the Viability of hGBM Cells without Affecting Microglial Viability

To analyze the effects of the flavonoid rutin in GL15 cell viability, which is derived from human GBM, and C20 cell viability, which is an immortalized human microglia cell, we conducted a study at different concentrations of the flavonoid (1–50 µM). The cell viability was determined by MTT, and the morphology of the cells well was analyzed by interference microscopy with phase contrast (Figure 1A–D). We observed that 24 h after the treatments, GBM cells treated with rutin at concentrations of 1, 5, and 10 µM presented morphology similar to the control. However, in the cultures treated with 30 and 50 µM rutin, there was a significant reduction in cell density and remaining adherent cells showed rounded morphology with contracted cytoplasm (Figure 1A), and there was a significant decrease (>50%) in cell viability in the treated cultures compared to the control (Figure 1B). On the other hand, no significant difference was observed in the morphology and viability in the cultures of C20 cells treated with rutin (Figure 1C,D).

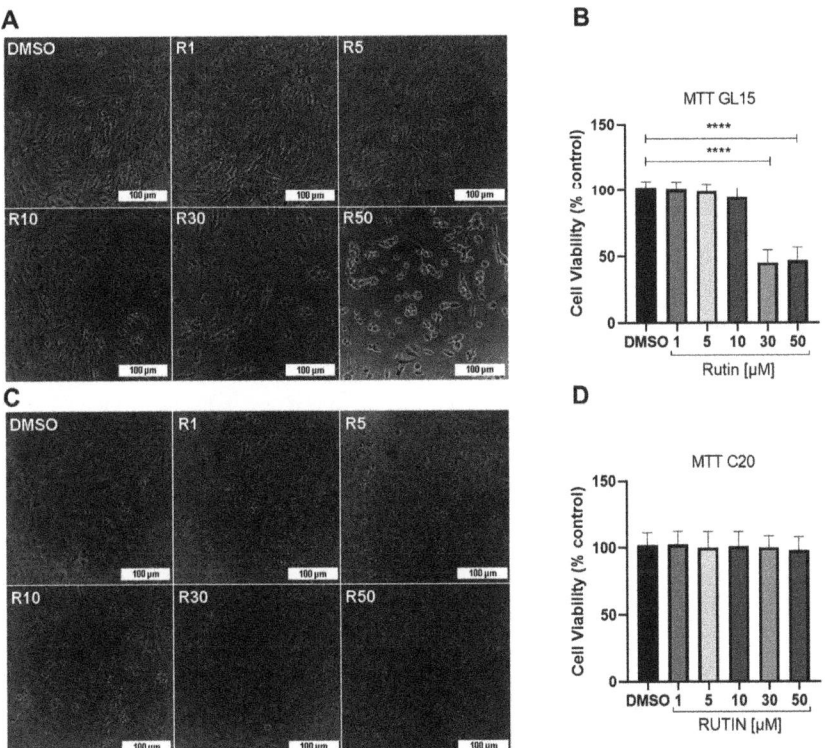

Figure 1. Effect of rutin on the viability of GL15 human glioblastoma cells and C20 human microglia. The cells were treated for 24 h with different concentrations of rutin (1, 5, 10, 30, and 50 µM) or maintained under control conditions (0.05% DMSO). (**A,C**) Phase contrast photomicrographs of GL15 and C20 cell cultures in different treatments; scale bar = 100 µm. (**B,D**) Analysis by MTT test of cell viability in GL15 and C20 cells in different treatments; values were expressed as the means ± SD ($n = 3$); the results were compared to controls (100%), and the significance was evaluated by a one-way ANOVA test followed by the Tukey test; **** $p < 0.0001$.

2.2. Rutin Regulates the Expression of miRNAs-125b in GBM Cells

We investigated the expression of miRNAs in GL15 cells at the intracellular level and in the extracellular matrix (secretome). Based on dose-dependent effects on the viability of GL15 GBM cells, the cells were treated with rutin at 30 µM or kept under control conditions (0.03% DMSO) and the expression of the onco miRNA-125b was analyzed after 24 h in the cells and in the secretome using RT-qPCR. We observed that GBM cells express and secrete miRNA-125b, and the treatment with rutin induces a highly significant reduction in the levels of this miRNA at both intracellular (** $p < 0.002$) and secretome (* $p < 0.02$), compared with control cultures (Figure 2).

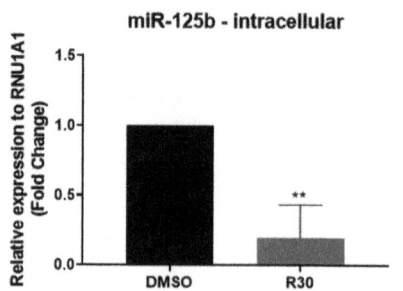 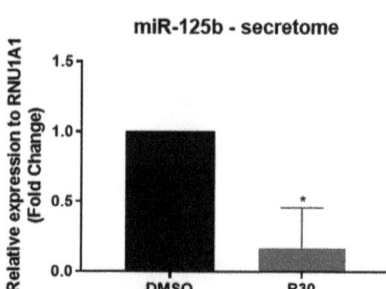

Figure 2. Effect of the flavonoid rutin on the regulation of miRNA-125b in GL15 human GBM cells. miRNA analyses using RT-qPCR. GL15 cells were treated for 24 h with rutin at 30 µM (R30) or maintained under control conditions (0.03% DMSO). The expression of intracellular miRNA-125b and the extracellular matrix (secretome) were analyzed. Values were expressed as means ± SD ($n = 3$); results expressed are relative to control and treatment; significance was determined by an unpaired t-test; ** $p < 0.002$; * $p < 0.02$.

2.3. Rutin Modulates the Expression of STAT3 in GBM Cells

To evaluate whether the STAT3 inflammatory signaling pathway is involved in the rutin effects on GBM cells, we analyzed the expression levels of STAT3 in GL15 cells treated with the flavonoid (30 µM) or maintained under control conditions (0.03% DMSO) after 24 h by Western blot technique. The data obtained indicated that the exposure of GL15 cells to rutin induced a significant (** $p < 0.002$) negative regulation in STAT3 protein expression (Figure 3).

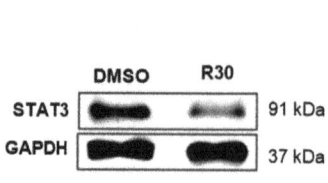 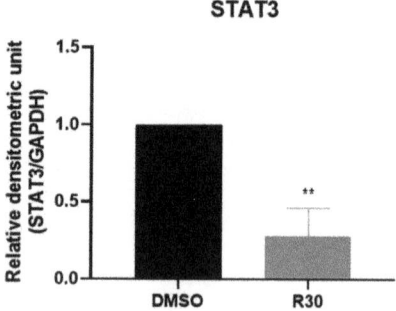

Figure 3. Effect of rutin on the regulation of STAT3 protein expression in GBM cells. GL15 cells were subjected to rutin treatment at a concentration of 30 µM (R30) or maintained under control conditions (0.03% DMSO), and STAT3 protein expression was evaluated by Western blot after 24 h. The results were normalized to the intensity of the reference protein, GAPDH, and significance was determined by an unpaired t-test; values were expressed as means ± SD ($n = 3$); ** $p < 0.002$.

2.4. The Treatment of GBM Cells with the Flavonoid Rutin Induces a Change in the Morphology of Microglia

To better understand the characterization of the microglial response to the exposure to the secretome of GBM cells, indirect interaction assays were performed. In these assays, cultures of human C20 microglia were exposed for 24 h to fresh medium as a negative control (NC), conditioned medium (CM) generated by GL15 cells under control conditions (CMGC), or conditioned medium generated after treatment with rutin at a concentration of 30 μM (CMGR). With phase contrast microscopy it was possible to analyze the morphology of C20 cells in different conditions, revealing a significant difference between the NC-, CMGC-, or CMGR-treated groups after 24 h (Figure 4). Only C20 microglia exposed to CMGR exhibited an elongated cell body and increased cellular processes, and the cellular layer showed some gaps juxtaposed with cells presenting this phenotype, suggesting a reactive response. However, this morphological pattern was not observed in C20 cells directly treated with rutin at the concentrations tested (1, 5, 10, 30, and 50 μM) (Figure 1C).

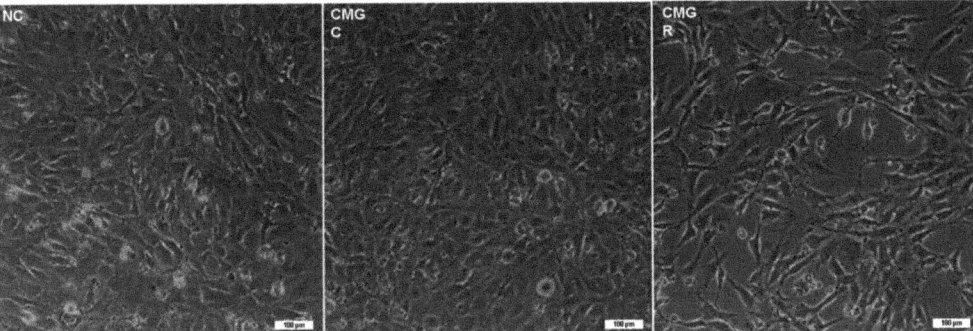

Figure 4. Effect of conditioned medium derived from GL15 GBM cells treated with the flavonoid rutin on the morphology of microglia C20. GL15 cells were treated for 24 h with rutin (30 μM) or maintained under control conditions (0.03% DMSO). C20 microglia were exposed to fresh medium including culture with fresh medium as a negative control (NC), to the culture medium from GL15 cells under control conditions treated with 0.03% DMSO (CMGC), or to the culture medium of GL15 cells treated with the flavonoid rutin at 30 μM (CMGR) for 24 h. The results represent three independent experiments. Phase-contrast photomicrographs of GL15 and C20 cells illustrate morphological differences between treatment and control; scale bar = 100 μm.

2.5. The Treatment of GBM Cells with Rutin Indirectly Regulates the Expression of Inflammatory Mediators in Microglia

We investigated the expression of inflammatory mediators (IL-6, IL-10, IL-1β, and TNF-α) by RT-qPCR in microglial cells (C20) in GL15 cells cultured for 24 h under negative control conditions, which was fresh medium without FBS(NC), treated with conditioned medium containing the secretome of GL15 cells under control conditions (CMGC) or treated with rutin at 30 μM (CMGR) for 24 h (Figure 5). We observed a significant reduction in the levels of the regulatory cytokine IL-10 in cultures treated with CMGR compared to the NC group and to the control conditioned medium (CMGC); however, there was no significant difference in cultures of C20 treated with control conditioned medium (CMGC) (**** $p < 0.0001$ and *** $p < 0.0002$, respectively) (Figure 5A). Under the same experimental conditions, we analyzed the expression of the inflammatory cytokines IL-6 and TNF-α. Remarkably, there was a significant reduction (**** $p < 0.0001$) in the expression of these cytokines when cells were exposed to CMGR compared to both CN and CMGC controls (Figure 5B,C). On the other hand, no statistically significant differences were observed in the expression of IL-1β under any of the treatment conditions (Figure 5D).

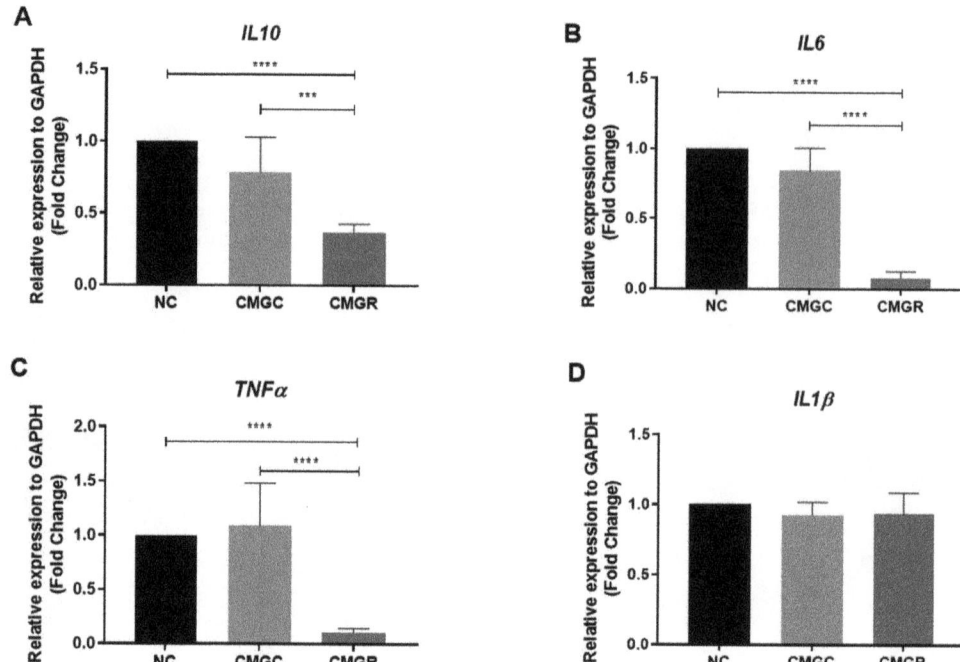

Figure 5. Effect of conditioned medium derived from glioblastoma GL15 cells treated with the flavonoid rutin on the expression of mRNA for cytokines IL10 (**A**), IL6 (**B**), TNFα (**C**) and IL1β (**D**) by C20 microglia. GL15 cells were treated for 24 h with rutin at a concentration of 30 μM (R30) or maintained under control conditions with (0.03% DMSO). C20 microglia were exposed to fresh medium as a negative control (NC), to the culture medium from GL15 cells under control conditions (treated with 0.03% DMSO, CMGC), or to the culture medium from GL15 cells treated with the flavonoid (CMGR). The cytokine expression was analyzed by RT-qPCR after 24 h. Values were expressed as means ± SD (n = 3). The significance was evaluated by a one-way ANOVA test followed by the Tukey test; **** $p < 0.0001$; *** $p < 0.0002$.

2.6. The Treatment of GBM Cells with the Flavonoid Rutin Negatively Regulates the Pro-Tumorigenic Signaling Pathway STAT3 in Microglia

We investigated the expression of STAT3 in C20 microglia using RT-qPCR and Western blot techniques with different experimental conditions, including culture with fresh medium as negative control (NC), treatment with conditioned medium containing the secretome of GL15 cells under control conditions using 0.03% DMSO (CMGC), and treatment with conditioned medium containing secretome from GL15 cells previously treated with 30 μM rutin (CMGR) (Figure 6). We observed that 24 h exposure of microglia to CMGC induced a significant increase (**** $p < 0.0001$) in STAT3 mRNA expression compared to NC. On the other hand, exposure to CMGR resulted in a significant reduction (**** $p < 0.0001$) in STAT3 mRNA expression in C20 cells (Figure 6A). Significant changes in STAT3 protein expression were also observed in the different conditions evaluated (Figure 6B). Therefore, treatment of hGBM cells with rutin for 24 h was able to induce a significant reduction (**** $p < 0.0001$) in the expression levels of both STAT3 mRNA and protein in microglia.

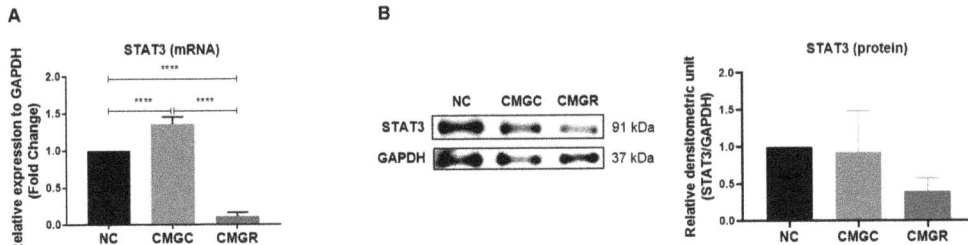

Figure 6. Effect of conditioned medium derived from glioblastoma GL15 cells treated with the flavonoid rutin on the mRNA and protein expression of STAT3. Assessments were made using RT-qPCR and Western blot techniques. C20 microglia were exposed to fresh medium as a negative control (NC), to the culture medium of GL15 cells under control conditions treated with 0.03% DMSO (CMGC), or to the culture medium of GL15 cells treated with the flavonoid rutin at 30 µM (CMGR) for 24 h. (**A**) STAT3 mRNA expression in microglia cells by RT-qPCR; (**B**) immunoreactive bands of STAT3 and GAPDH proteins in microglia and relative expression of STAT3 in microglia. Values were expressed as means ± SD (n = 3). The results were normalized to the intensity of the reference protein GAPDH. Significance was determined by a one-way ANOVA test followed by the Tukey test; **** $p < 0.0001$.

3. Discussion

The results obtained in this study are consistent with previous research using rutin, observing a significant reduction after 24 h treatment in the viability of rat C6 glioma cells and human GBM cells (GL15, U251, and TG1) at concentrations near or above 50 µM [22,25,26]. In this study, we conducted experiments with concentrations ranging from 1 to 50 µM and observed that the flavonoid at a concentration of 30 µM was sufficient to reduce the viability of human GL15 cells by around 50% within 24 h, without affecting the viability of C20 microglia cells.

Our research also aimed at contributing to the understanding of the complex interactions between GBM cells and other cells from the TME, providing valuable insights for future therapeutic approaches and research in brain cancer. Hence, we investigated the expression of miRNA-125b, considering that an in vitro study demonstrated that its positive expression stimulates the proliferation of human GBM cells while inhibiting apoptosis induced via Bcl-2 regulation [27]. Additionally, Smits et al. (2012) [28] showed that miRNA-125b expression induces angiogenesis, and Shi (2011) [29] observed its association with resistance to temozolomide in GBM treatment. Based on our results, we found that rutin reduced the expression levels of miRNA-125b in hGBM cells. This study represents, to our knowledge, the first evidence of the impact of rutin on the negative regulation of onco miRNAs. Signaling pathways play a crucial role in GBM biology, including the STAT3 and NFκB pathways. There is a significant interconnection between these pathways, resulting in complex crosstalk. This interaction may have a regulatory impact on pro-tumorigenic molecules [8,30]. In this context, as demonstrated by Parisi et al. (2016) [31], miRNA-125b is implicated in the regulation of the STAT3 signaling pathway and in the activation of microglia. Therefore, we analyzed the expression levels of STAT3 protein in GBM cells. A significant reduction in STAT3 protein was observed in the GL15 cells treated with the flavonoid rutin compared to the control. The reduction of STAT3 expression associated with the reduction of miRNA-125b suggests that rutin may influence the STAT3 and signaling pathways regulated by this miRNA.

Moreover, our investigation aimed to clarify whether rutin can modulate the microglia inflammatory profile during interaction with GBM cells and could have an impact on tumor sensibilization. As observed in previous studies, rutin has the potential to modulate the inflammatory profile of rat microglial cells in vitro, leading to significant changes after 24 h of treatment [23]. Based on the research conducted by da Silva et al. (2020) [25], which highlighted the ability of the flavonoid to modulate the inflammatory profile of microglia during interaction with rat glioma C6 cells, either through direct co-cultures or indirect interactions (via microglia secretome or C6 cells treated with the flavonoid), our current study aimed at gaining a deeper understanding of the microglial response to exposure to the secretome of human GBM cells (GL15). It became evident that when C20 microglia are treated with CMGR, changes in morphology occur, indicating possible glial reactivity. We also investigated the effects of this indirect interaction in the expression of cytokines IL-6, IL-10, IL-1β, and TNF-α, and in the STAT3 signaling protein in microglia subjected to a conditioned medium containing secretome from GBM cells treated or untreated with rutin, as well as under more homeostatic control conditions. We observed that the treatment of microglia with conditioned medium containing either control (CMGC) or rutin-treated (CMGR) secretome did not influence the mRNA expression of the cytokine IL-1β. IL-1β plays a relevant role in the activation of various signaling pathways, including the NFκB transcription factor, which regulates the production and release of pro-inflammatory mediators essential for the development and progression of glioma [32]. The lack of significant changes in IL-1β expression may indicate a highly controlled regulation or the influence of other factors on its expression. Furthermore, the modulation of IL-1β may depend on different regulators and cellular contexts, including other signaling pathways [33]. As revised by Nascimento et al. (2021) [34], in the GBM TME, IL-10 is positively regulated, and microglia shifts towards M2-like characteristics, contributing to the production of inflammatory cytokines. Through analysis, we observed a significant reduction in IL-10 mRNA levels in the CMGR-treated group compared to the NC group. However, no significance was found in the expression of IL-10 in microglia treated exclusively with CMGR. These results suggest that CMGR, composed of the secretome of GL15 cells after rutin treatment, may have the capacity to modulate IL-10 expression in microglia in a specific context, possibly mediated by complex interactions between secretome components and microglial cells. However, it is important to note that the lack of statistical significance in IL-10 expression in microglia treated exclusively with CMGR suggests that this influence may depend on additional factors or specific cellular interactions. On the other hand, we observed that CMGR can induce a significant reduction in mRNA expression for the cytokines IL-6 and TNF in microglia. These cytokines are associated with inflammatory regulation in the TME [30,35], and they may have important implications for modulating the immune and inflammatory response in the GBM environment, especially in immunomodulating the microglial profile. Our findings are in line with the results of Silva et al. (2020) [25], who demonstrated a reduction in the expression of IL-6 and IL-10 levels in rat microglia cultures treated with C6 glioma cell secretome exposed to rutin at 50 μM for 24 h. In contrast, an increase in IL-1β and TNF levels was observed in these same results. Differences in cell lines and the doses of rutin used may explain the differences in responses observed. These complexities highlight the importance of interpreting results, taking into account the specific contexts of each study.

STAT3 is highly activated in the TME, and besides its high expression in GBM cells, it is also associated with microglial modulation in this environment [36]. In the indirect interaction between GBM under control conditions (CMGC), we observed positive regulation in STAT3 mRNA expression in microglia. On the other hand, microglia exposed to CMGR showed a significant reduction in STAT3 mRNA and protein expression compared to microglia in the NC group. Considering the role of the signaling protein STAT3 in the expression of inflammatory cytokines [37], the reduction of its expression in CMGR-treated microglia may also be implicated in the negative regulation of hGBM cells' miRNA-125b, as well as IL-6 mRNA, which may be related to reductions in TNF mRNA expression in the context of change in the inflammatory profile. This observation highlights the complexity of the STAT3 pathway and the need to consider multiple aspects of the regulation of signaling pathways, such as the NFκB pathway, which is actively associated with inflammatory mediators in the GBM TME.

Although this evidence suggests the positive impact of rutin on anti-glioma actions, it is essential to conduct a more comprehensive and in-depth analysis of the dysregulation of specific molecules and the intricate mechanisms associated with GBM progression. The intrinsic heterogeneity of GBM, evidenced by the molecular diversity between different tumor lineages, justifies the need to include other GBM lineages in these investigations. This approach allows us to cover the different gene expressions, molecular profiles, and cellular responses, which are essential for a more complete understanding of the impact of rutin. Furthermore, the inclusion of analyses on explants from glioblastoma patients is also crucial, enabling the validation and contextualization of results in a scenario closer to real clinical conditions. Such diverse approaches would strengthen the scientific basis, enriching conclusions and contributing to a more comprehensive and translational approach in developing therapeutic strategies for GBM. The results of the present study, together with previous studies by us and others, consolidate the scientific basis for the use of rutin as an adjuvant in the treatment of GBM, which may be considered in other translational and clinical studies.

4. Materials and Methods

4.1. Cell Culture

The GL15 cell line (passages 120–130) established from a human GBM by Bocchini et al. (1991) [22,38] was chosen for its proliferation, migration, invasion, and resistance properties, and it was cultured in Dulbecco's Modified Eagle Medium (DMEM: Island Biological Company-GIBCO ®, Grand Island, NY, USA), containing 7 mmol/L glucose, 2 mmol/L L-glutamine, and 0.011 g/L pyruvic acid, as previously described by Santos et al. 2015 [22]. The immortalized primary human microglia C20 cell line, originally developed and characterized by Garcia-Mesa et al. (2017) [39] and kindly provided by Dr. Henning Ulrich from the Department of Biochemistry, Institute of Chemistry at the University of São Paulo (USP), was cultured in DMEM F12 50/50 medium as described by the authors [39]. Both cultures were supplemented with 10% fetal bovine serum (FBS) and antibiotics (100 U/mL penicillin and 100 µg/mL streptomycin, Gibco ®) and maintained in an incubator under standardized conditions of a humidified atmosphere with 5% CO_2 at a temperature of 37 °C. Cells were cultured in 100 mm polystyrene plates (TPP, Trasadingen, Switzerland), following the protocol described by Santos et al. (2015), until reaching the desired confluence. Upon reaching confluence, the medium was removed, and adherent cells were detached using a trypsin solution (0.05% trypsin and 0.02% EDTA in PBS) and seeded into 6- or 96-well polystyrene plates (Kasvi, São José dos Pinhais, SP, Brazil), according to the experiment, at a density of 5×10^4 cells/cm^2.

4.2. Treatment Drugs

Rutin (3-rutinoside of 3,3′,4′,5,6-pentahydroxyflavone) was obtained from Merck (Boston, MA, USA) (R5143) and dissolved in dimethyl sulfoxide (DMSO; Sigma, Tokyo, Japan) to form a 100 mM stock solution, which was stored and protected from light at −4 °C. At the time of treatments, GL15 cells were incubated for 24 h with rutin at concentrations varying between 1, 5, 10, 30, and 50 µM, depending on the experiment, in an attempt to investigate the most appropriate dose response. The vehicle for diluting flavonoids, dimethyl sulfoxide (DMSO), used to demonstrate cultivation under control conditions in a volume equivalent to the maximum concentration adopted in flavonoids (0.05%), was diluted directly in culture medium without fetal bovine serum (FBS) and did not show a significant effect on the parameters analyzed when compared to cultures that were not exposed to this solvent.

4.3. Cell Viability

To evaluate the viability of human glioblastoma GL15 and human microglia C20 cell lines, they were seeded in a 96-well plate (Kasvi) with an approximate cell density of 2.2×10^4 cells/cm^2, corresponding to approximately 8000 cells per well, and cultured in fresh medium DMEM or DMEM F12 properly supplemented with SFB. Thus, they were incubated for 24 h in standardized conditions of a humidified atmosphere with 5% CO_2 at a temperature of 37 °C. Cell viability was determined by the conversion of the yellow salt 3-(4,5-dimethylthiazol-2-yl)-2,5-diphenyl tetrazolium bromide (MTT) into formazan crystals (purple) by mitochondrial dehydrogenases of live cells. After 24 h of plating, cells were treated with the previously defined concentrations. After 24 h of treatment, cells were incubated with an MTT solution (Thermo Fisher, Waltham, MA, USA, 0.5 mg MTT per 1 mL) at 37 °C and 5% (v/v) CO_2 for 2 h. Subsequently, 100 µL of a lysis buffer containing 20% (w/v) sodium dodecyl sulfate (SDS), 50% (v/v) acetic acid, and 2.5% (v/v) 1 mol/L HCl were added, and the plates were incubated for 6 h. The optical density of the samples was measured using a spectrophotometer (Varioskan™ Flash Multimode Reader, Thermo Plate) at a wavelength of 540 nm. Three independent experiments with eight replicates for each variable were conducted, and the results were expressed as the percentage of viability of the treated groups relative to the control, which was considered 100%.

4.4. Culture with Indirect Interaction between GL15 and C20 Cells

For studies involving indirect interactions, cells were cultured in 6-well plates (Kasvi) at a density of 5×10^4 cells/cm². The GBM GL15 cells were cultured in fresh medium DMEM appropriately supplemented with FBS. Thus, they were incubated for 24 h under standardized conditions of a humidified atmosphere with 5% CO_2 at a temperature of 37 °C. After 24 h treating GL15 GBM cells under control conditions (0.03% DMSO) or with rutin (30 µM), the conditioned media (CM) of the cultures, containing the secretome produced by GL15 cells, were collected and centrifuged at $2000 \times g$ for 5 min to remove any cellular debris. The CM was immediately used to treat human microglia C20 cells (indirect interaction) at a 1:4 ratio (fresh medium:CM). GL15 cells were collected and prepared for miRNA extraction following the manufacturer's protocol using the miRNeasy kit (Qiagen, Hilden, Germany). After 24 h treating C20 cells with CM from GL15 cells treated with rutin (Rutin-treated GL15 conditioned medium—CMGR) or under control conditions (Control GL15 conditioned medium—CMGC), cells were collected for RNA extraction using Trizol®reagent (Invitrogen, Waltham, MA, USA, Life Technologies, Carlsbad, CA, USA, 15596026), following the manufacturer's protocol. The experiments were performed in triplicate.

4.5. Analysis of miRNA Expression by RT-qPCR

The pellet samples of GL15 human GBM cells containing approximately 1×10^6 cells were mixed with 700 µL of QIAzol Lysis Reagent from the miRNeasy kit (Qiagen). For the isolation of miRNAs from the cell culture supernatant, the miRNeasy Serum/Plasm Advanced kit (Qiagen) was used. For the supernatant, 5 times the volume of QIAzol Lysis Reagent provided by the manufacturer was added. The samples were vortexed for 1 min. Chloroform was added in the recommended volume for each kit, vigorously mixed for 15 s, and incubated for 3 min at room temperature. Subsequently, the samples were centrifuged for 15 min at $12,000 \times g$ at 4 °C. After centrifugation, the aqueous phase was collected and transferred to a new 1.5 mL tube (approximately 350 µL). Next, 1.5 times the volume (525 µL) of 100% ethanol was added and homogenized using a pipette for each sample. The samples were then transferred to a column (RNeasy MinElute spin column) provided by the manufacturer and centrifuged for 15 s at $\geq 10,000 \times g$ at room temperature. The liquid passing through the column of each sample was discarded, and the column was washed with 700 µL of Buffer RWT and centrifuged for another 15 s at $\geq 10,000 \times g$ at room temperature. Again, the liquid passing through the column of each sample was discarded, and the column was washed with 500 µL of Buffer RPE and centrifuged for 15 s at $\geq 10,000 \times g$ at room temperature. Then, the column of each sample was washed with 500 µL of 80% ethanol and centrifuged for 2 min at $\geq 10,000 \times g$ at room temperature. The columns were transferred to new properly labeled 1.5 mL tubes and left with the cap open for 5 min to evaporate residual ethanol. Thirty microliters of RNase-free ultrapure water provided by the manufacturer were added, followed by centrifugation for 1 min at maximum speed. The samples were stored at −80 °C until the next step. The experiments were conducted in triplicate. For the extraction of miRNAs from the cell culture supernatant, the miRNeasy Serum/Plasma kit (Qiagen) was used following the manufacturer's recommendations. For cDNA synthesis, the miScript II RT Kit (Qiagen) was used with 10 ng of RNA quantified by Nanodrop™ 2000 spectrophotometer (Thermo Fisher Scientific), according to the manufacturer's recommendations. The samples were incubated for 60 min at 37 °C, 95 °C for 5 min, and immediately placed on ice. Five microliters of diluted cDNA (1:20), 5 µL of SYBR™ Green PCR Master Mix (Thermo Fisher Scientific), and 1 µL of the commercial primer set miRCURY LNA (Qiagen) were used for a final volume of 10 µL. The amplification was performed on an ABI7500 FAST thermocycler (Applied Biosystem, Waltham, MA, USA). The endogenous control RNU1A1 was used for result normalization. The expression of miRNA levels was calculated using the $2^{-\Delta\Delta CT}$ method [40] and analyzed using GraphPad Prism v 9.1.1 2020 (La Jolla, CA, USA).

4.6. Analysis of mRNA Expression by RT-qPCR

To analyze the expression of inflammatory cytokines by C20 microglia under control conditions (fresh medium), or treated with the conditioned medium from GL15 cells cultured for 24 h under control conditions (CMGC), or treated with the conditioned medium from GL15 cells cultured for 24 h in the presence of the flavonoid rutin at 30 µM (CMGR), cells were cultured in 6-well plates (Kasvi) with a cell density of approximately 1×10^6 cells/cm^2 and incubated for 24 h under standardized conditions of a humidified atmosphere with 5% CO_2 at a temperature of 37 °C. After 24 h of treatments, the total RNA was extracted using Trizol® reagent (Thermo Fisher Scientific) following the recommended manufacturer's protocol. The experiment was performed in biological triplicate. RNA quantification was carried out using NanoDrop™ 2000 (Thermo Fisher Scientific). The samples were stored at −80 °C until further use. For the cDNA reaction, 1.5 µg of RNA and the commercial High-Capacity cDNA Reverse Transcription kit were used, following the manufacturer's recommendations (Thermo Fisher Scientific). The cDNA was stored at −20 °C until use. Subsequently, real-time quantitative PCR (RT-qPCR) was performed on the ABI7500 FAST instrument (Applied Biosystems) under standard Taqman thermal cycling conditions by the manufacturer. The expressions of mRNAs in treated samples and control conditions were evaluated using commercial TaqMan® probes: IL-6 (Hs00174131_m1), IL-10 (Hs00961622_m1), TNF-α (Hs00174128_m1), and IL-1β (Hs01555410_m1). The reference gene GAPDH (Hs99999905_m1) (Thermo Fisher Scientific) was used as a normalizer. The cDNA samples were diluted 1:100, 5 µL of TaqMan Universal Master Mix (Thermo Fisher Scientific) and 0.5 µL of specific TaqMan® probes for each monoplex reaction were added to achieve a final volume of 10 µL. Expression analyses of STAT3 were performed by RT-qPCR assays using SYBR™ Green PCR Master Mix and the following primers: STAT3 Forward (5′ to 3′): ACCAGCAGTATAGCCGCTTC, STAT3 Reverse (5′ to 3′): GCCACAATCCGGGCAATCT, and the endogenous control GAPDH Forward (5′ to 3′): GCCAGCATCGCCCCACTTG, GAPDH Reverse (5′ to 3′): GTGAAGGTCAACGGAT. The expression levels of mRNAs were calculated using the $2^{-\Delta\Delta CT}$ method (Schmittgen and Livak, 2008) [40] and analyzed using GraphPad Prism v 9.1.1 (2020).

4.7. Analysis of Signaling Pathways by Western Blot

The analysis of the effect of rutin on the expression of proteins involved in cellular signaling was conducted on human GL15 GBM cells treated directly with the flavonoid (30 µM), as well as on human C20 microglia cells under control conditions (fresh medium), or treated with the conditioned medium from GL15 cells cultured for 24 h under control conditions (CMGC), or treated with the conditioned medium from GL15 cells cultured for 24 h in the presence of rutin at 30 µM (CMGR). Cells were cultured in 6-well plates (Kasvi) with a cell density of approximately 5×10^5 cells/cm^2. After 24 h of treatments, total proteins were cold-extracted (with ice immersion) using a buffer containing 4 M urea,

2% SDS, 2 mM EGTA, 62.5 mM Tris-HCl pH 6.8, 2 mM EDTA, and 0.5% Triton X-100 and supplemented with 1 µL/mL of a protease inhibitor cocktail (Sigma-Aldrich, P8340). The experiments were performed in triplicate. The concentration of total proteins in the extracts obtained was quantified using the Lowry method. For Western blot analyses, proteins were separated by polyacrylamide gel electrophoresis and sodium dodecyl sulfate (SDS-PAGE) and electrotransferred to polyvinylidene difluoride (PVDF) membranes (Bio-Rad; Hercules, CA, USA). For immunodetection, the membranes were initially blocked in a buffer composed of 5% skim milk (Molico) in Tris-buffered saline with Tween 20 (TBS-T), containing 50 mM Tris-HCl, 150 mM NaCl, 0.05% Tween 20, and pH 7.4 (HCl) at 25 °C for 1 h. They were then incubated overnight at 4 °C with primary antibodies for STAT-3 (1:1000, Santa Cruz) and GAPDH (1:10,000, MERCK). The membranes were then washed three times with TBS-T and incubated for 1 h at room temperature with a secondary antibody anti-rabbit conjugated with peroxidase (1:5000; Molecular Probes, G21234) diluted in 5% skim milk TBS-T. After three washes with TBS-T and one wash with TBS, the membranes were incubated with the chemiluminescent substrate solution (ECL Plus Biorad Substrate Kit) for 5 min. Immunoreactive bands were then analyzed using the ImageQuant LAS 500 apparatus (GE Healthcare Life Sciences, Marlborough, MA, USA). The relative expression value of proteins was normalized according to the expression of GAPDH in the same sample. Quantification was obtained by densitometric scanning (ScanJet 4C, Hewlett Packard, Palo Alto, CA, USA) of three experiments and analyzed with ImageJ 1.33u software (Wayne Rasband, National Institutes of Health, Bethesda, MD, USA).

4.8. Statistical Analysis of Results

Data were statistically analyzed using GraphPad Prism 8 software (GraphPad, San Diego, CA, USA) for Windows. Experimental results are presented as means ± standard deviation (SD). To determine the statistical difference between the groups, analysis of variance was performed using a one-way ANOVA test, followed by Tukey's post-hoc test for multiple comparisons. Parametric statistical tests were employed for comparisons between treatment groups and control groups. Statistical differences were considered significant at $p \leq 0.05$. All experiments were repeated at least three times.

5. Conclusions

The results herein presented reinforce the anti-glioma potential of the flavonoid rutin and reveal its ability to modulate STAT3 signaling and the expression of onco miRNA-125b, which, through indirect interaction studies with microglia, is likely to impact the inflammatory profile of these cells towards a more antitumoral responsive phenotype. Rutin induced changes in the morphology of microglia in response to GBM cell treatment. Furthermore, the positive regulation of inflammatory mediators in microglia suggests a crucial role of rutin in modulating the local immune response. By negatively regulating the pro-tumorigenic signaling pathway STAT3 in microglia, rutin may have significant implications in suppressing tumor progression.

These findings provide valuable insights for the development of targeted therapies against GBM, which is known for its resistance to conventional treatments. The discoveries presented in this research indicate that rutin possesses properties capable of affecting multiple aspects of interactions between GBM cells and microglia, making it a promising substance for future investigations and the development of innovative therapeutic approaches.

Author Contributions: Conceptualization: I.S.L., B.L.d.S. and S.L.C.; Methodology: I.S.L., É.N.S., C.K.V.N. and B.L.d.S.; Formal analysis: I.S.L., B.L.d.S. and S.L.C.; Investigation: I.S.L., C.K.V.N. and B.L.d.S.; Resources: B.S.d.F.S.; Data curation: B.L.d.S., C.K.V.N. and S.L.C.; Writing—original draft: I.S.L., C.K.V.N., B.L.d.S. and S.L.C.; Writing—review and editing: B.L.d.S. and S.L.C.; Visualization: B.S.d.F.S.; Project administration: S.L.C.; Funding acquisition: S.L.C. All authors have read and agreed to the published version of the manuscript.

Funding: This work was supported by the Coordination of Personnel Improvement of Higher Level (CAPES, Process 88887.685766/2022-00 MPhil fellowship for I.S.L.) and the National Council for Scientific and Technological Development (CNPq) (Research Fellowship to SLC Process No. 307539/2018-0, National Institute for Translational Neuroscience Brazil).

Institutional Review Board Statement: Not applicable.

Informed Consent Statement: Not applicable.

Data Availability Statement: Data are contained within the article.

Acknowledgments: We would like to thank the Postgraduate Program in Immunology and the Laboratory of Neurochemistry and Cell Biology of the Federal University of Bahia.

Conflicts of Interest: The authors declare no conflicts of interest.

References

1. Wang, H.; Xu, T.; Huang, Q.; Jin, W.; Chen, J. Immunotherapy for Malignant Glioma: Current Status and Future Directions. *Trends Pharmacol. Sci.* **2020**, *41*, 123–138. [CrossRef]
2. Grochans, S.; Cybulska, A.M.; Simińska, D.; Korbecki, J.; Kojder, K.; Chlubek, D.; Baranowska-Bosiacka, I. Epidemiology of Glioblastoma Multiforme–Literature Review. *Cancers* **2022**, *14*, 2412. [CrossRef]
3. Virtuoso, A.; Giovannoni, R.; De Luca, C.; Gargano, F.; Cerasuolo, M.; Maggio, N.; Lavitrano, M.; Papa, M. The Glioblastoma Microenvironment: Morphology, Metabolism, and Molecular Signature of Glial Dynamics to Discover Metabolic Rewiring Sequence. *Int. J. Mol. Sci.* **2021**, *22*, 3301. [CrossRef]
4. Amici, S.A.; Dong, J.; Guerau-de-Arellano, M. Molecular Mechanisms Modulating the Phenotype of Macrophages and Microglia. *Front. Immunol.* **2017**, *8*, 1520. [CrossRef]
5. Rolle, C.E.; Sengupta, S.; Lesniak, M.S. Mechanisms of Immune Evasion by Gliomas. *Adv. Exp. Med. Biol.* **2012**, *746*, 53–76.
6. Solinas, G.; Germano, G.; Mantovani, A.; Allavena, P. Tumor-Associated Macrophages (TAM) as Major Players of the Cancer-Related Inflammation. *J. Leukoc. Biol.* **2009**, *86*, 1065–1073. [CrossRef]
7. Wei, J.; Gabrusiewicz, K.; Heimberger, A. The Controversial Role of Microglia in Malignant Gliomas. *Clin. Dev. Immunol.* **2013**, *2013*, 285246. [CrossRef]
8. Chang, N.; Ahn, S.H.; Kong, D.-S.; Lee, H.W.; Nam, D.-H. The Role of STAT3 in Glioblastoma Progression through Dual Influences on Tumor Cells and the Immune Microenvironment. *Mol. Cell Endocrinol.* **2017**, *451*, 53–65. [CrossRef]
9. Kim, J.; Patel, M.; Ruzevick, J.; Jackson, C.; Lim, M. STAT3 Activation in Glioblastoma: Biochemical and Therapeutic Implications. *Cancers* **2014**, *6*, 376–395. [CrossRef]
10. Wu, A.; Wei, J.; Kong, L.-Y.; Wang, Y.; Priebe, W.; Qiao, W.; Sawaya, R.; Heimberger, A.B. Glioma Cancer Stem Cells Induce Immunosuppressive Macrophages/Microglia. *Neuro Oncol.* **2010**, *12*, 1113–1125. [CrossRef]
11. Uddin, M.S.; Al Mamun, A.; Alghamdi, B.S.; Tewari, D.; Jeandet, P.; Sarwar, M.S.; Ashraf, G.M. Epigenetics of Glioblastoma Multiforme: From Molecular Mechanisms to Therapeutic Approaches. *Semin. Cancer Biol.* **2022**, *83*, 100–120. [CrossRef] [PubMed]
12. Shi, J. Regulatory Networks between Neurotrophins and MiRNAs in Brain Diseases and Cancers. *Acta Pharmacol. Sin.* **2015**, *36*, 149–157. [CrossRef] [PubMed]
13. Bartel, D.P. MicroRNAs. *Cell* **2004**, *116*, 281–297. [CrossRef] [PubMed]
14. Cao, Q.; Li, Y.-Y.; He, W.-F.; Zhang, Z.-Z.; Zhou, Q.; Liu, X.; Shen, Y.; Huang, T.-T. Interplay between MicroRNAs and the STAT3 Signaling Pathway in Human Cancers. *Physiol. Genom.* **2013**, *45*, 1206–1214. [CrossRef] [PubMed]
15. Buruiană, A.; Florian, Ș.I.; Florian, A.I.; Timiș, T.-L.; Mihu, C.M.; Miclăuș, M.; Oșan, S.; Hrapșa, I.; Cataniciu, R.C.; Farcaș, M.; et al. The Roles of MiRNA in Glioblastoma Tumor Cell Communication: Diplomatic and Aggressive Negotiations. *Int. J. Mol. Sci.* **2020**, *21*, 1950. [CrossRef] [PubMed]
16. Gentile, M.T.; Ciniglia, C.; Reccia, M.G.; Volpicelli, F.; Gatti, M.; Thellung, S.; Florio, T.; Melone, M.A.B.; Colucci-D'Amato, L.; Ruta Graveolens, L. Induces Death of Glioblastoma Cells and Neural Progenitors, but Not of Neurons, via ERK 1/2 and AKT Activation. *PLoS ONE* **2015**, *10*, e0118864. [CrossRef] [PubMed]
17. Ganeshpurkar, A.; Saluja, A.K. The Pharmacological Potential of Rutin. *Saudi Pharm. J.* **2017**, *25*, 149–164. [CrossRef] [PubMed]
18. Nasrabadi, N.P.; Zareian, S.; Nayeri, Z.; Salmanipour, R.; Parsafar, S.; Gharib, E.; Aghdaei, A.H.; Zali, M.R. A Detailed Image of Rutin Underlying Intracellular Signaling Pathways in Human SW480 Colorectal Cancer Cells Based on MiRNAs-lncRNAs-mRNAs-TFs Interactions. *J. Cell Physiol.* **2019**, *234*, 15570–15580. [CrossRef]
19. Imani, A.; Maleki, N.; Bohlouli, S.; Kouhsoltani, M.; Sharifi, S.; Maleki Dizaj, S. Molecular Mechanisms of Anticancer Effect of Rutin. *Phytother. Res.* **2021**, *35*, 2500–2513. [CrossRef]
20. Zhang, P.; Sun, S.; Li, N.; Ho, A.S.W.; Kiang, K.M.Y.; Zhang, X.; Cheng, Y.S.; Poon, M.W.; Lee, D.; Pu, J.K.S.; et al. Rutin Increases the Cytotoxicity of Temozolomide in Glioblastoma via Autophagy Inhibition. *J. Neurooncol* **2017**, *132*, 393–400. [CrossRef]
21. Lang, G.-P.; Li, C.; Han, Y.-Y. Rutin Pretreatment Promotes Microglial M1 to M2 Phenotype Polarization. *Neural Regen. Res.* **2021**, *16*, 2499. [CrossRef] [PubMed]

22. Santos, B.L.; Oliveira, M.N.; Coelho, P.L.C.; Pitanga, B.P.S.; da Silva, A.B.; Adelita, T.; Silva, V.D.A.; Costa, M.d.F.D.; El-Bachá, R.S.; Tardy, M.; et al. Flavonoids Suppress Human Glioblastoma Cell Growth by Inhibiting Cell Metabolism, Migration, and by Regulating Extracellular Matrix Proteins and Metalloproteinases Expression. *Chem. Biol. Interact.* **2015**, *242*, 123–138. [CrossRef] [PubMed]
23. da Silva, B.A.; Coelho, C.P.L.; Amparo, A.O.J.; de Almeida, A.M.M.C.; Borges, P.J.M.; dos Santos, C.S.; Costa, D.M.d.F.; Mecha, M.; Rodriguez, G.C.; da Silva, A.V.D.; et al. The Flavonoid Rutin Modulates Microglial/Macrophage Activation to a CD150/CD206 M2 Phenotype. *Chem. Biol. Interact.* **2017**, *274*, 89–99. [CrossRef] [PubMed]
24. de Amorim, V.C.M.; Júnior, M.S.O.; da Silva, A.B.; David, J.M.; David, J.P.L.; de Fátima, M.D.C.; Butt, A.M.; da Silva, V.D.A.; Costa, S.L. Agathisflavone Modulates Astrocytic Responses and Increases the Population of Neurons in an in Vitro Model of Traumatic Brain Injury. *Naunyn Schmiedebergs Arch. Pharmacol.* **2020**, *393*, 1921–1930. [CrossRef]
25. da Silva, A.B.; Coelho, C.P.L.; das Neves, M.O.; Oliveira, J.L.; Oliveira, J.A.A.; da Silva, K.C.; Soares, J.R.P.; Pitanga, B.P.S.; dos Santos, C.S.; de Faria, G.P.L.; et al. The Flavonoid Rutin and Its Aglycone Quercetin Modulate the Microglia Inflammatory Profile Improving Antiglioma Activity. *Brain Behav. Immun.* **2020**, *85*, 170–185. [CrossRef]
26. Santos, B.L.; Silva, A.R.; Pitanga, B.P.S.; Sousa, C.S.; Grangeiro, M.S.; Fragomeni, B.O.; Coelho, P.L.C.; Oliveira, M.N.; Menezes-Filho, N.J.; Costa, M.F.D.; et al. Antiproliferative, Proapoptotic and Morphogenic Effects of the Flavonoid Rutin on Human Glioblastoma Cells. *Food Chem.* **2011**, *127*, 404–411. [CrossRef] [PubMed]
27. Xia, H.-F.; He, T.-Z.; Liu, C.-M.; Cui, Y.; Song, P.-P.; Jin, X.-H.; Ma, X. MiR-125b Expression Affects the Proliferation and Apoptosis of Human Glioma Cells by Targeting *Bmf*. *Cell. Physiol. Biochem.* **2009**, *23*, 347–358. [CrossRef]
28. Smits, M.; Wurdinger, T.; Hof, B.; Drexhage, J.A.R.; Geerts, D.; Wesseling, P.; Noske, D.P.; Vandertop, W.P.; Vries, H.E.; Reijerkerk, A. Myc-associated Zinc Finger Protein (MAZ) Is Regulated by MiR-125b and Mediates VEGF-induced Angiogenesis in Glioblastoma. *FASEB J.* **2012**, *26*, 2639–2647. [CrossRef]
29. Shi, L. MicroRNA-125b-2 Confers Human Glioblastoma Stem Cells Resistance to Temozolomide through the Mitochondrial Pathway of Apoptosis. *Int. J. Oncol.* **2011**, *40*, 119–129. [CrossRef]
30. McFarland, B.C.; Hong, S.W.; Rajbhandari, R.; Twitter, G.B.; Gray, G.K.; Yu, H.; Benveniste, E.N.; Nozell, S.E. NF-KB-Induced IL-6 Ensures STAT3 Activation and Tumor Aggressiveness in Glioblastoma. *PLoS ONE* **2013**, *8*, e78728. [CrossRef]
31. Parisi, C.; Napoli, G.; Pelegrin, P.; Volonté, C. M1 and M2 Functional Imprinting of Primary Microglia: Role of P2X7 Activation and MiR-125b. *Mediat. Inflamm.* **2016**, *2016*. [CrossRef]
32. Kai, K.; Komohara, Y.; Esumi, S.; Fujiwara, Y.; Yamamoto, T.; Uekawa, K.; Ohta, K.; Takezaki, T.; Kuroda, J.; Shinojima, N.; et al. Macrophage/Microglia-Derived IL-1β Induces Glioblastoma Growth via the STAT3/NF-KB Pathway. *Hum. Cell* **2022**, *35*, 226–237. [CrossRef] [PubMed]
33. Sun, Y.; Liu, W.-Z.; Liu, T.; Feng, X.; Yang, N.; Zhou, H.-F. Signaling Pathway of MAPK/ERK in Cell Proliferation, Differentiation, Migration, Senescence and Apoptosis. *J. Recept. Signal Transduct.* **2015**, *35*, 600–604. [CrossRef]
34. Nascimento, R.P.; Santos, B.L.; Silva, K.C.; Amaral da Silva, V.D.; Fátima Costa, M.; David, J.M.; David, J.P.; Moura-Neto, V.; Oliveira, M.d.N.; Ulrich, H.; et al. Reverted Effect of Mesenchymal Stem Cells in Glioblastoma Treated with Agathisflavone and Its Selective Antitumoral Effect on Cell Viability, Migration, and Differentiation via STAT3. *J. Cell Physiol.* **2021**, *236*, 5022–5035. [CrossRef] [PubMed]
35. Rong, X.; Xu, J.; Jiang, Y.; Li, F.; Chen, Y.; Dou, Q.P.; Li, D. Citrus Peel Flavonoid Nobiletin Alleviates Lipopolysaccharide-Induced Inflammation by Activating IL-6/STAT3/FOXO3a-Mediated Autophagy. *Food Funct.* **2021**, *12*, 1305–1317. [CrossRef] [PubMed]
36. Andersen, R.S.; Anand, A.; Harwood, D.S.L.; Kristensen, B.W. Tumor-Associated Microglia and Macrophages in the Glioblastoma Microenvironment and Their Implications for Therapy. *Cancers* **2021**, *13*, 4255. [CrossRef] [PubMed]
37. Beurel, E.; Jope, R.S. Lipopolysaccharide-Induced Interleukin-6 Production Is Controlled by Glycogen Synthase Kinase-3 and STAT3 in the Brain. *J. Neuroinflam.* **2009**, *6*, 9. [CrossRef]
38. Bocchini, V.; Casalone, R.; Collini, P.; Rebel, G.; Curto, F. Lo Changes in Glial Fibrillary Acidic Protein and Karyotype during Culturing of Two Cell Lines Established from Human Glioblastoma Multiforme. *Cell Tissue Res.* **1991**, *265*, 73–81. [CrossRef]
39. Garcia-Mesa, Y.; Jay, T.R.; Checkley, M.A.; Luttge, B.; Dobrowolski, C.; Valadkhan, S.; Landreth, G.E.; Karn, J.; Alvarez-Carbonell, D. Immortalization of Primary Microglia: A New Platform to Study HIV Regulation in the Central Nervous System. *J. Neurovirol.* **2017**, *23*, 47–66. [CrossRef]
40. Schmittgen, T.D.; Livak, K.J. Analyzing real-time PCR data by the comparative CT method. *Nat. Protoc.* **2008**, *3*, 1101–1108. [CrossRef]

Disclaimer/Publisher's Note: The statements, opinions and data contained in all publications are solely those of the individual author(s) and contributor(s) and not of MDPI and/or the editor(s). MDPI and/or the editor(s) disclaim responsibility for any injury to people or property resulting from any ideas, methods, instructions or products referred to in the content.

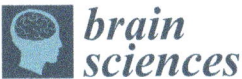

Article

Polymersomes for Sustained Delivery of a Chalcone Derivative Targeting Glioblastoma Cells

Ana Alves [1,2,3], Ana M. Silva [4], Joana Moreira [2,5], Claúdia Nunes [6], Salette Reis [6], Madalena Pinto [2,5], Honorina Cidade [2,5], Francisca Rodrigues [4], Domingos Ferreira [1,3], Paulo C. Costa [1,3] and Marta Correia-da-Silva [2,5,*]

1. UCIBIO—Applied Molecular Biosciences Unit, MedTech-Laboratory of Pharmaceutical Technology, Faculty of Pharmacy, University of Porto, Rua Jorge Viterbo Ferreira 228, 4050-313 Porto, Portugal; pccosta@ff.up.pt (P.C.C.)
2. Laboratory of Organic and Pharmaceutical Chemistry, Department of Chemical Sciences, Faculty of Pharmacy, University of Porto, Rua Jorge Viterbo Ferreira 228, 4050-313 Porto, Portugal
3. Associate Laboratory i4HB—Institute for Health and Bioeconomy, Faculty of Pharmacy, University of Porto, 4050-313 Porto, Portugal
4. REQUIMTE/LAQV, ISEP, Polytechnic of Porto, Rua Dr. António Bernardino de Almeida, 431, 4200-072 Porto, Portugal
5. Interdisciplinary Center of Marine and Environment Research (CIIMAR), University of Porto, Terminal dos Cruzeiros do Porto de Leixões, Avenida General Norton de Matos P, 4450-208 Matosinhos, Portugal
6. LAQV, REQUIMTE—Associated Laboratory for Green Chemistry, Department of Chemical Sciences, Faculty of Pharmacy, University of Porto, Rua Viterbo Ferreira 228, 4050-313 Porto, Portugal
* Correspondence: m_correiadasilva@ff.up.pt; Tel.: +351-22-042-8689

Abstract: Glioblastoma (GBM) is a primary malignant tumor of the central nervous system responsible for the most deaths among patients with primary brain tumors. Current therapies for GBM are not effective, with the average survival of GBM patients after diagnosis being limited to a few months. Chemotherapy is difficult in this case due to the heterogeneity of GBM and the high efficacy of the blood–brain barrier, which makes drug absorption into the brain extremely difficult. In a previous study, 3′,4′,3,4,5-trimethoxychalcone (MB) showed antiproliferative and anti-invasion activities toward GBM cells. Polymersomes (PMs) are an attractive, new type of nanoparticle for drug administration, due to their high stability, enhanced circulation time, biodegradability, and sustained drug release. In the present study, different MB formulations, PEG2000-PCL and PEG5000-PCL, were synthesized, characterized, and compared in terms of 14-day stability and in vitro cytotoxicity (hCMEC/D3 and U-373 MG).

Keywords: synthesis; chalcones; glioblastoma; nanotechnology; polymersomes

1. Introduction

More than 10 million cancer cases are reported each year, and cancer is one of the most devastating diseases [1]. Concerning brain cancer [2], approximately 189,000 individuals die annually on a global scale, and glioblastoma (GBM) is the most common and aggressive form of central nervous system tumor [3–6]. The median overall survival for GBM patients remains around 15 months [5,6]. The prognosis tends to be poor due to some treatment limitations and particularities of this disease, such as being highly invasive and non-localized, having diffuse characteristics, and poorly responding to local drug activity [4–6]. The prevalence of this ailment is more commonly observed in males over the age of 45 years than in females and younger ages [7].

The available chemotherapy is not successful due to the blood–brain barrier (BBB) efficacy as well as the heterogeneity of brain cancers [8]. The first step in the treatment of GBM is surgery, followed by radiation and combined therapy with temozolomide (TMZ). TMZ is the standard drug for chemotherapy in GBM [9], reaching "blockbuster" status in

2010 [10], after being approved by the Food and Drug Administration (FDA) in 2005 [11]. TMZ has been already incorporated into liposomes for the treatment of brain tumors [12], with nanocarriers being considered a promising strategy to treat GBM [13]. A new generation of drug delivery system (DDS), namely, polymersomes (PMs), was reported for the first time by Hammer and Discher [14], who described the physical properties of polymeric structures of poly (ethylene oxide)-block-poly (ethylene) di-block copolymers (PEO-b-PEE) that are self-assembled in aqueous environments. PMs are hollow vesicles with an internal environment that is separated from the surrounding aqueous medium by a bilayer of amphiphilic polymers [15]. PMs have emerged as a compelling novel category of nanoparticles in the field of drug delivery owing to their ability to encapsulate both hydrophilic and hydrophobic molecules within their aqueous cavity or hydrophobic membrane. These particles have better physicochemical properties than liposomes, including higher stability, enhanced circulation time, biodegradability, and sustained drug release [14]. Moreover, they can vary in dimensions and charge, and some have been already demonstrated to be biocompatible and biodegradable [16]. PMs can contain chemical groups available on their surface for conjugation with targeting moieties, without compromising their functionality. The anti-cancer drugs doxorubicin and paclitaxel were simultaneously loaded within PMs composed of poly(ethylene glycol)-poly(ε-caprolactone) PEG-PCL and poly(ethylene glycol)-poly-lactic acid PEG-PLA copolymers [17,18]. These PMs delivered these drugs to tumors implanted in mice, and a 50% size reduction in tumors was reported five days after the drug injection. Besides cancer therapy, PMs can be utilized as carriers for gene delivery, enabling the transport of genetic material such as DNA or RNA into cells. The encapsulation of nucleic acids within PMs protects them from degradation and facilitates their efficient uptake into cells, enabling gene therapy applications [19,20].

Natural and synthetic chalcones have attracted the scientific community's attention due to their broad array of reported biological activities, including antitumor activity, which is produced through the inhibition of diverse molecular targets [21–25]. Our research group has identified several chalcones with notable growth-inhibitory activities in human tumor cell lines [26–28]. Among them, 3',4',3,4,5-trimethoxychalcone (MB) was found to be one of the most potent in vitro growth inhibitors of several cancer cell lines [27]. In particular, 3',4',3,4,5-trimethoxychalcone (MB) displayed potent antiproliferative activity against different cancer cells, and this effect was associated with antimitotic activity [27]. In another work, chalcone MB inhibited the cell metabolic activity of two GBM cell cultures, i.e., human glioblastoma astrocytoma (U87) and murine glioma (GL261), more effectively than other structurally related chalcones [28]. Moreover, the non-tumor endothelial cell line bEnd.3 showed high resistance toward chalcone MB, with a decrease in metabolic activity only at 100 µM, demonstrating some selectivity of MB to GBM cell cultures and not non-tumor cell line bEnd.3 [28]. Another study assessed its ability to reduce the critical hallmark features of GBM and to induce apoptosis and cell cycle arrest and showed that MB successfully reduced the invasion and proliferation capacity of tumor cells, promoting G2/M cell cycle arrest and apoptosis in GBM cell lines [28]. Interestingly, the incorporation of MB into liposomes maintained the inhibitory activity against U 87 [28]. Nevertheless, as liposomes have some disadvantages such as low encapsulation efficiency and poor physical and chemical stability, PMs were developed in this study as alternative DDSs for the inclusion and sustained delivery of this promising anti-GBM compound. For the preparation of PMs, PEG-PCL copolymers were synthesized based on previous research methods published on the preparation of PMs and the encapsulation of anti-cancer drugs such as paclitaxel [29], docetaxel [30], and doxorubicin [31]. After the characterization of the prepared PMs, their cytotoxic effects on the growth of the most representative GBM cell line [32], U-373 MG, and on the growth of a healthy brain endothelial cell line (hCMEC/D3) were evaluated. In this study, free MB was also evaluated for the first time against these two cell lines.

2. Materials and Methods

2.1. General Information

Chalcone MB was synthesized and characterized by the Laboratory of Organic and Pharmaceutical Chemistry, Department of Chemical Sciences, Faculty of Pharmacy/CIIMAR research group, as previously described [27]. Methoxy PEG 2000, Methoxy PEG 5000, ε-caprolactone, and Sn(oct)$_2$ were acquired from Sigma-Aldrich Co. (Sintra, Portugal) and methanol (HPLC grade) from VWR chemicals. IR spectra were obtained in a KBr microplate in an FTIR spectrometer Nicolet iS 10 from Thermo Scientific with the Smart OMNI-Transmission accessory (Software OMNIC 8.3, Thermo Scientific, Madison, WI, USA). ^{1}H and ^{13}C NMR spectra were recorded in the Department of Chemistry at the University of Aveiro, Portugal, on a Bruker Avance 300 instrument (Bruker Biosciences Corporation, Billerica, MA, USA) (^{1}H: 300.13 MHz; ^{13}C: 75.47 MHz). ^{13}C NMR assignments were made in bidimensional HSQC and HMBC experiments (long-range C, H coupling constants were optimized to 7 and 1 Hz). Chemical shifts are expressed in ppm values relative to tetramethylsilane (TMS) as an internal reference and coupling constants are reported in hertz (Hz). HPLC was performed on a Dionex Ultimate 3000 (Thermo Scientific, Darmstadt, Germany).

2.2. Synthesis and Preparation of Polymersomes

The amphiphilic PEG-PCL diblock copolymer was synthesized via ring-opening polymerization using a microwave-assisted procedure. Briefly, the reaction was carried out under microwave irradiation: firstly, 2.5 g of PEG2000 and methoxyPEG5000 was dried at 120 °C and 1000 w for 10 min; then, 6.55 g ε-Caprolactone (PCL) and 10 µL Sn(oct)$_2$ were added to the dried methoxyPEG; the reaction continued at 130 °C for 25 min while stirred at 30 rpm and under 1000 w irradiation. For purification, the synthesized copolymer was dissolved in chloroform and then precipitated by adding an adequate amount of diethyl ether. This procedure was repeated three times and then the precipitate was freeze-dried to remove residual water; following that, the obtained copolymer was kept at −20 °C. The NMR spectrum of PEG-PCL diblock was acquired at room temperature in CDCl$_3$.

Self-assembled structures were prepared using the film rehydration method. Briefly, 20 mg of the copolymer and 5 mg of MB in 2 mL of dichloromethane were transferred into a round-bottomed flask. The solvent was evaporated under vacuum using a rotary evaporator. The thin, dried polymer film was hydrated through the addition of 2 mL distilled water at 60 °C and stirred continuously overnight under 1250 rpm. The polymer dispersion was sonicated for 30 min at 25 °C followed by extrusion 20 times through a homogenizer (FPG12800 Pressure Cell Homogeniser, Unit 5 New Horizon Business Center Barrows Road Harlow Essex CM19 5FN UK).

2.3. Characterization of Polymersomes

2.3.1. Particle Size and Polydispersion Index

We prepared 40 µL of PMs in 1960 µL purified water and analyzed the samples using dynamic light scattering (DLS) with a ZetaPALS apparatus (Brookhaven Instruments Corporation, Holtsville, NY, USA). The data collected, mean diameter and PDI, through PALS Particle Sizing Software (Version 5, Brookhaven Instruments Corporation, Holtsville, NY, USA) were expressed as mean ± standard deviation.

2.3.2. Thermal Behavior

MB–excipient and excipient–excipient compatibility studies were performed using a DSC 200 F3 Maia (Netzsh–Gerätebau GmbH, Selb, Germany). MB, excipients, and formulations of PMs were weighed directly in DSC aluminum pans and scanned in a range of temperatures of −40 to 340 °C under a nitrogen atmosphere with a 40 mL/min flow. A heating rate of 10 °C/min was used, and the thermograms obtained were observed for any interaction. An empty aluminum pan was used as a reference. The onset and peak maximum temperatures were calculated using Proteus Analysis software (Version 6.1,

Netzsh-Gerätebau GmbH, Selb, Germany). The DSC cell was calibrated (sensitivity and temperature) with Hg (m.p. −38.8 °C), In (m.p. 156.6 °C), Sn (m.p. 231.9 °C), Bi (m.p. 271.4 °C), Zn (m.p. 419.5 °C), and CsCl (m.p. 476.0 °C) as standards.

2.3.3. Negative-Staining Transmission Electronic Microscopy

For negative-staining transmission electron microscopy, 10 µL of samples was mounted on Formvar/carbon film-coated mesh nickel grids (Electron Microscopy Sciences, Hatfield, PA, USA) and left standing for 2 min. The liquid in excess was removed with filter paper, and 10 µL of 1% uranyl acetate was added to the grids and left standing for 10 seconds, after which the liquid in excess was removed with filter paper. Visualization was carried out on a JEOL JEM 1400 TEM at 120 kV (Tokyo, Japan). Images were digitally recorded using a CCD digital camera Orious 1100W Tokyo, Japan at the HEMS/i3S of the University of Porto. Transmission electronic microscopy was performed at the HEMS core facility at i3S, University of Porto, Portugal.

2.3.4. Entrapment Efficiency

The obtained formulations were centrifuged (4500 rpm for 15 min) (Model 5804, Eppendorf, Hauppauge, NY, USA). The supernatants were diluted in methanol (1:2) to promote the release of MB encapsulated in PMs. The obtained samples were analysed with HPLC. Chromeleon 7.2 software was used for data acquisition. The chromatographic conditions included a commercially available Acclaim^{TM} 120 C18 (100 × 4.6 mm) column with a particle size of 5 µm from Thermo Fisher Scientific (Bremen, Germany). The optimized mobile phase was water: methanol (25:75, v:v) following an isocratic flow of 1.0 mL/min for 10 min, and the temperature of the column was set at room temperature. The injection volume was 10 µL, and the detection was performed at 238 nm. A calibration curve for MB was prepared in methanol from five standard solutions: 28 µg/mL, 32 µg/mL, 40 µg/mL, 56 µg/mL and 61 µg/mL. Through interpolation of the calibration curve, the MB concentration in the supernatant was obtained. The theoretical concentration of MB was calculated considering the initial amount of MB added and the dilutions performed throughout the procedure. Thus, the encapsulation efficiency (EE) was calculated as follows:

$$EE(\%) = \frac{NPC}{TC} \times 100$$

where TC is the theoretical concentration of the MB if the entrapment efficiency is 100% (µg/mL) and NPC is the final concentration of the MB in the nanoparticle (µg/mL).

2.3.5. Stability Study

A stability study was performed for the PM formulations with and without MB. Samples were periodically evaluated regarding mean diameter and PDI at time 0 and after 1, 7 and 14 days at 4 °C.

2.3.6. MTT Cell Viability Assay

Cell reagents were purchased from Gibco (Invitrogen Corporation, Life Technologies, Renfrew, UK). Immortalized human brain capillary endothelial cells (hCMEC/D3 cell line) were kindly donated by Dr. PO Couraud (INSERM, Paris, France). The human astrocytoma U-87 MG cell line was purchased from the American Type Culture Collection (ATCC). The human glioblastoma astrocytoma derived from a malignant tumor (U-373 MG) was obtained from Sigma-Aldrich. For hCMEC/D3, U-87 MG, and U-373 MG, passages 48–49, 53–56 and 16–17 were used, respectively. Cells were cultivated as reported by and Teixeira et al. [33].

For the 3-(4,5-dimethylthiazol-2-yl)-2,5-diphenyltetrazolium bromide (MTT) assay, cells were seeded in 96-well plates (25 × 10^3 cells/mL) and exposed to different concentrations (0.1, 1, 10, 100 µM) of PEG2000-PCL, PEG5000-PCL, PEG2000-PCL-MB, PEG5000-PCL-MB, and MB for 24 h. Following the removal of the formulations from each well, cells were washed with HBSS. The number of viable cells was determined by adding MTT reagent and incubating for 3 h at 37 °C. DMSO was used to solubilize the crystals. Triton X-100 1% (w/v) and culture medium were used as negative and positive controls, respectively. The absorbance was read at 590 nm with background subtraction at 630 nm. Results were expressed as percentages of cell viability.

2.3.7. In Vitro Chalcone MB Release

In vitro chalcone MB release studies were performed using a cellulose dialysis bag diffusion technique (Spectra/Por 3 molecular porous membrane tubing) filled with 1 mL of PEG5000-PCL-MB in isotonic phosphate buffer solution (PBS) at pH 6.3. The dialysis membranes were placed in 80 mL of PBS under magnetic stirring at 100 rpm, maintained at 37 °C for 24 h. At fixed time intervals (T0, T1, T2, T3, T4, T5, T24 h), 1 mL of the PBS solutions was withdrawn and the solution obtained was analyzed using HPLC (same conditions described in Section 2.3.4). A calibration curve was prepared from seven standard solutions of MB in methanol (0.02 µg/mL, 0.05 µg/mL, 0.083 µg/mL, 0.12 µg/mL, 0.23 µg/mL, 0.55 µg/mL, and 1.32 µg/mL).

The same procedure was applied to free MB. The studies were performed in triplicate and the cumulative percentage of the released compound was determined by calculating the mean, indicating the standard deviations.

2.4. Statistical Analysis

The results are shown as the mean ± standard deviation of three batches of the same formulation (n = 3). The results of mean diameter, EE, and cell viability were statistically analyzed using ANOVA, after confirming the normality and homogeneity of the variance with the Shapiro–Wilk and Levene tests. Significance was set at $p < 0.05$. Differences between groups for ANOVA were compared with a post hoc test (Tukey's HSD), and different letters in the same sample represent significant differences between different concentrations. All the statistical analyses were performed with IBM SPSS Statistics for Windows (Version 28.0., IBM Co., Armonk, NY, USA).

3. Results

3.1. Synthesis and Characterization of PEG-PCL Diblock Copolymer

The amphiphilic PEG2000-PCL and PEG5000-PCL diblock copolymers were obtained using the ring-opening polymerization (ROP) method (Scheme 1). The most commonly used catalyst, stannous octoate ($Sn(Oct)_2$), was selected [34,35]. The macroinitiator, methoxy polyethylene glycol (methoxyPEG2000 and methoxyPEG2000), was dried at 120 °C with microwave irradiation [36] and ε-caprolactone (PCL) was then added [37–39].

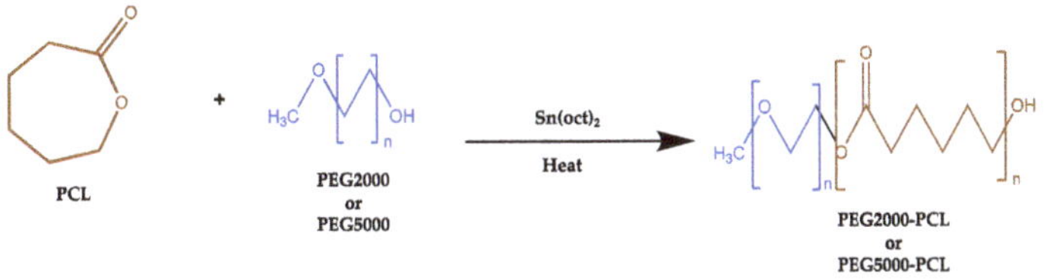

Scheme 1. Synthesis of PEG2000-PCL and PEG5000-PCL through ring-opening polymerization. PCL, ε-caprolactone.

The structure of the diblock copolymers was established using ^{1}H and ^{13}C NMR (Figure 1), according to Zavvar, T. et al. [40]. The characteristic OCH_2CH_2O of the PEG block was assigned to the chemical shift at δ_H 3.6 ppm (green, Figure 1). The triplet at δ_H 4.1 ppm was assigned to the CH_2 alpha carbonyl of the PCL block (blue, Figure 1). The -CH_2 CH_2 CH_2- protons of the PCL block appeared at δ_H 1.6 (grey, Figure 1) and 1.4 ppm (purple, Figure 1) as multiplets. Figure 2 shows the ^{13}C NMR spectrum of the

PEG5000-PCL di-block. Regarding the PEG segment, the aliphatic carbons were detected at δ_C 77.4 and 77.3 ppm (green, Figure 2) and the methylene carbon at δ_C 64.2 ppm (yellow). Regarding the PCL segment, the signals at δ_C 173.6 (red), 76.8 (grey), and 34.2 (blue) ppm were assigned to the carbonyl of the ester -COO-, the carbon linked to the hydroxy, and the CH_2 alpha carbonyl groups, respectively. The signals of aliphatic carbons were observed at δ_C 28.4, 25.6, and 24.7 ppm (pink).

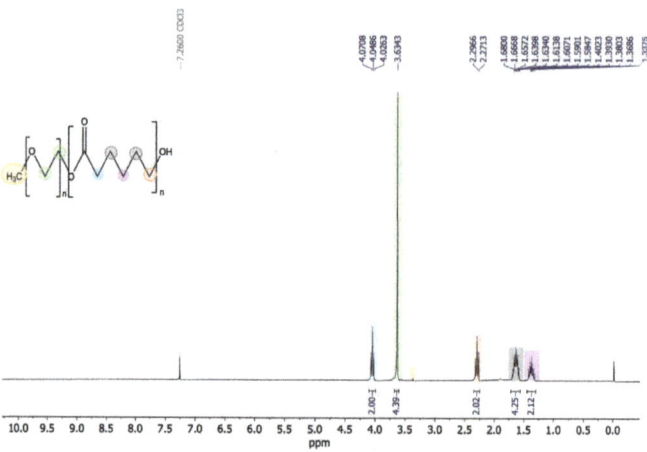

Figure 1. ^{1}H NMR spectrum (CDCl$_3$) of PEG5000-PCL copolymers.

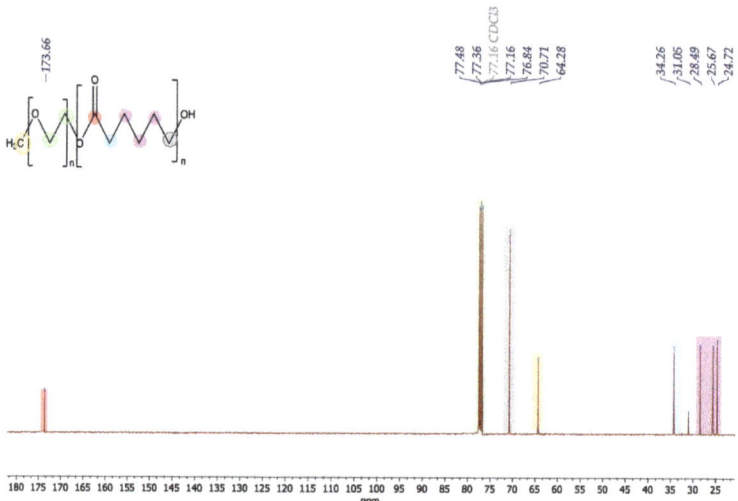

Figure 2. ^{13}C NMR spectrum (CDCl$_3$) of PEG5000-PCL copolymers.

When using Equation (2) to calculate the number of monomers (NMs), we can see that the reaction proceeded successfully, with PEG2000-PCL presenting 45 monomers of PEG2000 and 83 monomers of PCL, while PEG5000-PCL presents 114 monomers of PEG5000 and 108 of PCL. This shows that the polymerization of ε-caprolactone occurred.

$$NM = (\int CL)/[(\text{Protons of CL}/\text{Protons of PEG}) \times \int PEG] \times Mw\ PCL$$

where $\int CL$ = sum of NMR signals of CL (10.39); Mw PCL = molecular weight of PCL (114 g/mol); Protons of CL = number of theoretical protons of one unit of CL (10); Protons of PEG = number of theoretical protons of one unit of PEG (4); $\int PEG$ = sum of NMR signals of PEG (4.39).

3.2. Particle Size and Polydispersion Index

The mean diameter and polydispersion index (PDI) of PMs are summarized in Table 1. Overall, the mean diameter was less than 200 nm. Empty PEG2000-PCL PMs were larger than PEG5000-PCL PMs, at 128.56 nm and 112.13 nm, respectively. The presence of MB in the PEG5000-PCL and PEG2000-PCL PMs increased the mean diameter of the particles ($p > 0.05$). The ability of particles to effectively travel to the interstitial space through tumor vessel walls depends on the particle size/opening size ratio. In general, the decrease in the particle size improves the transport through tumor vessel walls. A decrease in nanoparticle size is observed with higher molecular weight of the polymer, due to lipophilicity increase in the polymer with the molecular weight [41,42]. Due to the rapid and irregular angiogenesis of tumor tissues, fenestrations and deterioration of blood vessels are common [43,44]. These are open doors for smaller particles; therefore, the smaller the PMs, the greater the possibility of leaking into the tumor interstitial fluid, leading to accumulation and eventually destruction of tumor cells.

Table 1. Effective mean diameter and PDI for PM particles of diblock copolymers prepared using the film rehydration method.

Formulation	Effective Mean Diameter (nm)	PDI
PEG2000-PCL	129 ± 2	0.369 ± 0.002
PEG2000-PCL-MB	192 ± 7	0.317 ± 0.010
PEG5000-PCL	112.1 ± 0.9	0.168 ± 0.009
PEG5000-PCL-MB	224 ± 6	0.284 ± 0.001

PEG = methoxy polyethylene glycol; PCL = ε-caprolactone; PDI = polydispersion index. Values are expressed as mean ± standard deviation (n = 3).

The PDI values of 0.1 to 0.3 represent nearly monodisperse preparation, whereas PDI > 0.4 suggests a broad distribution of macromolecular sizes in solution [45]. For all formulations studied, the PDI was less than or around 0.3, which is generally indicated as a limit for monodisperse preparations.

3.2.1. Thermal Behavior

DSC thermograms of the PM components are shown in Figure 3A. For the PEG2000 and PEG5000, the onset temperatures were 52 °C and 60 °C and the maximum temperature peaks were 59 °C and 67 °C, respectively. Regarding PCL, the onset was −11 °C and the maximum temperature peak was 3 °C. For the PEG2000-PCL copolymer, the onset and maximum temperatures for the first peak were 32 °C and 44 °C, respectively, and for the second peak were 51 °C and 53 °C, respectively. For PEG5000-PCL, the onset temperatures were 52 °C and 55 °C and the maximum peak temperatures were 52 °C and 59 °C. Here, the different onsets indicate that the crystalline structure was modified for both PCL and PEG. The onset of pure MB was 126 °C and the maximum temperature peak was 130 °C. The PM formulations with MB are shown in Figure 3B. PEG2000-PCL-MB and PEG5000-PCL-MB presented only a peak with the onset, at 48 °C and 53 °C, respectively. These results suggest that MB is molecularly dispersed in the formulations, which can be attested by the absence of its maximum peak. Overall, there was a significant change in the crystalline forms of PEG2000-PCL and PEG5000-PCL with the inclusion of MB.

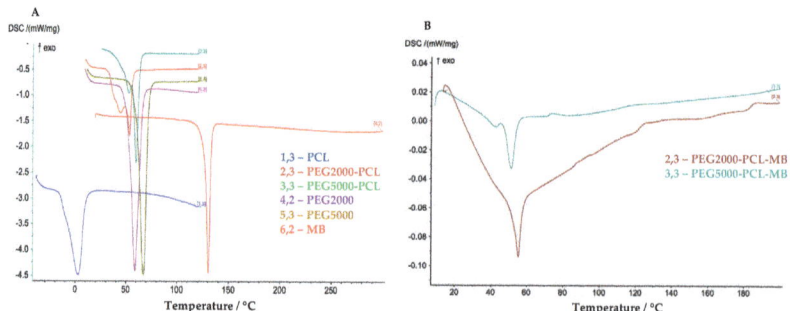

Figure 3. A mixture of empty diblock PMs and their constituents (**A**) and diblock PMs with MB (**B**). PCL—ε-caprolactone; MB—3′,4′,3,4,5-trimethoxychalcone.

3.2.2. Negative-Staining Transmission Electron Microscopic Study

The transmission electron microscopy (TEM) technique was used for imaging the PMs prepared with the film rehydration method to evaluate their morphology.

Figure 4A shows a circular shape for the PEG5000-PCL PMs. The size was verified using DLS. In Figure 4B, it is possible to observe that the inclusion of MB does not interfere with the shape or size of the PMs.

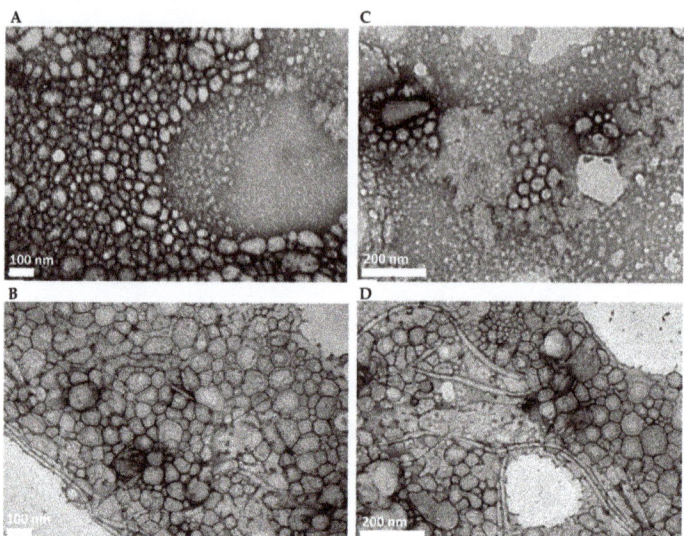

Figure 4. TEM images of PMs formed through film rehydration: (**A**) PEG5000-PCL; (**B**) PEG5000-PCL-MB; (**C**) PEG2000-PCL; (**D**) PEG2000-PCL-MB.

Regarding the PEG2000-PCL (Figure 4C) and the PEG2000-PCL-MB (Figure 4D) PMs, the morphology of the particles remains spherical and there is no evidence that MB alters their shape.

3.2.3. Entrapment Efficiency

The entrapment efficiency (EE) of chalcone MB in PMs was determined through indirect measurement of the compound that was encapsulated in the formulation, as conducted via HPLC. Data were fitted to the least squares linear regression, and a calibration curve was obtained: $y = 0.0534x - 0.8284$. The correlation coefficient was 0.9997, which demonstrates the good linearity in the tested range for MB. Both PMs of PEG5000-PCL-MB and PEG2000-PCL-MB had high EE (98% and 83%, respectively).

3.2.4. Stability Study

The aqueous formulations were stored at 4 °C and showed no relevant change after 1, 7 and 14 days, indicating the stability of the prepared PMs (Figure 5).

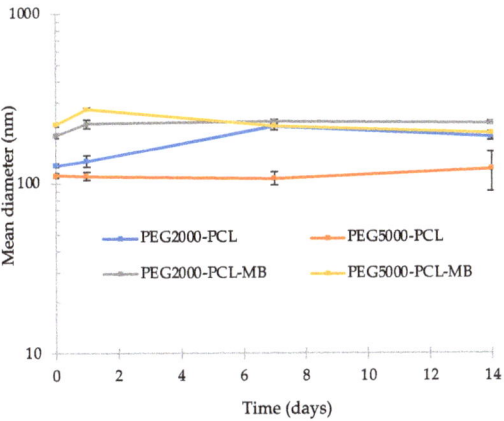

Figure 5. Effective diameter of diblock copolymers PMs, with and without MB, from the day of their production to 1, 7, and 14 days at 4 °C. Values are expressed as mean ± standard deviation (n = 3).

After 1 day, the PEG5000-PCL-MB PMs increased in mean diameter from 223.83 nm to 277.27 nm (p = 0.0002), while after 7 days, a mean diameter of 218.87 nm (p = 0.0013) was observed. Nevertheless, after 14 days, the particles with and without MB showed sizes of 199.10 nm (p = 0.050) and 122.06 nm (p = 0.482), respectively. For the PEG5000-PCL PMs, the mean diameter without MB did not show significant differences over time (p = 0.444).

Concerning PEG2000-PCL-MB PMs, after 1 day of their preparation, the mean diameter increased from 191.87 nm to 225.77 nm (p = 0.014); after 7 days, the formulations showed a mean diameter of 232.37 nm (p = 0.478); and after 14 days, the mean diameter was 227.83 nm (p = 0.398). PEG2000-PCL PMs without MB did not present significant differences (p = 0.323) after 1 day of their preparation. However, after 7 days, the mean diameter increased from 135.83 nm to 218.73 nm (p = 0.0006). After 14 days, the particles then showed a mean diameter of 165.87 nm (p = 0.155).

3.2.5. Cell Viability Assay

The viability of the glioblastoma U-373 MG cell line and brain endothelial cell line hCMEC/D3 after exposure to PEG2000-PCL and PEG5000-PCL PMs, with and without MB, was evaluated using an MTT assay and compared with the free compound. The U-373 MG cell line was selected for this work since it is a more representative cellular line of the GBM compared to U87 [32].

The free compound decreased the viability of the glioblastoma cell line at all tested concentrations (0.1 μM (18.41% ± 4.77), 1 μM (10.70% ± 3.81), 10 μM (8.67% ± 4.37), and 100 μM (3.01% ± 1.91)), while we only observed a decrease in the brain endothelial cell viability at the highest concentrations tested (10 μM (50.54% ± 9.06) and 100 μM (26.15% ± 3.15)) (Figure 6).

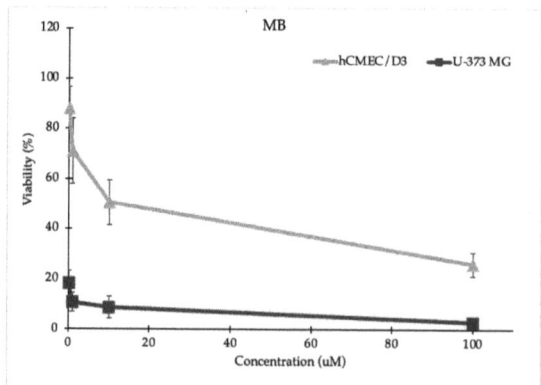

Figure 6. Viability of hCMEC/D3 and U-373MG cell lines (MTT assay) after exposure to different concentrations of MB. Values are expressed as mean ± standard deviation (n = 3).

The encapsulation of MB on PMs of PEG2000-PCL and PEG5000-PCL protected the brain endothelial cells from the cytotoxic effect of MB (Figure 7A), while the cell growth of glioblastoma cells decreased significantly at concentrations $\geq$ 0.01 mg/mL (Figure 7B). The IC$_{50}$ values of PEG2000-PCL-MB and PEG5000-PCL-MB PMs for U-373 MG were 0.093 mg/mL and 0.067 mg/mL, respectively. It is important to highlight that the cell growth of brain endothelial cell lines was not affected in the presence of empty PMs, at any concentration.

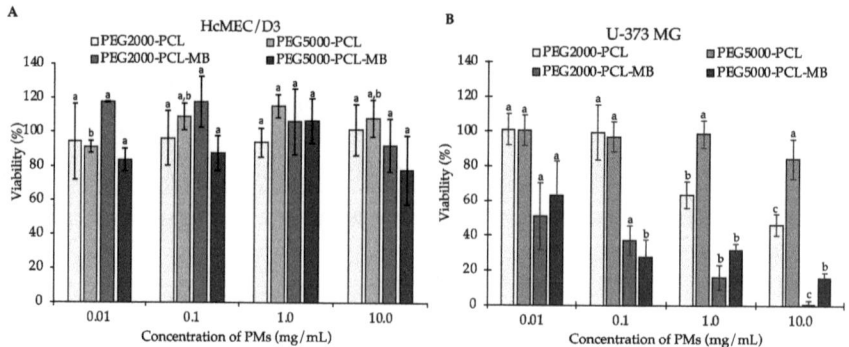

Figure 7. Viability of hCMEC/D3 and U-373MG cell lines (MTT assay) after exposure to different concentrations of PMs with and without MB on the viability of hCMEC/D3 (**A**) and U-373 MG (**B**) cell lines. Values are expressed as mean ± standard deviation (n = 3). Different letters (a,b,c) in the same sample represent significant differences ($p < 0.05$) between different concentrations, according to Tukey's HSD test.

Overall, the prepared PMs were able to preserve the viability of the hCMEC/D3 brain endothelial cell lines, which were affected in the presence of free MB, increasing the selectivity for the glioblastoma cell line.

3.2.6. In Vitro Chalcone MB Release

An in vitro release study of chalcone MB was performed to evaluate the release of the compound from PMs of PEG5000-PCL at pH 6.3 (GBM pHs) over time up to 24 h. Between 0 h and 5 h, slowly increasing amounts of free MB were detected in the outer phase of the membrane bag containing PEG5000-PCL-MB (Figure 8). Moreover, the amount of MB detected in the outer phase of the membrane bag containing PEG5000-PCL-MB was lower than the amount detected when free MB was placed in the bag. The sustained release of lipophilic drugs, such as MB, can be attributed to its entrapment in the hydrophobic part of the PMs (Figure 9) [46]. In vitro studies have shown that drug release depends on the block length of the hydrophobic segment and the crystallinity of the copolymer [47]. PMs have a much slower drug release rate, which is dependent on block length. Certain drugs have been found to release up to 90% after 20 days [47]. Another study showed that the maximum drug release was obtained after a period of 120 h [48].

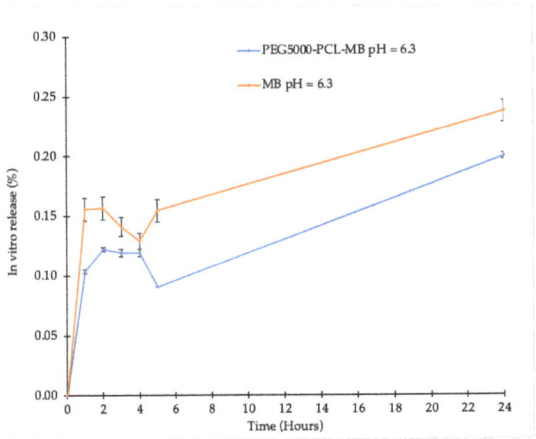

Figure 8. Chalcone MB detected through HPLC in the outer phase of dialysis bags containing free MB or PEG5000-PCL PMs, at pH = 6.3 and 37 °C. Values are expressed as mean ± standard deviation ($n = 3$).

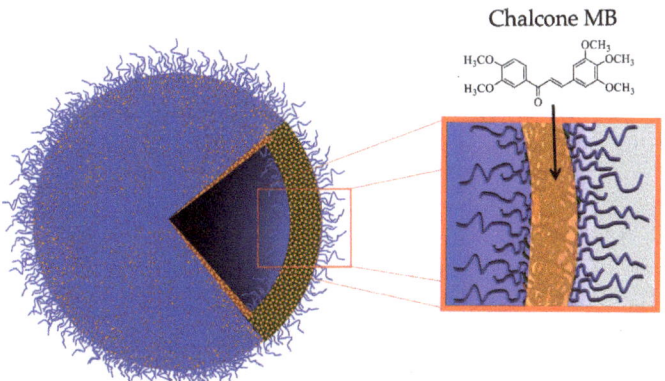

Figure 9. Representation of PM and the chalcone MB.

4. Conclusions

In a previous work, the chalcone derivative MB was successfully incorporated into liposomes, while maintaining an inhibitory activity against glioblastoma cell lines. Considering that liposomes have some disadvantages related to low encapsulation efficiency, poor physical and chemical stability, as well as low chemical versatility, more stable particles were obtained in this work—polymersomes (PMs). Diblocks were successfully synthesized via ROP. PEG5000-PCL and PEG2000-PCL PMs showed a mean diameter of about 200 nm. The stability of PMs was tested, and PEG5000-PCL PMs showed no significant changes after 1, 7, and 14 days, while PEG2000-PCL PMs were slightly modified over time. Both formulations presented spherical particles, with a uniform morphology and similar size. Moreover, both formulations exhibited high EE. The chalcone MB displayed cytotoxicity at 10 and 100 µM in the HcMEC/D3 cell line, while the PEG2000-PCL and PEG5000-PCL PMs, with and without MB, did not show any cytotoxicity for this healthy brain endothelial cell line. On the other hand, the PEG2000-PCL-MB and PEG5000-PCL-MB PMs maintained cytotoxicity against the U-373MG glioblastoma cell line at all tested concentrations. Therefore, the prepared PMs with MB were highly selective for the glioblastoma cell line. PMs with the chalcone MB released this compound at pH 6.3; however, a sustained release was observed. This can be attributed to the drug entrapment in the hydrophobic part of the PM.

Overall, the prepared PMs seem highly attractive nanocarriers for the sustained release of MB. In the future, the crossing of the BBB by these PMs may be studied and, if needed, BBB permeation can be optimized by functionalizing these PMs with transferrin.

Author Contributions: Conceptualization, P.C.C. and M.C.-d.-S.; methodology, C.N., S.R., F.R., H.C., M.P., P.C.C. and M.C.-d.-S.; validation, A.A., F.R., P.C.C. and M.C.-d.-S.; formal analysis, A.A., F.R., P.C.C. and M.C.-d.-S.; investigation, A.A., A.M.S. and J.M.; data curation, A.A., A.M.S. and J.M.; writing—original draft preparation, A.A., F.R., C.N., P.C.C. and M.C.-d.-S.; writing—review and editing, F.R., H.C., M.C.-d.-S., P.C.C., D.F., S.R. and M.P.; supervision, M.C.-d.-S., P.C.C. and D.F.; project administration, M.C.-d.-S.; funding acquisition, D.F. All authors have read and agreed to the published version of the manuscript.

Funding: This research was funded by national funds from FCT—Fundação para a Ciência e a Tecnologia (I.P.) in the scope of the projects UIDP/04378/2020 and UIDB/04378/2020 (Marine Natural Products and Medicinal Chemistry Group_CIIMAR), of the Research Unit on Applied Molecular Biosciences—UCIBIO, and the project LA/P/0140/2020 of the Associate Laboratory Institute for Health and Bioeconomy—i4HB. A.A. acknowledges FCT for its PhD scholarship (grant number SFRH/BD/144607/2019) and A.M.S. is thankful for its PhD grant (SFRH/BD/144994/2019). Francisca Rodrigues (CEECIND/01886/2020) is thankful for her contract financed by FCT/MCTES (CEEC Individual Program Contract). The authors acknowledge the support of the i3S Scientific Platform HEMS, which is part of the national infrastructure PPBI—Portuguese Platform of Bioimaging (PPBI-POCI-01-0145-FEDER-022122).

Institutional Review Board Statement: Not applicable.

Informed Consent Statement: Not applicable.

Data Availability Statement: Data are contained within this article.

Acknowledgments: The authors acknowledge Ana Rita Malheiro and Rui Fernandes for their assistance with TEM performance (HEMS core facility at i3S, University of Porto, Portugal).

Conflicts of Interest: The authors declare no conflicts of interest.

References

1. Petersen, P.E. Oral cancer prevention and control—The approach of the World Health Organization. *Oral Oncol.* **2009**, *45*, 454–460. [CrossRef] [PubMed]
2. Ferlay, J.; Soerjomataram, I.; Dikshit, R.; Eser, S.; Mathers, C.; Rebelo, M.; Parkin, D.M.; Forman, D.; Bray, F. Cancer incidence and mortality worldwide: Sources, methods and major patterns in GLOBOCAN 2012. *Int. J. Cancer* **2015**, *136*, E359–E386. [CrossRef] [PubMed]
3. Louis, D.N.; Perry, A.; Reifenberger, G.; Von Deimling, A.; Figarella-Branger, D.; Cavenee, W.K.; Ohgaki, H.; Wiestler, O.D.; Kleihues, P.; Ellison, D.W. The 2016 World Health Organization Classification of Tumors of the Central Nervous System: A summary. *Acta Neuropathol.* **2016**, *131*, 803–820. [CrossRef] [PubMed]
4. Martins, S.M.; Sarmento, B.; Nunes, C.; Lucio, M.; Reis, S.; Ferreira, D.C. Brain targeting effect of camptothecin-loaded solid lipid nanoparticles in rat after intravenous administration. *Eur. J. Pharm. Biopharm.* **2013**, *85*, 488–502. [CrossRef] [PubMed]
5. Vieira de Castro, J.; Gomes, E.D.; Granja, S.; Anjo, S.I.; Baltazar, F.; Manadas, B.; Salgado, A.J.; Costa, B.M. Impact of mesenchymal stem cells' secretome on glioblastoma pathophysiology. *J. Transl. Med.* **2017**, *15*, 200. [CrossRef]
6. Goncalves, C.S.; Vieira de Castro, J.; Pojo, M.; Martins, E.P.; Queiros, S.; Chautard, E.; Taipa, R.; Pires, M.M.; Pinto, A.A.; Pardal, F.; et al. WNT6 is a novel oncogenic prognostic biomarker in human glioblastoma. *Theranostics* **2018**, *8*, 4805–4823. [CrossRef]
7. Chandana, S.R.; Movva, S.; Arora, M.; Singh, T. Primary brain tumors in adults. *Am. Fam. Physician* **2008**, *77*, 1423–1430.

8. Yan, H.; Wang, L.; Wang, J.; Weng, X.; Lei, H.; Wang, X.; Jiang, L.; Zhu, J.; Lu, W.; Wei, X.; et al. Two-order targeted brain tumor imaging by using an optical/paramagnetic nanoprobe across the blood brain barrier. *ACS Nano* **2012**, *6*, 410–420. [CrossRef]
9. Arora, A.; Somasundaram, K. Glioblastoma vs temozolomide: Can the red queen race be won? *Cancer Biol. Ther.* **2019**, *20*, 1083–1090. [CrossRef]
10. Moody, C.L.; Wheelhouse, R.T. The medicinal chemistry of imidazotetrazine prodrugs. *Pharmaceuticals* **2014**, *7*, 797–838. [CrossRef]
11. Jatyan, R.; Singh, P.; Sahel, D.K.; Karthik, Y.G.; Mittal, A.; Chitkara, D. Polymeric and small molecule-conjugates of temozolomide as improved therapeutic agents for glioblastoma multiforme. *J. Control. Release Off. J. Control. Release Soc.* **2022**, *350*, 494–513. [CrossRef] [PubMed]
12. Zhan, W. Delivery of liposome encapsulated temozolomide to brain tumour: Understanding the drug transport for optimisation. *Int. J. Pharm.* **2019**, *557*, 280–292. [CrossRef] [PubMed]
13. Glaser, T.; Han, I.; Wu, L.; Zeng, X. Targeted Nanotechnology in Glioblastoma Multiforme. *Front. Pharmacol.* **2017**, *8*, 166. [CrossRef] [PubMed]
14. Discher, B.M.; Won, Y.Y.; Ege, D.S.; Lee, J.C.; Bates, F.S.; Discher, D.E.; Hammer, D.A. Polymersomes: Tough vesicles made from diblock copolymers. *Science* **1999**, *284*, 1143–1146. [CrossRef]
15. Figueiredo, P.; Balasubramanian, V.; Shahbazi, M.A.; Correia, A.; Wu, D.; Palivan, C.G.; Hirvonen, J.T.; Santos, H.A. Angiopep2-functionalized polymersomes for targeted doxorubicin delivery to glioblastoma cells. *Int. J. Pharm.* **2016**, *511*, 794–803. [CrossRef]
16. Lee, J.S.; Feijen, J. Polymersomes for drug delivery: Design, formation and characterization. *J. Control. Release Off. J. Control. Release Soc.* **2012**, *161*, 473–483. [CrossRef]
17. Ahmed, F.; Pakunlu, R.I.; Srinivas, G.; Brannan, A.; Bates, F.; Klein, M.L.; Minko, T.; Discher, D.E. Shrinkage of a rapidly growing tumor by drug-loaded polymersomes: pH-triggered release through copolymer degradation. *Mol. Pharm.* **2006**, *3*, 340–350. [CrossRef]
18. Ahmed, F.; Pakunlu, R.I.; Brannan, A.; Bates, F.; Minko, T.; Discher, D.E. Biodegradable polymersomes loaded with both paclitaxel and doxorubicin permeate and shrink tumors, inducing apoptosis in proportion to accumulated drug. *J. Control. Release Off. J. Control. Release Soc.* **2006**, *116*, 150–158. [CrossRef]
19. Spain, S.G.; Yaşayan, G.; Soliman, M.; Heath, F.; Saeed, A.O.; Alexander, C. 4.424—Nanoparticles for Nucleic Acid Delivery. In *Comprehensive Biomaterials*; Ducheyne, P., Ed.; Elsevier: Oxford, UK, 2011; pp. 389–410.
20. Aguilar, Z.P. Chapter 5—Targeted Drug Delivery. In *Nanomaterials for Medical Applications*; Aguilar, Z.P., Ed.; Elsevier: Amsterdam, The Netherlands, 2013; pp. 181–234.
21. Moreira, J.; Almeida, J.; Saraiva, L.; Cidade, H.; Pinto, M. Chalcones as Promising Antitumor Agents by Targeting the p53 Pathway: An Overview and New Insights in Drug-Likeness. *Molecules* **2021**, *26*, 3737. [CrossRef]
22. Thapa, P.; Upadhyay, S.P.; Suo, W.Z.; Singh, V.; Gurung, P.; Lee, E.S.; Sharma, R.; Sharma, M. Chalcone and its analogs: Therapeutic and diagnostic applications in Alzheimer's disease. *Bioorg. Chem.* **2021**, *108*, 104681. [CrossRef]
23. Kar Mahapatra, D.; Asati, V.; Bharti, S.K. An updated patent review of therapeutic applications of chalcone derivatives (2014-present). *Expert. Opin. Ther. Pat.* **2019**, *29*, 385–406. [CrossRef] [PubMed]
24. Rammohan, A.; Reddy, J.S.; Sravya, G.; Rao, C.N.; Zyryanov, G.V. Chalcone synthesis, properties and medicinal applications: A review. *Environ. Chem. Lett.* **2020**, *18*, 433–458. [CrossRef]
25. Jasim, H.A.; Nahar, L.; Jasim, M.A.; Moore, S.A.; Ritchie, K.J.; Sarker, S.D. Chalcones: Synthetic Chemistry Follows Where Nature Leads. *Biomolecules* **2021**, *11*, 1203. [CrossRef]
26. Fonseca, J.; Marques, S.; Silva, P.M.; Brandão, P.; Cidade, H.; Pinto, M.M.; Bousbaa, H. Prenylated Chalcone 2 Acts as an Antimitotic Agent and Enhances the Chemosensitivity of Tumor Cells to Paclitaxel. *Molecules* **2016**, *21*, 982. [CrossRef]
27. Pinto, P.; Machado, C.M.; Moreira, J.; Almeida, J.D.P.; Silva, P.M.A.; Henriques, A.C.; Soares, J.X.; Salvador, J.A.R.; Afonso, C.; Pinto, M.; et al. Chalcone derivatives targeting mitosis: Synthesis, evaluation of antitumor activity and lipophilicity. *Eur. J. Med. Chem.* **2019**, *184*, 111752. [CrossRef] [PubMed]
28. Mendanha, D.; Vieira de Castro, J.; Moreira, J.; Costa, B.M.; Cidade, H.; Pinto, M.; Ferreira, H.; Neves, N.M. A New Chalcone Derivative with Promising Antiproliferative and Anti-Invasion Activities in Glioblastoma Cells. *Molecules* **2021**, *26*, 3383. [CrossRef] [PubMed]
29. Zhang, L.; Zhu, D.; Dong, X.; Sun, H.; Song, C.; Wang, C.; Kong, D. Folate-modified lipid-polymer hybrid nanoparticles for targeted paclitaxel delivery. *Int. J. Nanomed.* **2015**, *10*, 2101–2114. [CrossRef]
30. Conte, C.; Moret, F.; Esposito, D.; Dal Poggetto, G.; Avitabile, C.; Ungaro, F.; Romanelli, A.; Laurienzo, P.; Reddi, E.; Quaglia, F. Biodegradable nanoparticles exposing a short anti-FLT1 peptide as antiangiogenic platform to complement docetaxel anticancer activity. *Mater. Sci. Eng. C* **2019**, *102*, 876–886. [CrossRef]
31. Hu, C.; Fan, F.; Qin, Y.; Huang, C.; Zhang, Z.; Guo, Q.; Zhang, X.; Pang, X.; Ou-Yang, W.; Zhao, K.; et al. Redox-Sensitive Folate-Conjugated Polymeric Nanoparticles for Combined Chemotherapy and Photothermal Therapy Against Breast Cancer. *J. Biomed. Nanotechnol.* **2018**, *14*, 2018–2030. [CrossRef]
32. Allen, M.; Bjerke, M.; Edlund, H.; Nelander, S.; Westermark, B. Origin of the U87MG glioma cell line: Good news and bad news. *Sci. Transl. Med.* **2016**, *8*, 354re353. [CrossRef]
33. Teixeira, M.I.; Lopes, C.M.; Gonçalves, H.; Catita, J.; Silva, A.M.; Rodrigues, F.; Amaral, M.H.; Costa, P.C. Formulation, Characterization, and Cytotoxicity Evaluation of Lactoferrin Functionalized Lipid Nanoparticles for Riluzole Delivery to the Brain. *Pharmaceutics* **2022**, *14*, 185. [CrossRef] [PubMed]

34. Alibolandi, M.; Sadeghi, F.; Sazmand, S.H.; Shahrokhi, S.M.; Seifi, M.; Hadizadeh, F. Synthesis and self-assembly of biodegradable polyethylene glycol-poly (lactic acid) diblock copolymers as polymersomes for preparation of sustained release system of doxorubicin. *Int. J. Pharm. Investig.* **2015**, *5*, 134–141. [CrossRef] [PubMed]
35. Deng, Y.; Chen, H.; Tao, X.; Trépout, S.; Ling, J.; Li, M.-H. Synthesis and self-assembly of poly(ethylene glycol)-block-poly(N-3-(methylthio)propyl glycine) and their oxidation-sensitive polymersomes. *Chin. Chem. Lett.* **2019**, *31*, 1931–1935. [CrossRef]
36. Meng, F.; Engbers, G.H.M.; Feijen, J. Biodegradable polymersomes as a basis for artificial cells: Encapsulation, release and targeting. *J. Control. Release* **2005**, *101*, 187–198. [CrossRef] [PubMed]
37. Ahmed, F.; Hategan, A.; Discher, D.E.; Discher, B.M. Block Copolymer Assemblies with Cross-Link Stabilization: From Single-Component Monolayers to Bilayer Blends with PEO−PLA. *Langmuir* **2003**, *19*, 6505–6511. [CrossRef]
38. Hruska, Z.; Hurtrez, G.; Walter, S.; Riess, G. An improved technique of the cumylpotassium preparation: Application in the synthesis of spectroscopically pure polystyrene-poly(ethylene oxide) diblock copolymers. *Polymer* **1992**, *33*, 2447–2449. [CrossRef]
39. Shahriari, M.; Taghdisi, S.M.; Abnous, K.; Ramezani, M.; Alibolandi, M. Synthesis of hyaluronic acid-based polymersomes for doxorubicin delivery to metastatic breast cancer. *Int. J. Pharm.* **2019**, *572*, 118835. [CrossRef]
40. Zavvar, T.; Babaei, M.; Abnous, K.; Taghdisi, S.M.; Nekooei, S.; Ramezani, M.; Alibolandi, M. Synthesis of multimodal polymersomes for targeted drug delivery and MR/fluorescence imaging in metastatic breast cancer model. *Int. J. Pharm.* **2020**, *578*, 119091. [CrossRef]
41. Altmeyer, C.; Karam, T.K.; Khalil, N.M.; Mainardes, R.M. Tamoxifen-loaded poly(L-lactide) nanoparticles: Development, characterization and in vitro evaluation of cytotoxicity. *Mater. Sci. Eng. C Mater. Biol. Appl.* **2016**, *60*, 135–142. [CrossRef]
42. Musumeci, T.; Ventura, C.A.; Giannone, I.; Ruozi, B.; Montenegro, L.; Pignatello, R.; Puglisi, G. PLA/PLGA nanoparticles for sustained release of docetaxel. *Int. J. Pharm.* **2006**, *325*, 172–179. [CrossRef]
43. Adepu, S.; Ramakrishna, S. Controlled Drug Delivery Systems: Current Status and Future Directions. *Molecules* **2021**, *26*, 5905. [CrossRef] [PubMed]
44. Kargozar, S.; Baino, F.; Hamzehlou, S.; Hamblin, M.R.; Mozafari, M. Nanotechnology for angiogenesis: Opportunities and challenges. *Chem. Soc. Rev.* **2020**, *49*, 5008–5057. [CrossRef] [PubMed]
45. Bartenstein, J.E.; Robertson, J.; Battaglia, G.; Briscoe, W.H. Stability of polymersomes prepared by size exclusion chromatography and extrusion. *Colloids Surf. A Physicochem. Eng. Asp.* **2016**, *506*, 739–746. [CrossRef]
46. Wu, D.Q.; Chu, C.C. Biodegradable hydrophobic-hydrophilic hybrid hydrogels: Swelling behavior and controlled drug release. *J. Biomater. Sci. Polym. Ed.* **2008**, *19*, 411–429. [CrossRef]
47. Tamboli, V.; Mishra, G.P.; Mitra, A.K. Novel pentablock copolymer (PLA-PCL-PEG-PCL-PLA) based nanoparticles for controlled drug delivery: Effect of copolymer compositions on the crystallinity of copolymers and in vitro drug release profile from nanoparticles. *Colloid. Polym. Sci.* **2013**, *291*, 1235–1245. [CrossRef]
48. Danafar, H. Preparation and Characterization of PCL-PEG-PCL Copolymeric Nanoparticles as Polymersomes for Delivery Hydrophilic Drugs. *Iran. J. Pharm. Sci.* **2018**, *14*, 21–32. [CrossRef]

Disclaimer/Publisher's Note: The statements, opinions and data contained in all publications are solely those of the individual author(s) and contributor(s) and not of MDPI and/or the editor(s). MDPI and/or the editor(s) disclaim responsibility for any injury to people or property resulting from any ideas, methods, instructions or products referred to in the content.

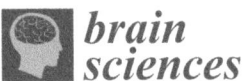

Article

Actin Alpha 2, Smooth Muscle (ACTA2) Is Involved in the Migratory Potential of Malignant Gliomas, and Its Increased Expression at Recurrence Is a Significant Adverse Prognostic Factor

Takumi Hoshimaru [1], Naosuke Nonoguchi [1,*], Takuya Kosaka [1], Motomasa Furuse [1], Shinji Kawabata [1], Ryokichi Yagi [1], Yoshitaka Kurisu [2], Hideki Kashiwagi [1], Masahiro Kameda [1], Toshihiro Takami [1], Yuko Kataoka-Sasaki [3], Masanori Sasaki [3], Osamu Honmou [3], Ryo Hiramatsu [1,†] and Masahiko Wanibuchi [1,†]

1 Department of Neurosurgery, Osaka Medical and Pharmaceutical University, Osaka 569-8686, Japan
2 Department of Pathology, Osaka Medical and Pharmaceutical University, Osaka 569-8686, Japan
3 Department of Neural Regenerative Medicine, Research Institute for Frontier Medicine, Sapporo Medical University School of Medicine, Hokkaido 060-8556, Japan
* Correspondence: naosuke.nonoguchi@ompu.ac.jp; Tel.: +81-72-683-1221
† These authors contributed equally to this work.

Abstract: Malignant glioma is a highly invasive tumor, and elucidating the glioma invasion mechanism is essential for developing novel therapies. We aimed to highlight actin alpha 2, smooth muscle (ACTA2) as potential biomarkers of brain invasion and distant recurrence in malignant gliomas. Using the human malignant glioma cell line, U251MG, we generated ACTA2 knockdown (KD) cells treated with small interfering RNA, and the cell motility and proliferation of the ACTA2 KD group were analyzed. Furthermore, tumor samples from 12 glioma patients who underwent reoperation at the time of tumor recurrence were utilized to measure ACTA2 expression in the tumors before and after recurrence. Thereafter, we examined how ACTA2 expression correlates with the time to tumor recurrence and the mode of recurrence. The results showed that the ACTA2 KD group demonstrated a decline in the mean motion distance and proliferative capacity compared to the control group. In the clinical glioma samples, ACTA2 expression was remarkably increased in recurrent samples compared to the primary samples from the same patients, and the higher the change in ACTCA2 expression from the start to relapse, the shorter the progression-free survival. In conclusion, ACTA2 may be involved in distant recurrence in clinical gliomas.

Keywords: high-grade glioma; actin alpha 2; smooth muscle (ACTA2); actin alpha; cardiac muscle 1 (ACTC1); cytoskeleton; cell migration; recurrence

1. Introduction

Malignant gliomas are characterized by aggressive tumor cell proliferation and a poor prognosis despite treatments, such as surgical resection, radiotherapy, and chemotherapy, with reported 5-year survival rates of approximately 4.7–10.1% for World Health Organization (WHO) grade 4 glioblastomas (GBM) [1,2]. Patients with malignant gliomas present with frequent recurrences not only locally but also in distant areas of the brain [3]. One of the factors limiting complete surgical resection and causing poor prognosis is attributed to glioma cell infiltration. Many studies have reported on the invasion of malignant gliomas; for example, malignant glioma cells modify the extracellular matrix (ECM) by releasing matrix metalloproteinases (MMPs) and coding and non-coding RNAs via extracellular vesicles, thereby remodeling it into an environment more stable for invasion [4–6]. Elucidating the mechanisms controlling the invasion and recurrence of malignant gliomas holds great promise for improving prognosis.

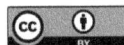

In this study, we focused on actin family genes as potential biomarkers of brain invasion and distant recurrence of gliomas. The major components of the cytoskeleton are actin filaments, which are also essential functional proteins that form the molecular apparatus responsible for cell motility and intracellular material transport [7]. In terms of glioma cell invasion described in the previous example, malignant glioma cells need to modify their contacts with the ECM, which involves the actin cytoskeleton [6]. Six isoforms of actin derived from six paralog genes exist, and numerous associations have been reported between actin isoform expression in varying cancers and prognosis or resistance to cancer drug treatment [8]. One of these isoforms, high expression of actin alpha, cardiac muscle 1 (ACTC1), is a significant poor prognostic factor in malignant gliomas [9]. We previously reported that ACTC1 knockdown (KD) in a human malignant glioma cell line inhibited cell migration ability [10].

Thus, we hypothesize that actin isoforms other than ACTC1 also involve cell migration and recurrence in malignant gliomas. Actin alpha 2, smooth muscle (ACTA2), one of the actin isoforms, is mainly found in the smooth muscle of the vascular system and is involved in its contractility [11]. This study aimed to investigate the role of ACTA2 in cell migration of glioma cells and determine the impact of ACTA2 expression level on prognosis and recurrence in glioma patients.

2. Materials and Methods

2.1. Cell Culture

U251MG, a human GBM cell line, was purchased from the Japan Collection of Research Bioresources Cell Bank (National Institutes of Biomedical Innovation, Health, and Nutrition, Osaka, Japan). The cells were cultured in Dulbecco's Modified Eagle's Medium supplemented with 10% fetal bovine serum, penicillin, streptomycin, and amphotericin B at 37 °C in an atmosphere of 5% CO_2.

2.2. Droplet Digital Polymerase Chain Reaction (dd-PCR)

According to the manufacturer's protocol, total RNA was extracted using the RNeasy Mini Kit (Qiagen, Hilden, Germany). A NanoDrop Lite spectrophotometer (Thermo Fisher Scientific Inc., Waltham, MA, USA) was used to measure the total RNA concentration and A260/A280 ratio. Samples with A260/A280 ratios < 1.8 were excluded. The QuantiTect Reverse Transcription Kit (Qiagen) was used for cDNA synthesis via RNA reverse transcription. A water/oil emulsion droplet in combination with a microfluidic device was used to conduct the dd-PCR analysis. To measure the ACTC1 expression levels, PCR mixtures with a final volume of 20 µL were prepared using 8 µL DNA (dilution: 2:6), 10 µL Digital PCR Supermix for Probes (Bio-Rad, Hercules, CA, USA), and 1 µL Bio-Rad Prime PCR primer assays for ribosomal protein L37 (RPL37) (dHsaCPE5037980; Bio-Rad) and ACTC1 (dHsaCPE5049966; Bio-Rad). To measure ACTA2 expression levels, PCR mixtures of 20 µL final volume were prepared using 8 µL DNA (dilution: 1:7), 10 µL Digital PCR Supermix for Probes (Bio-Rad), and 1 µL PCR primer assays for ribosomal protein L37 (RPL37) (dHsaCPE5037980; Bio-Rad) and ACTA2 (dHsaCPE5051320; Bio-Rad). Each droplet was amplified using PCR (C1000 Touch Thermal Cycler; Bio-Rad) after each sample was divided using a droplet generator. The thermal cycling conditions were the following: 95 °C for 10 min, 39 cycles of extension at 95 °C for 30 s/cycle, and 57 °C for 1 min, followed by 98 °C for 10 min. The target gene concentration was assessed by loading a 96-well PCR plate onto a QX200 droplet reader (Bio-Rad) after amplification. PCR data were analyzed to measure the number of droplets positive or negative for the ACTC1, ACTA2, and RPL37 probe in each sample using QuantaSoft (version 1.7.4, 2014) (Bio-Rad) analysis software. Using a Poisson algorithm to determine the target concentration, we calculated the proportion of target positive droplets. RPL37 was used as the reference gene for quantitative evaluation, and the results were expressed as the ratio of ACTC1 to RPL37 or ACTA2 to RPL37.

2.3. Small Interfering RNA Transfection

Lipofectamine™ RNAiMAX (Thermo Fisher Scientific Inc.) transfection reagent was utilized to transfect ACTC1-specific siRNA (sc-105181; Santa Cruz Biotechnology, Dallas, TX, USA) or/and ACTA2-specific siRNA (sc-43590; Santa Cruz Biotechnology) into U251MG following the manufacturer's protocol. ACTC1 knockdown alone (ACTC1-KD) cells were transfected using 3 µL ACTC1-specific siRNA, ACTA2 knockdown alone (ACTA2-KD) cells were transfected using 3 µL ACTA2-specific siRNA, and simultaneous knockdown of ACTC1 and ACTA2 (ACTC1/ACTA2-KD) cells were transfected using 3 µL each of ACTC1- and ACTA2-specific siRNA, respectively. As a negative control (NC), equal amounts of scrambled siRNA (sc-37007; Santa Cruz Biotechnology) and Lipofectamine™ RNAiMAX transfection reagent were used.

2.4. Proliferation Assay

At 24 h after completion of the siRNA transfection protocol, cells were detached and seeded in 6-well plates at 1.0×10^5 cells per well. The number of cells was measured using Countess® II FL (Thermo Fisher Scientific Inc.) after the cells were incubated at 37 °C in a 5% CO_2 atmosphere for 72 h. The doubling time for each cell was calculated through the measurement of the cell count after 72 h of incubation.

2.5. Migration Assay

Cells were seeded into 6-well plates at a density of 5.0×10^4 cells per well 24 h after the knockdown process. Following an additional 24 h incubation period, time-lapse imaging was conducted every 10 min for 18 h while cells were incubated at 37 °C in a 5% CO_2 atmosphere. For each group, eight regions of interest (ROIs) were defined, and the movement of cells within each ROI was analyzed using the Live Cell Imaging System SI8000 (Sony, Tokyo, Japan).

2.6. Immunohistochemistry

U251MG cells were immunostained using an ACTC1 antibody (GTX101876; GeneTex, Inc., Irvine, CA, USA) at a dilution of 1:500 and ACTA2 monoclonal antibody (1A4, eBioscience™; Thermo Fisher Scientific Inc.) at a dilution of 1:500, following the manufacturer's protocol. After three washes in phosphate-buffered saline (PBS), sections were incubated using the following secondary antibodies: goat anti-mouse IgG (H + L); Alexa Fluor 488-conjugated; A-11001 (Thermo Fisher Scientific Inc.) diluted at 1:200 and goat anti-rabbit IgG (H + L); Alexa Fluor 546-conjugated; and A-11010 (Thermo Fisher Scientific Inc.) diluted at 1:200. Incubation with secondary antibodies was performed for 2 h at 37 °C in a 5% CO_2 atmosphere. Subsequently, sections were washed three times with PBS, and the nuclei were stained with ibidi mounting medium with 4′,6-diamidino-2-phenylindole (DAPI) (ib50011; NIPPON Genetics Co, Ltd. Tokyo, Japan). Finally, using a confocal laser microscope (STELLARIS 8; Leica Microsystems GmbH, Wetzlar, Germany), the sections were mounted on coverslips and observed.

2.7. Clinical Tumor Samples and Medical Information

A total of 50 samples were acquired from consecutive patients who underwent a brain tumor resection at our hospital between 2014 and 2017 and were initially diagnosed with WHO grade 3 or 4 gliomas. Moreover, 24 samples were collected from 12 patients who underwent surgery at our hospital between 2014 and 2022. These patients were initially diagnosed with WHO grade 3 or 4 gliomas, manifested tumor recurrence, and subsequently underwent tumor resection because of relapse at our hospital during the same periods. All samples were cryopreserved at −80 °C in an ultra-low-temperature freezer immediately after resection. Using the method described earlier (Section 2.2), we determined the ACTA2 expression levels in the cryopreserved samples. Clinical information of these patients, such as age, sex, pathology, progression-free survival (PFS), overall survival (OS), characteristics of initial magnetic resonance imaging (MRI) findings, and postoperative therapy information, was extracted from their medical records. The institutional ethics committee approved this retrospective observational study (Osaka Medical and Pharmaceutical University 2022-189). An opt-out method was used to obtain patient consent for this study because of the retrospective nature of this study and the use of anonymized clinical data. Written informed consent for treatment was obtained from each patient.

2.8. Validation Using Data from the TCGA Database's Cohort of Glioma Patients

To investigate the correlation between ACTA2 expression levels and the prognosis of recurrent gliomas, we analyzed an independent patient cohort from the TCGA Research Network (https://www.cancer.gov/tcga: accessed on 31 August 2023), distinct from our dataset. The data were retrieved and analyzed through the GlioVis database (http://gliovis.bioinfo.cnio.es: accessed on 31 August 2023) [12]. First, "TCGA_GBMLGG", a WHO grade 2–4 clinical glioma dataset consisting of 667 samples, was used. All patients were adults, and samples were not differentiated by histology, tumor subtype, gender, and IDH status. Next, "TCGA_GBM" was used as a dataset confined to WHO grade 4, which contained 357 and 12 samples of primary and recurrent GBM, respectively. Samples used for analysis were restricted to IDH-wildtype and were not differentiated by tumor subtype or gender. HG-U113A was selected as the platform for gene expression.

We evaluated the impact of ACTA2 expression on the overall survival (OS) of glioma patients by categorizing them into two groups: ACTA2 high and ACTA2 low expression groups. Maximum selection rank statistics were employed to determine the optimal cut-off values of ACTA2 expression for these groupings.

2.9. Statistical Analysis

The data were subjected to statistical analysis and reported as mean values ± standard deviation or median with range. All statistical analyses were performed using JMP Pro (version 16.2.0) software (SAS Institute Inc., Cary, NC, USA). Statistical significance was determined at a threshold of $p < 0.05$.

3. Results

3.1. ACTC1 and ACTA2 KD through siRNA Transfection

The dd-PCR analysis demonstrated that the cells treated with ACTC1 and/or ACTA2 siRNA exhibited a decreased expression of each respective gene compared to the NC cells at 48 h post-transfection (Figure 1A,B, $p \leq 0.001$), which confirmed the successful KD of each gene via siRNA transfection. Additionally, ACTA2-KD cells showed increased ACTC1 expression compared to NC cells at 96 h post-transfection (Figure 1C, $p < 0.001$). Conversely, ACTC1-KD cells exhibited an increased ACTA2 expression at 96 h post-transfection (Figure 1D, $p < 0.001$).

3.2. Cell Proliferation of U251MG

ACTC1-KD cells showed a shorter doubling time than NC cells ($p = 0.027$), and ACTA2-KD and ACTC1/ACTA2-KD cells revealed longer doubling times compared to that of NC cells (Figure 2A, $p < 0.001$, $p = 0.006$, respectively). No significant difference was found in doubling times between ACTA2-KD and ACTC1/ACTA2-KD cells.

3.3. Cell Migration of U251MG

A decrease in cell motion velocity was observed compared to NC cells in ACTC1-KD cells, ACTA2-KD cells, and ACTC1/ACTA2-KD cells (Figure 2B). Similarly, compared to the NC cells, a remarkable reduction in motion distance was noted in the KD cells ($p < 0.001$). When comparing the motion distances between the KD groups, ACTC1-KD cells showed a significantly longer motion distance ($p = 0.009$). However, no significant difference was found in motion distances between ACTA2-KD cells and ACTC1/ACTA2-KD cells (Figure 2C).

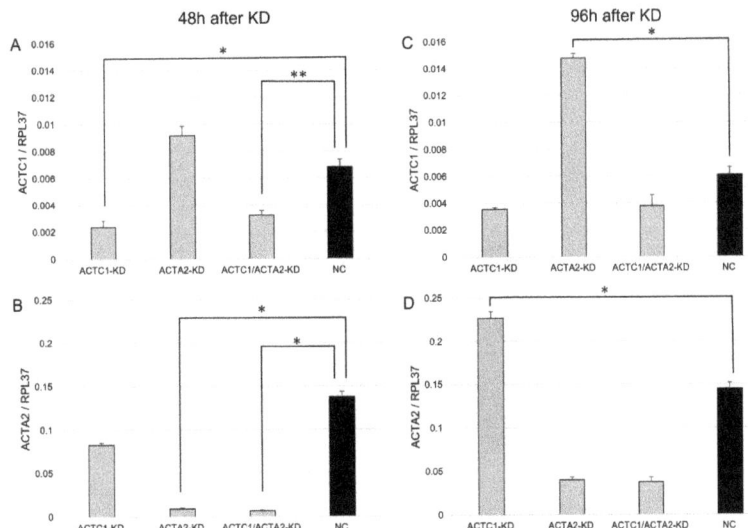

Figure 1. Droplet digital PCR analysis of actin alpha, cardiac muscle 1 (ACTC1) and actin alpha 2, smooth muscle (ACTA2) expression in U251MG cells. (**A**) ACTC1 siRNA-treated cells (ACTC1-KD and ACTC1/ACTA2-KD) demonstrated a significant decline in ACTC1 gene expression compared to negative control (NC) cells at 48 h after transfection. (**B**) ACTA2 siRNA-treated cells (ACTA2-KD and ACTC1/ACTA2-KD) revealed a significant decrease in ACTA2 gene expression compared to NC cells at 48 h after transfection. (**C**) ACTA2-KD cells revealed an increased ACTC1 gene expression compared to NC cells at 96 h after transfection. (**D**) ACTC1-KD cells showed increased ACTA2 gene expression compared to NC cells at 96 h after transfection. *, $p < 0.001$. **, $p = 0.001$. The Student's t-test was used to determine the p-values.

3.4. Immunohistochemistry

Lamellipodia are cell membrane protrusions at the leading edge of a cell that extend and migrate parallel to the substrate and are composed of a network of actin filaments [13]. In our study, we noted that ACTC1 exhibited accumulation specifically at the tips of the fan-shaped lamellipodia, while the ACTA2 accumulation in lamellipodia was less pronounced compared to ACTC1 (Figure 3A). The distinct differences in ACTC1 and ACTA2 localization within lamellipodia in U251MG cells are confirmed by these findings.

3.5. Lamellipodia Formation of U251MG

The proportion of cells showing lamellipodia formation, as observed in the simultaneously captured bright-field images, was compared among the KD cells and the NC cells. The results indicated that ACTC1-KD, ACTA2-KD, and ACTC1/ACTA2-KD cells revealed a reduced lamellipodia formation occurrence compared to NC cells (Figure 3B, $p \leq 0.001$).

3.6. Clinical Data of Malignant Glioma Patients

The median age at diagnosis was 64.5 years, ranging from 21 to 89 years, among 50 patients with primary malignant glioma. Of these patients, 64% were male. Among the cases, 11 were classified as WHO grade 3, while 39 were stratified as grade 4 gliomas. The median PFS was 9 months, with a range of 1 to 104 months. The median OS was 19 months, also ranging from 1 to 104 months. At the initial presentation, approximately 16% of the patients showed remotely enhanced lesions on Gd contrast-enhanced MRI that were not connected to the fluid-attenuated inversion recovery hyperintense lesions surrounding the main lesion.

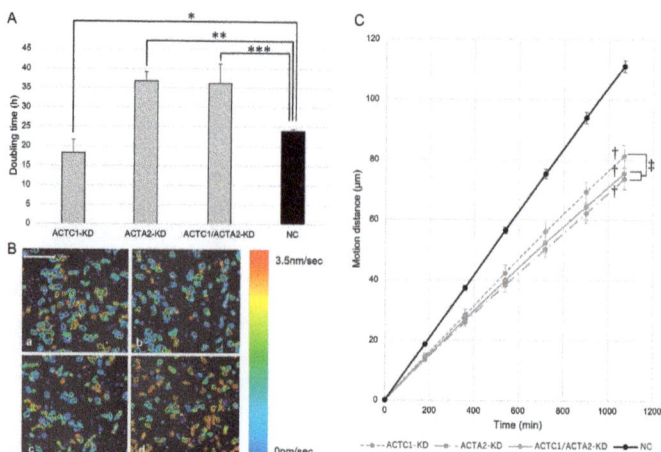

Figure 2. (**A**) The doubling time of each group was calculated. Among the NC and KD cells, the ACTC1-KD cells showed a shorter doubling time (*, $p = 0.027$). Conversely, the ACTA2-KD and ACTC1/ACTA2-KD cells revealed longer doubling times (**, $p < 0.001$, ***, $p = 0.006$). The Student's t-test was used to perform the statistical analysis. (**B**) The cell motions of each cell were analyzed using time-lapse images acquired using the Live Cell Imaging System SI8000. Areas where movement was detected are color-coded based on movement speed. A visual comparison of knockdown cells (a: ACTC1-KD; b: ACTA2-KD; c: ACTC1/ACTA2-KD) with the NC cells (d) indicated a reduction in the speed of movement in the knockdown cells. Scar bar = 500 μm. (**C**) Significant decreases in KD cells compared to NC cells were noted when calculating the motion distance during the observation period based on the motion velocity (†, $p < 0.001$, Student's t-test). The ACTC1-KD cells demonstrated a significantly longer motion distance than the other knockdown cells (‡, $p = 0.009$, analysis of variance). No significant differences were found between ACTA2-KD and ACTC1/ACTA2-KD cells (Student's t-test).

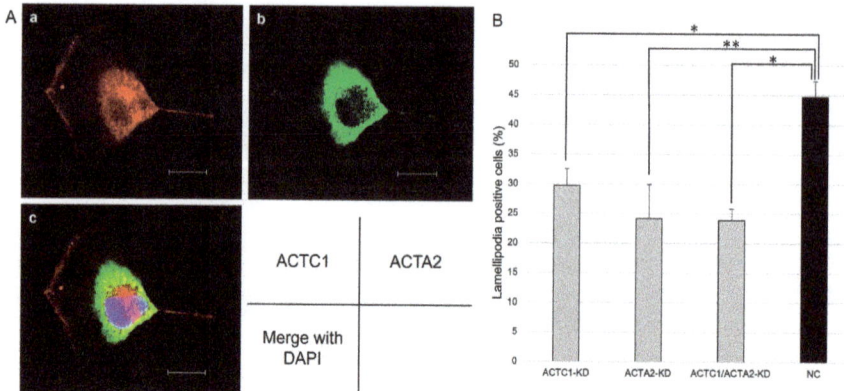

Figure 3. (**A**) Immunocytochemical staining of ACTC1 and ACTA2 in U251MG was visualized via a confocal laser microscope. ACTC1 was noted to accumulate at the lamellipodia, while ACTA2 accumulation at the lamellipodia was less prominent compared to ACTC1 (a: ACTC1 immunostaining; b: ACTA2 immunostaining; c: overlay with DAPI [blue], 600× magnification each). Scar bar = 20 μm (**B**) The rates of lamellipodia formation in each cell were calculated based on the bright-field images obtained simultaneously. ACTC1-KD, ACTA2-KD, and ACTC1/ACTA2-KD cells revealed a reduced lamellipodia formation compared to NC cells. *, $p < 0.001$. **, $p = 0.001$. Statistical analysis was conducted using the Student's t-test to determine the p-value.

Among the 12 patients diagnosed with recurrent malignant glioma, the median age at diagnosis was 48 years, ranging from 30 to 80 years. Of these patients, 75% were male. Among the cases, five were WHO grade 3, while seven were grade 4 gliomas. The median PFS was 8 months, with a range of 4 to 31 months. The median OS was 31.5 months, ranging from 11 to 80 months.

In 11 out of 12 patients, concurrent chemoradiotherapy with 60 Gy of X-ray radiation therapy together with temozolomide was initiated between the initial operation and reoperation, while one patient only received chemotherapy using temozolomide. Malignant glioma patient characteristics are summarized in Table 1.

Table 1. Malignant glioma patient characteristics.

		Primary Malignant Glioma ($n = 50$)	Recurrent Malignant Glioma ($n = 12$)
Age at diagnosis, median (range)		64.5 (19–91)	48 (30–80)
Sex			
	Male	32 (64%)	9 (75%)
	Female	18 (36%)	3 (25%)
WHO grade			
	3	11 (22%)	5 (42%)
	4	39 (78%)	7 (58%)
PFS (month), median (range)		9 (1–104)	8 (4–31)
OS (month), median (range)		19 (1–104)	31.5 (11–80)
Postoperative therapy			
	Radiotherapy	48 (96%)	11 (92%)
	Chemotherapy	48 (96%)	12 (100%)

3.7. ACTA2 Expression in Primary Malignant Glioma

A significant difference was noted when comparing ACTA2 expression levels between WHO grade 3 and grade 4 gliomas: the ACTA2/RPL37 ratio was approximately fourfold higher in grade 4 gliomas, with a median of 1.31 (range: 0.11–11.35) compared to a median of 0.28 (range: 0.04–2.09) in grade 3 gliomas (Figure 4A, $p = 0.002$). Moreover, the ACTA2 high expression group ($n = 16$) revealed a significantly higher proportion of distant lesions, accounting for 31.3% of the brain MRI findings at the initial visit, compared to 8.8% in the ACTA2 low expression group ($n = 34$) (Figure S1, $p = 0.044$).

In the validation cohort study using the TCGA database, WHO grade 4 gliomas ($n = 153$) had significantly higher ACTA2 gene expression than lower-grade gliomas of WHO grades 2 ($n = 226$) and 3 gliomas ($n = 244$) (Figure S2, $p < 0.001$).

When these glioma patients (grades 2–4: $n = 667$) were divided into two groups by ACTA2 expression, those with high ACTA2 expression ($n = 285$) had a significantly worse prognosis than those with low expression ($n = 382$) (Figure S3A, $p < 0.01$). In primary IDH-wildtype GBM, the ACTA2 high expression group ($n = 138$) also had a worse prognosis than the low expression group ($n = 219$) (Figure S3B, $p = 0.008$).

3.8. ACTA2 Expression in Recurrent Malignant Glioma

Comparing ACTA2 expression in initial and recurrent samples from the same glioma patients, we noted that ACTA2/RPL37 increased nearly twofold in recurrent cases (median value: 2.05, range: 0.12–17.39) compared to initial cases (median value: 0.90, range: 0.04–4.10). Specifically, 10 out of 12 patients showed an increased ACTA2 expression from the primary tumors to their corresponding relapsed tumors (Figure 4B, $p = 0.012$). When the PFS from initial disease to relapse was investigated, it was found that the high ACTA2 expression change group ($n = 6$) showed a median PFS of 5.5 months (range: 4–13), which was significantly shorter than a median of 13.5 months (range: 8–31) in the low ACTA2 expression change group ($n = 6$) (Figure 5A, $p = 0.011$). Similarly, when restricting the analysis to grade 4 gliomas, a significantly shorter PFS was noted in the group with a higher change in ACTA2 expression (high change group ($n = 4$): median 5 months (range: 4–7); low change group ($n = 3$): median 17 months (range: 10–31)) (Figure 5B, $p = 0.017$).

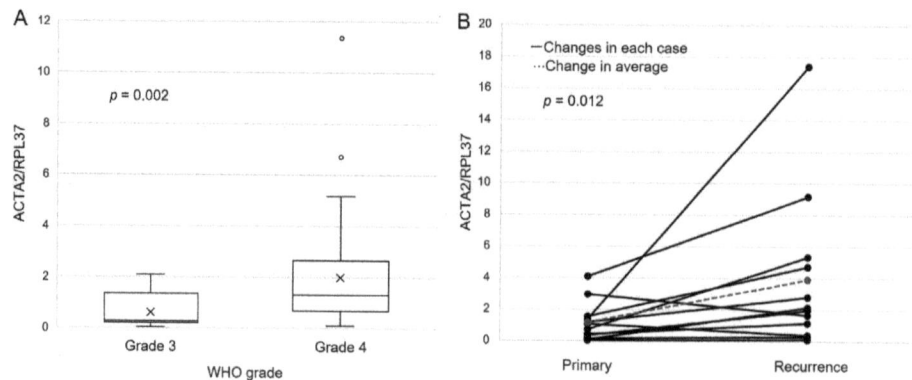

Figure 4. (**A**): ACTA2 expression was assessed in patients with grade 3 primary glioma ($n = 11$) and grade 4 ($n = 39$) patients. ACTA2/RPL37 ratio was significantly higher in grade 4 gliomas. The p-values were determined using the Wilcoxon signed-rank test. (**B**): ACTA2 expression changes from the initial diagnosis to recurrence in malignant glioma patients ($n = 12$) were measured. The ACTA2/RPL37 ratio was significantly higher in recurrent malignant glioma than in primary malignant glioma. Moreover, 10 out of 12 cases revealed increased ACTA2 expression during re-currence. Using paired-samples Wilcoxon signed-rank test, p-values were determined.

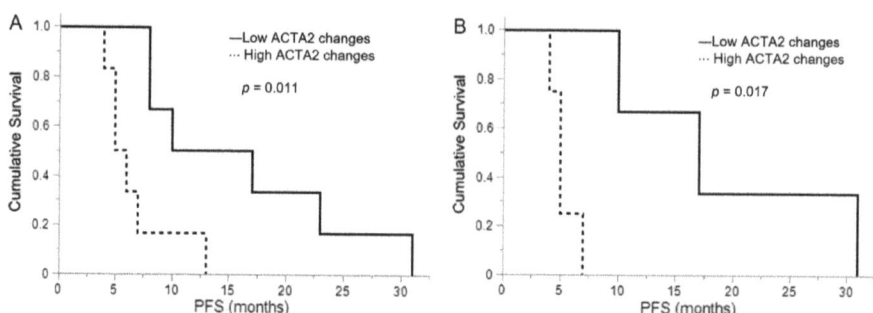

Figure 5. (**A**) The Kaplan–Meier method was used to compare progression-free survival (PFS) between the high and low ACTA2 changes from initial malignant glioma to recurrence. In malignant glioma patients ($n = 12$), the PFS in the high ACTA2 expression change group ($n = 6$) was remarkably shorter than the PFS in the low ACTA2 expression change group ($n = 6$). (**B**) In grade 4 glioma patients ($n = 7$), the PFS in the high ACTA2 expression change group ($n = 4$) was significantly shorter than the PFS in the low ACTA2 expression change group ($n = 3$). Statistical analysis was conducted using the log–rank test to determine the p-values.

In IDH-wildtype GBM in the TCGA database, the group with high expression of ACTA2 at the time of recurrence ($n = 7$) had a significantly worse prognosis than the group with low expression ($n = 5$) (Figure S3C, $p = 0.001$).

4. Discussion

In this study, KD of either ACTC1 or ACTA2 in the U251MG glioma cell line led to shorter cell motion distance. Mesenchymal migration, induced by lamellipodia formation, is a type of cancer cell migration [13,14], and we verified that either ACTC1 or ACTA2 KD significantly reduced lamellipodia formation. Previously, we reported that ACTC1 KD in a malignant glioma cell line reduced cell migration [10], and the study results suggest that ACTA2 is also involved in glioma cell migration. ACTA2 was highly expressed in grade 4 gliomas compared to grade 3 gliomas in clinical malignant glioma specimens, and multiple distant brain lesions were more common in the ACTA2 high expression group. These results suggest that ACTA2 may be a therapeutic target in controlling glioma migration and distant recurrence.

ATCA2 has been reported to be a migration-related factor in other cancers and nervous system cells. Furthermore, ACTA2 expression is associated with distant metastasis and poor prognosis in human epidermal growth factor receptor-positive breast, bladder, and colorectal cancers [15–17]. Lee et al. elucidated that a significant positive correlation was found between brain metastasis and ACTA2 gene amplification in lung adenocarcinoma and that a high ACTA2 expression is a poor prognostic factor [18]. They also revealed that ACTA2 is involved in metastasis via migration and invasion in lung adenocarcinoma from in vitro and in vivo assays and that ACTA2 silencing suppresses the EMT-related gene, FAK, and c-MET expression [19]. Zhang et al. also reported that ACTA2 downregulation in neural stem cells reduced cell migration [20].

The study revealed that ACTA2 expression was increased in most recurrent cases and that the higher the increase, the shorter the PFS. These results suggest that ACTA2 is involved in malignant glioma recurrence. Several hypotheses were generated regarding the underlying mechanism by which ACTC2 is involved in malignant glioma recurrence.

Malignant gliomas present with a poor prognosis, which is attributed in part to deep brain invasion, limiting complete surgical resection. As mentioned above, one of the migration factors in malignant gliomas is ACTA2, and one hypothesis for the involvement of ACTA2 in recurrence is that cells showing a higher ACTA2 expression may migrate and invade deeper into the brain and escape surgical resection.

Additionally, most of the patients in this study received a combination of anti-cancer drugs (temozolomide) and radiotherapy, referred to as the Stupp regimen, between the initial surgery and reoperation [21]. Another hypothesis is that ACTA2 is involved in resistance to the Stupp regimen. A number of reports exist elucidating actin and resistance to anti-cancer drugs: Che et al. reported that a high ACTC1 expression is associated with low sensitivity to the mitogenic inhibitor paclitaxel in non-small cell lung cancer [22], and Yang et al. reported that ACTC1 is a hub gene conferring chemotherapy resistance to a variety of tumors and its expression is upregulated in multidrug-resistant breast cancer cells [23]. Although one of the standard postoperative treatments for malignant gliomas is the Stupp regimen, which has been shown to prolong PFS and OS, malignant gliomas have also been reported to have a poor prognosis even after receiving the Stupp regimen [24]. Thus, understanding the mechanisms of resistance to radio-chemotherapy in malignant gliomas is crucial.

The present study shows that ACTA2 expression is a factor in the mechanism of malignant glioma recurrence and represents a challenge for future elucidation of the mechanism of malignant glioma recurrence and control.

In this study, we initially generated U251MG glioma cells in which one of the two α-actin paralog genes, ACTC1 and ACTA2, was knocked down. Interestingly, KD of either α-actin resulted in a remarkable upregulation of the expression of the other α-actin gene. Accordingly, ACTC1-KD cells demonstrated a suppressed ACTC1 expression and enhanced ACTA2 expression compared to control cells, while ACTA2-KD cells demonstrated a suppressed ACTA2 expression and enhanced ACTC1 expression. This fact implies that the ACTC1 and ACTA2 gene expression is controlled by a complementary expression regulation system, suggesting that there may be some biologically purposive reason for compensating for the decline in one α-actin through the increased expression of the other. We added U251MG glioma cells with a simultaneous KD of the ACTC1 and ACTA2 genes as "ACTC1/ACTA2-KD cells" in vitro assays to explore the significance of this complementary regulation of ACTC1 and ACTA2 expression.

The evaluation results of ACTC1 gene expression, ACTA2 gene expression, cell proliferation ability, cell migration capacity, and lamellipodia formation ability in the three KD cell lines compared to control cells (sham-KD) are summarized in Table 2.

Table 2. Summary of in vitro study.

	ACTC1 Expression	ACTA2 Expression	Cell Proliferation	Cell Motility	Lamellipodia Formation
ACTC1-KD	↓	↑	↑	↓	↓
ACTA2-KD	↑	↓	↓	↓	↓
ACTC1/ACTA2 double KD	↓	↓	↓	↓	↓

In evaluating cellular proliferative capacity, ACTC1-KD cells demonstrated an increased proliferative capacity, while ACTA2-KD and double KD cells showed a significantly decreased proliferative capacity. Among these three types of KD cells, only ACTC1-KD cells with a significantly increased expression of ACTA2 compared to control cells revealed increased cell proliferation, while ACTA2-KD and ACTC1/ACTA2-KD cells with a suppressed ACTA2 expression demonstrated a significantly decreased cell proliferation. These results suggest that ACTA2 has a stimulatory effect on glioma cell proliferation, while ACTC1 expression has a minimal effect on cell proliferation.

It has been reported that ACTC1 is not involved in cell proliferation in malignant glioma [9]. The acquisition of ACTA2 expression has been reported in activated cancer-associated fibroblasts in oral and pancreatic cancer, which are known to be involved in cancer cell proliferation [25–27], and it is conceivable that ACTA2 is also involved in cell proliferation in malignant glioma through a similar mechanism.

Knockdown of either ACTC1 or ACTA2 also inhibited lamellipodia formation, but immunocytochemistry revealed differences in the distribution of ACTC1 and ACTA2 in lamellipodia. This result suggests that each may play an independent role in lamellipodia formation. Taken together, our data suggest that the regulation of ACTC1 and ACTA2 expression is complementary but that their biological roles are not identical.

Six actin isoforms (paralog genes) exist, and the tissues in which they are significantly expressed vary by isoform [8,28]. The interaction between expression and function among actin isoforms has already been reported in several cases: actin gamma 2, smooth muscle (ACTG2) is overexpressed in ACTC1 knockout mice [29]. Moreover, it has also been reported that transgenic ACTC1 expression in actin alpha skeletal muscle (ACTA1) knockout mice restores lethality and muscle weakness associated with ACTA1 loss [30]. Elucidating the mechanisms of interaction between actin isoforms will provide a springboard to explore the mechanisms of cancer migration and proliferation, including in malignant gliomas.

This study has limitations that include the retrospective nature of the study. Another limitation is the limited number of cases where initial and recurrent samples were available from the same patient.

5. Conclusions

The present study revealed that ACTA2 is an important migratory factor in malignant gliomas and is involved in recurrence. Elucidation of the migration mechanism in malignant gliomas is crucial in developing future therapeutic regimens, and ACTA2 is a promising candidate as a therapeutic target. Additionally, the interaction between actin isoforms in cancer can be confirmed via the present study and previous reports. Exploring the mechanisms of interaction between actin isoforms may provide a clue to understanding the migration and proliferation mechanisms of cancers, including malignant gliomas.

Supplementary Materials: The following supporting information can be downloaded at https://www.mdpi.com/article/10.3390/brainsci13101477/s1: Figure S1: Relationship between distant disease at first presentation and ACTA2 expression level; Figure S2: ACTA2 gene expression level by grade in WHO grade 2–4 clinical gliomas in the TCGA cohort; Figure S3: The Relationship between ACTA2 gene expression and survival prognosis of gliomas in the TCGA.

Author Contributions: Conceptualization, N.N., Y.K.-S., M.S., O.H. and M.W.; methodology, T.H., N.N., T.K., M.F., S.K., T.T., Y.K.-S., M.S., O.H., R.H. and M.W.; validation, T.H., N.N. and T.K.; formal analysis, T.H.; investigation, T.H. and N.N.; resources, T.H., N.N., T.K., M.F., S.K., R.Y., Y.K., H.K., M.K. and M.W.; data curation, T.H. and N.N.; writing—original draft preparation, T.H.; writing—review and editing, N.N.; visualization, T.H. and N.N.; supervision, N.N., O.H., R.H. and M.W.; project administration, M.W.; funding acquisition, M.W. All authors have read and agreed to the published version of the manuscript.

Funding: This work was partly funded by Grants-in-Aid for Scientific Research (C) (No. 20K09359 M.W.) from the Japan Society for the Promotion of Science (JSPS) KAKENHI. Funding sources did not have any role in study design, data collection and analysis, the decision to submit for publication, or manuscript preparation.

Institutional Review Board Statement: The institutional ethics committee approved this retrospective observational study (Osaka Medical and Pharmaceutical University 2022-189).

Informed Consent Statement: Owing to the retrospective nature of this study and the utilization of anonymized clinical data, an opt-out method was used to obtain patient consent for this study. Each patient provided written consent for treatment.

Data Availability Statement: All of the data analyzed in this study are available on reasonable request from the corresponding author.

Acknowledgments: We extend our thanks to Shinobu Ohba and Teruo Ueno from the Center for Medical Research & Development at Osaka Medical and Pharmaceutical University for their technical support and guidance.

Conflicts of Interest: The authors declare no conflict of interest.

References

1. Ostrom, Q.T.; Cioffi, G.; Waite, K.; Kruchko, C.; Barnholtz-Sloan, J.S. CBTRUS statistical report: Primary brain and other central nervous system tumors diagnosed in the United States in 2014–2018. *Neuro Oncol.* **2021**, *23*, iii1–iii105. [CrossRef] [PubMed]
2. Narita, Y.; Shibui, S.; Committee of Brain Tumor Registry of Japan Supported by the Japan Neurosurgical Society. Trends and outcomes in the treatment of gliomas based on data during 2001–2004 from the Brain Tumor Registry of Japan. *Neurol. Med. Chir.* **2015**, *55*, 286–295. [CrossRef] [PubMed]
3. Claes, A.; Idema, A.J.; Wesseling, P. Diffuse glioma growth: A guerilla war. *Acta Neuropathol.* **2007**, *114*, 443–458. [CrossRef]
4. de Vrij, J.; Maas, S.L.; Kwappenberg, K.M.; Schnoor, R.; Kleijn, A.; Dekker, L.; Luider, T.M.; de Witte, L.D.; Litjens, M.; van Strien, M.E.; et al. Glioblastoma-derived extracellular vesicles modify the phenotype of monocytic cells. *Int. J. Cancer* **2015**, *137*, 1630–1642. [CrossRef] [PubMed]
5. Schiera, G.; Di Liegro, C.M.; Di Liegro, I. Extracellular Membrane Vesicles as Vehicles for Brain Cell-to-Cell Interactions in Physiological as well as Pathological Conditions. *Biomed. Res. Int.* **2015**, *2015*, 152926. [CrossRef] [PubMed]
6. Schiera, G.; Di Liegro, C.M.; Di Liegro, I. Molecular Determinants of Malignant Brain Cancers: From Intracellular Alterations to Invasion Mediated by Extracellular Vesicles. *Int. J. Mol. Sci.* **2017**, *18*, 2774. [CrossRef]
7. Pollard, T.D.; Cooper, J.A. Actin, a central player in cell shape and movement. *Science* **2009**, *326*, 1208–1212. [CrossRef]
8. Suresh, R.; Diaz, R.J. The remodeling of actin composition as a hallmark of cancer. *Transl. Oncol.* **2021**, *14*, 101051. [CrossRef]
9. Ohtaki, S.; Wanibuchi, M.; Kataoka-Sasaki, Y.; Sasaki, M.; Oka, S.; Noshiro, S.; Akiyama, Y.; Mikami, T.; Mikuni, N.; Kocsis, J.D.; et al. ACTC1 as an invasion and prognosis marker in glioma. *J. Neurosurg.* **2017**, *126*, 467–475. [CrossRef]
10. Wanibuchi, M.; Ohtaki, S.; Ookawa, S.; Kataoka-Sasaki, Y.; Sasaki, M.; Oka, S.; Kimura, Y.; Akiyama, Y.; Mikami, T.; Mikuni, N.; et al. Actin, alpha, cardiac muscle 1 (ACTC1) knockdown inhibits the migration of glioblastoma cells in vitro. *J. Neurol. Sci.* **2018**, *392*, 117–121. [CrossRef]
11. Yuan, S.M. α-smooth muscle actin and ACTA2 gene expressions in vasculopathies. *Braz. J. Cardiovasc. Surg.* **2015**, *30*, 644–649. [CrossRef] [PubMed]

12. Bowman, R.L.; Wang, Q.; Carro, A.; Verhaak, R.G.; Squatrito, M. GlioVis data portal for visualization and analysis of brain tumor expression datasets. *Neuro Oncol.* **2017**, *19*, 139–141. [CrossRef] [PubMed]
13. Small, J.V.; Stradal, T.; Vignal, E.; Rottner, K. The lamellipodium: Where motility begins. *Trends Cell Biol.* **2002**, *12*, 112–120. [CrossRef]
14. Yamazaki, D.; Kurisu, S.; Takenawa, T. Regulation of cancer cell motility through actin reorganization. *Cancer Sci.* **2005**, *96*, 379–386. [CrossRef]
15. Jeon, M.; You, D.; Bae, S.Y.; Kim, S.W.; Nam, S.J.; Kim, H.H.; Kim, S.; Lee, J.E. Dimerization of EGFR and HER2 induces breast cancer cell motility through STAT1-dependent ACTA2 induction. *Oncotarget* **2017**, *8*, 50570–50581. [CrossRef] [PubMed]
16. Gao, X.; Chen, Y.; Chen, M.; Wang, S.; Wen, X.; Zhang, S. Identification of key candidate genes and biological pathways in bladder cancer. *PeerJ.* **2018**, *6*, e6036. [CrossRef]
17. Zhao, B.; Baloch, Z.; Ma, Y.; Wan, Z.; Huo, Y.; Li, F.; Zhao, Y. Identification of potential key genes and pathways in early-onset colorectal cancer through bioinformatics analysis. *Cancer Control.* **2019**, *26*, 1073274819831260. [CrossRef]
18. Lee, H.W.; Seol, H.J.; Choi, Y.L.; Ju, H.J.; Joo, K.M.; Ko, Y.H.; Lee, J.I.; Nam, D.H. Genomic copy number alterations associated with the early brain metastasis of non-small cell lung cancer. *Int. J. Oncol.* **2012**, *41*, 2013–2020. [CrossRef]
19. Lee, H.W.; Park, Y.M.; Lee, S.J.; Cho, H.J.; Kim, D.H.; Lee, J.I.; Kang, M.S.; Seol, H.J.; Shim, Y.M.; Nam, D.H.; et al. Alpha-smooth muscle actin (ACTA2) is required for metastatic potential of human lung adenocarcinoma. *Clin. Cancer Res.* **2013**, *19*, 5879–5889. [CrossRef]
20. Zhang, J.; Jiang, X.; Zhang, C.; Zhong, J.; Fang, X.; Li, H.; Xie, F.; Huang, X.; Zhang, X.; Hu, Q.; et al. Actin alpha 2 (ACTA2) downregulation inhibits neural stem cell migration through rho GTPase activation. *Stem Cells Int.* **2020**, *2020*, 4764012. [CrossRef]
21. Stupp, R.; Mason, W.P.; van den Bent, M.J.; Weller, M.; Fisher, B.; Taphoorn, M.J.; Belanger, K.; Brandes, A.A.; Marosi, C.; Bogdahn, U.; et al. Radiotherapy plus concomitant and adjuvant temozolomide for glioblastoma. *N. Engl. J. Med.* **2005**, *352*, 987–996. [CrossRef] [PubMed]
22. Che, C.L.; Zhang, Y.M.; Zhang, H.H.; Sang, Y.L.; Lu, B.; Dong, F.S.; Zhang, L.J.; Lv, F.Z. DNA microarray reveals different pathways responding to paclitaxel and docetaxel in non-small cell lung cancer cell line. *Int. J. Clin. Exp. Pathol.* **2013**, *6*, 1538–1548. [PubMed]
23. Yang, M.; Li, H.; Li, Y.; Ruan, Y.; Quan, C. Identification of genes and pathways associated with MDR in MCF-7/MDR breast cancer cells by RNA-seq analysis. *Mol. Med. Rep.* **2018**, *17*, 6211–6226. [CrossRef]
24. Stupp, R.; Hegi, M.E.; Mason, W.P.; van den Bent, M.J.; Taphoorn, M.J.; Janzer, R.C.; Ludwin, S.K.; Allgeier, A.; Fisher, B.; Belanger, K.; et al. Effects of radiotherapy with concomitant and adjuvant temozolomide versus radiotherapy alone on survival in glioblastoma in a randomized phase III study: 5-year analysis of the EORTC-NCIC trial. *Lancet Oncol.* **2009**, *10*, 459–466. [CrossRef] [PubMed]
25. Marsh, D.; Suchak, K.; Moutasim, K.A.; Vallath, S.; Hopper, C.; Jerjes, W.; Upile, T.; Kalavrezos, N.; Violette, S.M.; Weinreb, P.H.; et al. Stromal features are predictive of disease mortality in oral cancer patients. *J. Pathol.* **2011**, *223*, 470–481. [CrossRef]
26. Öhlund, D.; Handly-Santana, A.; Biffi, G.; Elyada, E.; Almeida, A.S.; Ponz-Sarvise, M.; Corbo, V.; Oni, T.E.; Hearn, S.A.; Lee, E.J.; et al. Distinct populations of inflammatory fibroblasts and myofibroblasts in pancreatic cancer. *J. Exp. Med.* **2017**, *214*, 579–596. [CrossRef]
27. Lavie, D.; Ben-Shmuel, A.; Erez, N.; Scherz-Shouval, R. Cancer-associated fibroblasts in the single-cell era. *Nat. Cancer* **2022**, *3*, 793–807. [CrossRef]
28. Vedula, P.; Kashina, A. The makings of the "actin code": Regulation of actin's biological function at the amino acid and nucleotide level. *J. Cell Sci.* **2018**, *131*, jcs215509. [CrossRef]
29. Kumar, A.; Crawford, K.; Close, L.; Madison, M.; Lorenz, J.; Doetschman, T.; Pawlowski, S.; Duffy, J.; Neumann, J.; Robbins, J.; et al. Rescue of cardiac alpha-actin-deficient mice by enteric smooth muscle gamma-actin. *Proc. Natl. Acad. Sci. USA* **1997**, *94*, 4406–4411. [CrossRef]
30. Nowak, K.J.; Ravenscroft, G.; Jackaman, C.; Filipovska, A.; Davies, S.M.; Lim, E.M.; Squire, S.E.; Potter, A.C.; Baker, E.; Clément, S.; et al. Rescue of skeletal muscle alpha-actin-null mice by cardiac (fetal) alpha-actin. *J. Cell Biol.* **2009**, *185*, 903–915. [CrossRef]

Disclaimer/Publisher's Note: The statements, opinions and data contained in all publications are solely those of the individual author(s) and contributor(s) and not of MDPI and/or the editor(s). MDPI and/or the editor(s) disclaim responsibility for any injury to people or property resulting from any ideas, methods, instructions or products referred to in the content.

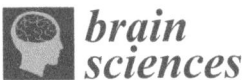

Article

The Role of Ketone Bodies in Treatment Individualization of Glioblastoma Patients

Corina Tamas [1,2,3], Flaviu Tamas [1,2,3,*], Attila Kovecsi [4,5], Georgiana Serban [1,6], Cristian Boeriu [7,8] and Adrian Balasa [2,3]

[1] Doctoral School, "George Emil Palade" University of Medicine, Pharmacy, Science and Technology, 540142 Targu Mures, Romania; corina.hurghis@umfst.ro (C.T.); georgiana.serban94@yahoo.com (G.S.)
[2] Neurosurgery Department, Emergency Clinical County Hospital, 540136 Targu Mures, Romania; adrian.balasa@yahoo.fr
[3] Department of Neurosurgery, "George Emil Palade" University of Medicine, Pharmacy, Science and Technology, 540142 Targu Mures, Romania
[4] Department of Morphopathology, "George Emil Palade" University of Medicine, Pharmacy, Science and Technology, 540142 Targu Mures, Romania; kovecsiattila@gmail.com
[5] Department of Morphopathology, Emergency Clinical County Hospital, 540136 Targu Mures, Romania
[6] Department of Anesthesiology and Intensive Care, Emergency Clinical County Hospital, 540136 Targu Mures, Romania
[7] Department of Emergency Medicine, George Emil Palade University of Medicine, Pharmacy, Science, and Technology, 540142 Targu Mures, Romania; cristian.boeriu@umfst.ro
[8] Department of Emergency Medicine, Emergency Clinical County Hospital, 540136 Targu Mures, Romania
* Correspondence: flaviu.tamas@umfst.ro; Tel.: +40729368150

Abstract: Glioblastoma is the most common and aggressive primary brain tumor in adults. According to the 2021 WHO CNS, glioblastoma is assigned to the IDH wild-type classification, fulfilling the specific characteristic histopathology. We have conducted a prospective observational study to identify the glucose levels, ketone bodies, and the glucose-ketone index in three groups of subjects: two tumoral groups of patients with histopathological confirmation of glioblastoma (9 male patients, 7 female patients, mean age 55.6 years old) or grade 4 astrocytoma (4 male patients, 2 female patients, mean age 48.1 years old) and a control group (13 male patients, 9 female patients, mean age 53.9 years old) consisting of subjects with no personal pathological history. There were statistically significant differences between the mean values of glycemia (p value = 0.0003), ketones (p value = 0.0061), and glucose-ketone index (p value = 0.008) between the groups of patients. Mortality at 3 months in glioblastoma patients was 0% if the ketone levels were below 0.2 mM and 100% if ketones were over 0.5 mM. Patients with grade 4 astrocytoma and the control subjects all presented with ketone values of less than 0.2 mM and 0.0% mortality. In conclusion, highlighting new biomarkers which are more feasible to determine such as ketones or glucose-ketone index represents an essential step toward personalized medicine and survival prolongation in patients suffering from glioblastoma and grade 4 astrocytoma.

Keywords: astrocytoma; glioblastoma; glucose; ketones; metabolism; diet

1. Introduction

Glioblastoma (GBM) is the most common and aggressive primary brain tumor in adults accounting for up to 45.2% of the primary cerebral malignancies [1–6]. The Central Brain Tumor Registry of the United States reports an average annual incidence of 3.19/100,000 people, while the United Kingdom Office of National Statistics reports a doubling of the number of cases from 2.4 to 5.0/100,000 between the years 1995 and 2015, with the current numbers having increased from 983 to 2531 cases per year [7–9]. The incidence of GBM increases with age, reaching a peak among individuals between 75 and 84 years old, with a higher prevalence in men (1.57% more than in women) [6,8,10,11].

The previous "World Health Organization Classification of Tumors of the Central Nervous System" (WHO CNS), 2016, based on histopathological diagnosis, used the term glioblastoma, which is divided into three subclasses: Isocitrate Dehydrogenase (IDH) mutant (10%), IDH wild-type (90%), and IDH with not otherwise specified (NOS), each of which presents with a completely different biology and prognosis [12]. According to the WHO CNS 2021 classification, the term glioblastoma is assigned only to the IDH wild-type subclass, fulfilling the specific histopathological characteristics of diffuse astrocytoma but with one or more genetic modifications (Telomerase reverse transcriptase-TERT promoter mutation, chromosome 7 or chromosome 10 damage (+7/−10), or Epidermal Growth Factor Receptor-EGFR gene amplification). IDH mutant astrocytomas are considered one single subtype of varying degrees (WHO 2,3, or 4). The presence of the homozygous deletion Cyclin-dependent Kinase Inhibitor-CDKN2A/B without histopathological findings of necrosis or microvascular proliferation defines WHO grade 4 astrocytoma (ASTRO G4) [13].

Most studies focus on the mechanisms of tumor cell invasion into the brain's microenvironment (Rho GTPases, Casein Kinase 2, and Ephrin receptors as major invasion factors) [14–16]. Recent studies have highlighted the reprogramming process of the cellular metabolism, which has a definitive role in preparing the cellular microenvironment for tumor invasion [17–19]. One of the defining characteristics of tumor development at the bioenergetic level is the ability of tumor cells to exploit the glycolytic metabolism independent of the presence of oxygen, a phenomenon known as the Warburg effect [5,6,20–22]. Many recent studies have questioned the possibility of using other energy sources such as ketone bodies (KBs) by GBM to generate energy [23–25].

Fatty acids and glucose are metabolized to acetyl coenzyme A (acetyl-CoA) inside the hepatocyte mitochondria. Acetyl-CoA enters the citric acid cycle by condensation with oxaloacetate. Glycolysis produces pyruvate, which is a precursor of oxaloacetate. If there is a significant decrease in glycolysis, oxaloacetate is preferentially used in the process of gluconeogenesis, becoming unavailable for condensation with acetyl-CoA produced through the degradation of fatty acids. In this case, acetyl-CoA deviates from the citric acid cycle to the formation of KBs (Figure 1) [22,26–28].

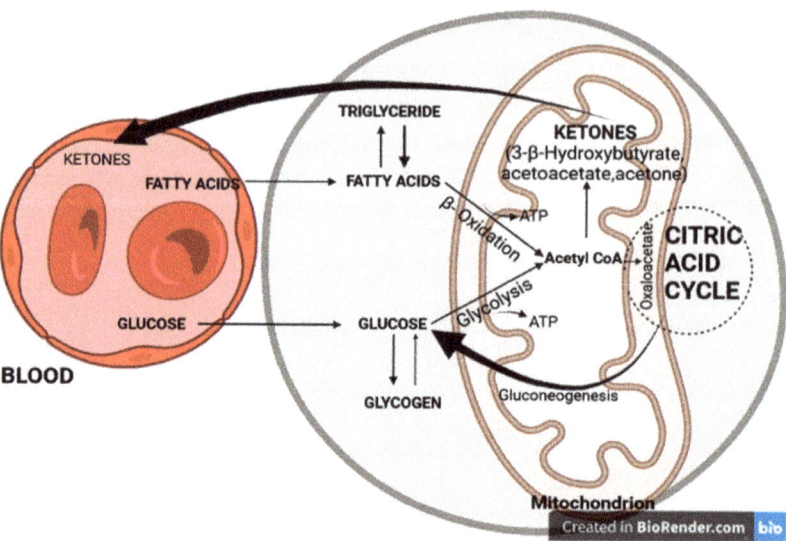

Figure 1. Glucose and fatty acid metabolism in hepatocyte mitochondria.

KBs are made up of three molecules: 3-β-hydroxybutyrate, acetoacetate, and acetone. 3-β-hydroxybutyrate results from the reduction of acetoacetate at the mitochondrial level and is the main transporter of energy from the liver to other tissues, of which the brain is the most important. Most tissues can use fatty acids as a source of energy during periods of severe hypoglycemia. The brain does not benefit from this adaptive mechanism and therefore, KBs are an essential alternative source of energy [29–34].

2. Materials and Methods

2.1. Aims and Scope

By using commercially available kits, we aimed to highlight the differences in blood glucose levels and KB values from the peripheral blood between three groups of patients: two tumoral groups with GBM/ASTRO G4 and a control group of healthy subjects, without influencing their diets.

By analyzing the differences between these groups, we aimed to determine if it is possible to use KBs and the glucose-ketone index (GKI) as prognostic factors of tumoral aggression.

2.2. Patients

This prospective observational study was conducted in the Neurosurgery Department of the Emergency Clinical Hospital of Targu Mures between January 2021 and June 2022 in accordance with the Declaration of Helsinki. The included patients were adults (>34 years old) who provided informed consent. The protocol of this study was approved by the Hospital's Ethics Committee. Three groups of subjects were included in the study: two groups of patients with histopathological confirmation of GBM or ASTRO G4 and a control group of subjects without a personal history of malignant pathologies.

Patients who were on a certain diet (such as ketogenic diets or similar) or had dietary restrictions and patients suffering from diabetes or other metabolic diseases were excluded. From the tumoral groups, patients who underwent biopsy or partial resection, and patients presenting with a Karnofski Performance Score (KPS) less than 80 were excluded. From the control group, subjects with a known personal pathological history such as metabolic diseases, benignant or malignant non-glial brain tumors, or systemic cancer were excluded [35].

2.3. Parameters Measured

In all of the three groups, a jeun glycemia and KBs (3-β-hydroxybutyrate) from the peripheral blood were measured using available commercial kits (Medical Device NOVA PRO GLU KET CONTROL, NOVA BIOMEDICAL, Product Code 47292, Category Code W0101060108). Fasting blood sampling was performed in the early morning of the second day after admission.

Based on the glycemic values and KB levels, the GKI was calculated. By determining the GKI, a single value that expresses the relationship between glucose (major fermentable tumor fuel) and KBs (non-fermentable fuel) was obtained. As most commercial kits express blood glucose in mg/dL and ketones in mM (including the kits used in this study), glucose units were converted to mM using the following formula [36]:

$$\text{GKI (mM)} = [\text{Glucose (mg/dL)}/18.016 \ (g \times dL/moL)]/\text{Ketone (mM)}$$

The weight and height of the included patients were also considered, and the body mass index (BMI) was calculated according to the following formula: weight (kg)/[height (m)]^2.

2.4. Assessment of the Clinical Condition

The Motor Assessment Scale was used to assess motor deficits and the Glasgow Coma Scale was used to assess consciousness [37,38]. The KPS was used to assess the functional status of patients both before and after the surgery.

2.5. Neuroimaging Evaluation

Preoperative magnetic resonance imaging (MRI) scans and immediate postoperative cranial computer tomography (CT) scans were performed for all patients. Follow-up MRIs were performed every 3 months during the patient's lifetime. Tumor mass was measured based on the following formula: (maximum axial diameter × maximum coronal diameter × maximum sagittal diameter)/2 [39]. Perilesional edema has been defined as the T2 hypersignal area surrounding the tumor. The size of the edema was estimated based on the ratio of the minimum and maximum distances from the edge of the tumor to the outer edge of the edema on the axial scans.

The histopathological diagnosis could be suspected after analyzing the imaging aspects of the tumors: GBM was characterized by peripheral contrast enhancement and the central hyposignal area in the T1C+ sequence (Figure 2a–c). ASTRO G4 is sometimes difficult to categorize based on imaging aspects. It is characterized by the heterogeneity of contrast enhancement in the T1C+ sequence and a hypo/isosignal in the T1 sequence. Figure 2d–f shows the MRI aspects of a patient from the tumoral group with a confirmed histopathological diagnosis of ASTRO G4; the T1C + hyposignal area represents the area of tumoral tissue and not the area of perilesional edema.

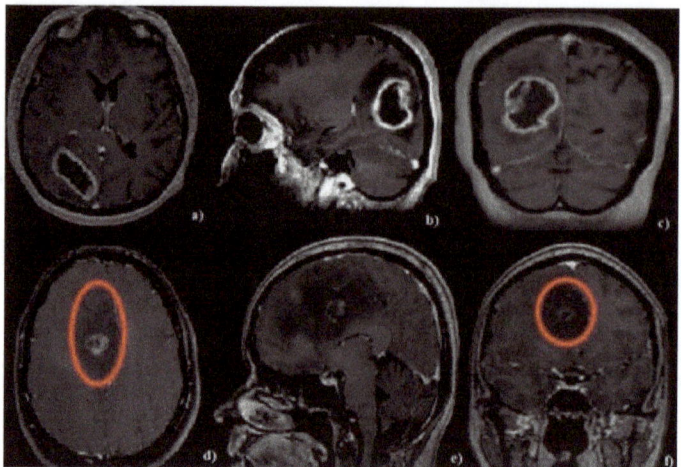

Figure 2. Cerebral MRI, T1C+ sequence: (**a–c**) showing a glioblastoma patient. (**d–f**) showing a grade 4 astrocytoma patient. Red circle (**d,f**) shows tumor boundaries.

2.6. Specific Medical Management

All patients included in the tumoral groups received dexamethasone at a dose of 4 to 16 mg per day according to the current treatment protocols. Preoperative medication was administered for between 1 and 5 days. Patients who survived for more than 1 month received postoperative chemotherapy and radiation therapy in accordance with the STUPP protocol [40].

2.7. Surgical Management

All surgical interventions were performed under general anesthesia. The surgical approaches were guided by the neuronavigation system (Curve 2.1; Brainlab, 81829 Munich, Germany) allowing us to perform minimal invasive craniotomies centered on the tumor's locations. In tumors located near eloquent areas, the image injection option of our surgical microscope (Captiview; Leica Microsystems, 35578 Wetzlar, Germany) was used in conjunction with the neuronavigation system (Figure 3).

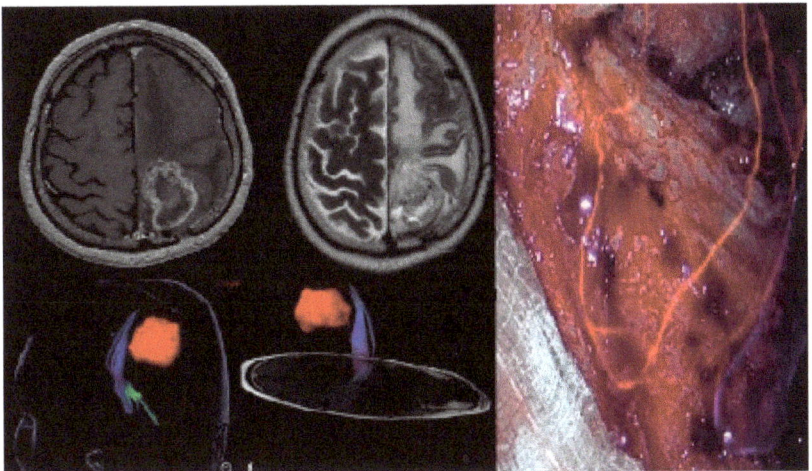

Figure 3. Postcentral GBM (cerebral MRI, T1C+, and T2 sequences). Tractography showing the pyramidal tracts and image injection into the surgical microscope (Captiview, Leica Microsystems GmbH 35578 Wetzlar Germany).

The trajectories of approach were chosen to be as short as possible by using transsylvian or transsulcal approaches while simultaneously avoiding eloquent areas. The use of retractors was avoided; instead, "dynamic retraction" technique described by Spetzler et al. [41] was used, paying significant attention to sulcal and fissure dissections to minimize the surgical sacrifice of the brain parenchyma.

Total resection (considered over 90%) was performed under the operating microscope (Leica Microsystems, 35578 Wetzlar, Germany). The extent of the resection was assessed by the main operator and an experienced radiologist.

2.8. Histopathological Analysis

The histopathological diagnosis was established within the Pathological Anatomy Department of our institute in accordance with the WHO 2016 and 2021 classification standards for tumors of the central nervous system.

2.9. Statistical Analysis

Statistical analysis included elements of descriptive statistics (mean, median, and standard deviation) and inferential statistics. The Shapiro–Wilk test was applied to determine the distribution of the analyzed data series.

The t-Student parametric test for unpaired data was applied to compare means and the non-parametric Mann–Whitney test was applied to compare medians. The significance threshold value chosen for p was 0.05 with a confidence interval of 95%. Statistical analysis was performed using the GraphPad Prism trial version utility.

3. Results

3.1. General Clinical Features

Out of a total of 22 patients with brain tumors, 27.3% had ASTRO G4. IDH mutation was present in 100% of ASTRO G4 patients. Men accounted for 59.1% of the patients and the mean age was 56.3 years (range: 34 to 74 years).

The control group had similar characteristics to the tumor groups: 59.1% of the subjects were male, with an average age of 53.9 years (range: 36 to 78 years). There was no statistically significant difference in the mean age between the three groups ($p > 0.05$ using the t-Student test, Table 1).

Table 1. General and specific characteristics.

		Tumor Group		Standard Deviation		Control Group	p-Value
		ASTRO G4	GBM	**General Characteristics**			
				Tumor group	Control group		
Gender	Male	66.7 (4)	56.3 (9)			59.1 (13)	
% (N)	Female	33.3 (2)	43.7 (7)			40.9 (9)	
Years	Average age	48.1	55.6			53.9	0.512
	Age range	34–66	44–78	56.09 ± 12.33	53.45 ± 14.10	36–78	
				Specific Characteristics (average)			
	Wight (kg)	80	89.6	85.00 ± 12.72	82.23 ± 16.70	82.2	0.538
	Height (cm)	169.8	175	173.6 ± 7.681	171.2 ± 10.13	171.2	0.379
	BMI	27.8	28.3	28.15 ± 3.867	28.02 ± 4.136	28.0	0.914
	Ketone Bodies (mM)	0.13	0.26	0.227 ± 0.2004	0.0773 ± 0.0812	0.08	0.0061
	Glycemia (mg/dL)	138.5	129.6	132.0 ± 39.43	96.73 ± 11.78	96.7	0.0003
	GKI (mM)	63.7	29.3	38.68 ± 29.80	16.85 ± 21.37	18.0	0.0080
	Clinical debut (weeks)	12.7	2.9	85.00 ± 12.72	82.23 ± 16.70	82.2	0.538
	Headache	83.3	93.7				
	Motor deficit	33.3	56.3				
%	Confusion	16.7	50				
	Seizures	16.7	25				
	Aphasia	16.7	12.5				

3.2. Specific Clinical Features

In the tumor groups, the average BMI (body-mass index) was 28.1%, the average GKI was 38.7%, and the average KB value was 0.2%. The median time interval from the onset of symptoms to the diagnosis of GBM or ASTRO G4 (cranial MRI examination) was 6 weeks. Headache was the main onset sign, present in 90.1% of patients, followed by motor deficit and confusion in 45.4% and 40.9% of cases, respectively.

The control group showed an average BMI of 28.0%, an average GKI of 16.8%, and an average KB value of 0.08%. Regarding KBs, the values were less than 0.2 mM in patients with ASTRO G4, similar to the control group.

There were no statistically significant differences (p-value < 0.05; CI 95%) in the mean height, weight, and BMI between the three groups of subjects as per the t-Student test (Table 1). The mean values of glycemia, KBs, and GKI showed statistically significant differences between the three groups (p-value < 0.05 using the Mann–Whitney test, Table 1).

3.3. Tumor Characteristics

Most tumors were located in the left frontal lobe both for GBM (54.5%) and ASTRO G4 (50% of the total number of patients). The maximum/minimum diameter was 68/24 mm for GBM and 54/21 mm for ASTRO G4, and the maximum/minimum diameter of the area of perilesional edema was 60/0.2 mm for GBM and 40/0.1 mm for ASTRO G4 (Table 2).

Table 2. Imaging and histopathological characteristics.

		ASTRO G4 (%)	GBM (%)
Tumor location	Frontal	50	50
	Temporal	33.3	31.2
	Parietal	16.7	37.5
	Occipital	16.7	31.2
	Insular	0.0	12.5
Cerebral hemisphere	Left	33.3	37.5
	Right	66.7	62.5

Table 2. Cont.

		ASTRO G4 (%)	GBM (%)
Tumor size (mm)		40.1/30.2	48.4/39.6
Size of the perilesional edema (mm)		23.6/3.5	23/2.4
Ki-67 index	≤15	50	18.7
	15–30	16.7	37.5
	≥30	33.3	43.8
P53 +		83.3	50

3.4. Histopathological Features

Tumor tissue consisted of atypical glial tumor cells with increased mitotic activity and variable cellularity with infiltrative character. No myxoid character or microcyst formation was noted. Tumoral cells had rounded or elongated hyperchromic nuclei with variable pleomorphism and fine, eosinophilic fibrillar processes. Tumor cells with marked pleomorphism were characterized by larger nuclei with lobed, vesicular character, sometimes with bizarre shapes. Foci of necrosis have been identified in all cases, sometimes with palisading of the surrounding nuclei, and microvascular hyperplasia with hyperplastic endothelial cells, often with the presence of "glomeruloid" bodies (Figure 4, Table 2) [42].

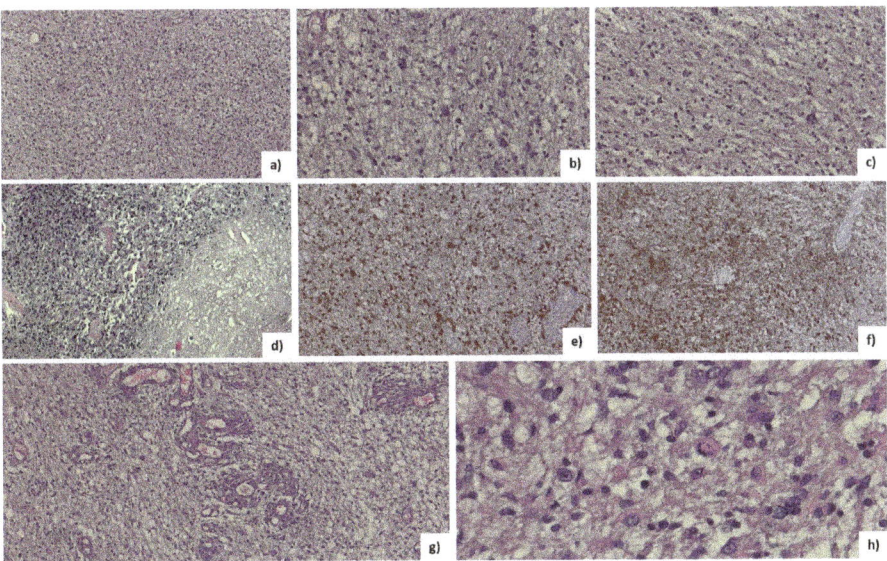

Figure 4. (**a**) Hematoxylin-Eosin (HE) GBM (10×); (**b**,**c**) nuclear pleomorphism (HE, 20×); (**d**) tumor and necrosis (HE, 20×); (**e**,**f**) positive IDH 1-R132H mutation on immunohistochemistry (HE, 20×); (**g**) microvascular proliferation with hyperplastic endothelia (HE, 20×); (**h**) atypical mitosis (HE, 40×).

3.5. Postoperative Death

The 3-month death rate was 0.0% in patients with ASTRO G4 and 43.75% in patients with GBM. At 1 month, the death rate was 12.5% in patients with GBM. The rate of postoperative complications was 16.7% in patients with ASTRO G4 and 18.75% in those with GBM. Postoperative complications have not led to death (Table 3).

Table 3. Ketone body values and mortality at 3 months after the surgical intervention.

	Ketone Bodies	Tumor Group ASTRO G4 (%)	Tumor Group GBM (%)	Control Group (%)
	≤0.2 mM	100	56.25	100
	>0.2 mM	0.0	43.75	0.0
MORTALITY AT 3 MONTHS	≤0.2 mM	0.0	0.0	
	0.2–0.5 mM	0.0	85.7	
	≥0.5 mM	0.0	100	

4. Discussion

Due to the low survival rate of patients with GBM/ASTRO G4, there is an urgent need for adjuvant therapies that increase survival and quality of life. In this context, cellular metabolism, especially glucose and KB metabolism, represents a therapeutic target and a broad topic of research [10,26,30,43,44].

KBs play essential roles in various metabolic pathways such as β-oxidation (Fatty Acid Oxidation), the biosynthesis of sterols, the tricarboxylic acid cycle, de novo lipogenesis, and gluconeogenesis [45–47]. They are a vital alternative for fueling the brain during periods of nutrient deprivation. KBs are mainly produced inside the liver from acetyl-CoA and are transported to extrahepatic tissues for terminal oxidation [22,26,29]. Normally, the blood levels of KBs are situated below 0.5 mM. Values between 0.5 and 1.0 mM are considered slightly higher, while values between 1.0 and 3.0 mM are considered moderately high [18,27,48,49].

The current treatment protocol for GBM and malignant astrocytomas consists of surgery, followed by radiotherapy and chemotherapy (temozolomide) [40,50–52]. However, the average survival duration is still less than 15 months, and the 5-year survival is below 10% [6,8,10,11]. These patients also have an increased risk of suicide, possibly due to the poor prognosis of this pathology and because of treatment-related side effects, such as mood-altering steroids [53]. Establishing new treatment regimens based on different peripheral markers that are easy to determine from the patient's peripheral blood, such as KBs, and introducing adjuvant therapies based on these parameters, such as ketogenic diets, and thus essentially individualizing treatments, may result in an increase in the survival rate. In this context, tumoral cellular metabolism may be a new therapeutic target that warrants attention.

Most studies have revealed that brain tumor cells are dependent on glucose for survival and KBs cannot be used effectively as alternative fuels [29,46]. Therefore, this "metabolic management area," defined by decreasing the blood glucose levels and increasing KB levels, may result in the improvement of the survival rate in patients suffering from high-grade malignancies [6,33,36,54]. It is well known that during physical exercise, fasting, carbohydrate restriction, or insulin deficiency, KB levels increase, and even if ketoacidosis is a pathological condition with serious repercussions, mild ketonemia can have beneficial effects in cancer [55–57]. Unfortunately, in GBM, this theory may not be applicable [26,58].

Certain oncogenic mutations such as Phosphatidylinositol-3-kinase (PI3K)/Protein kinase B (AKT)/Mammalian target of rapamycin (mTOR) significantly influence GBM metabolism by promoting the use of glucose as an energy substrate and promoting the synthesis of FAs [14,20,26,46,59]. These mutations induce the "glucose dependence" of tumor cells, which would be directly targeted by glucose deprivation [6,23,29]. Unfortunately, GBM is characterized by high heterogeneity and has even raised the hypothesis that it could use FAs as a substrate for generating new tumor blocks [29,60]. Metabolic reprogramming takes place, with a defining role in all stages of GBM development. Due to this high individualized heterogeneity of GBM, it is very difficult to establish certain easily determinable biological markers that can predict the degree of tumor aggressiveness, the response to oncological treatment, and even the need to administer adjuvant treatments, such as ketogenic diets [21,30,31,61].

In this prospective study, we explored the possibility of using KBs and GKI for predicting tumor aggressiveness in patients with GBM or ASTRO G4. We aimed to highlight the possibility of establishing individualized treatment protocols based on these parameters, which are easy to determine from samples of the patient's peripheral blood by using cheap commercial kits.

We have established that mortality rates at three months following the surgical intervention were 85.7% in patients presenting with KB values between 0.2 and 0.5 mM, and 100% in patients with KB values above 0.5 mM (Table 3). Additionally, we want to highlight that KB values over 0.2 mM were recorded only in patients with GBM, suggesting the fact that this aggressive, heterogeneous tumor may benefit from an extremely complex adaptive metabolic mechanism, and dietary changes or medication administration for reaching the "metabolic management area" could be ineffective in this category of patients [6,33,36,54]. In contrast, KB values of less than 0.2 mM were recorded in patients with ASTRO G4, which were similar values to healthy subjects.

Most studies that present the use of ketogenic diets as adjuvant therapies in glioma patients do not take into consideration the histopathological classification, therefore, the results are often contradictory [5,30,62].

Sargaço et al. tried to establish the effects of ketogenic diets in patients with gliomas in a systematic review. They found nine relevant studies showing an overall survival increase (in half of the analyzed studies), as well as the quality of life (in 25% of cases), in patients who were administered ketogenic diets, and only in one quarter of the cases the quality of life decreased [63]. Unfortunately, the analyzed studies established the histopathological diagnosis of GBM or astrocytoma grade 2, 3, or 4 without mentioning the molecular subtype or other histopathological details of the included cases. Based on our results, we want to highlight the need of viewing GBM and ASTRO G4 as two distinct pathologies characterized by their tumoral heterogeneity.

Sperry et al. demonstrated that U87 glioma cell lines as well as cell culture lines derived from GBM patients, including those with mutations in the mTOR/AKT/PI3K/IDH1 signaling pathways, can use KBs for tumor growth under standard and physiological culture conditions. Furthermore, it has been shown that the administration of ketogenic diets to tumor-bearing animals does not decrease the rate of tumor growth or improve the survival of these animals, proving the metabolic plasticity of GBM [29]. The drawback of this study is the lack of correlation of the obtained results with the blood values of KBs.

Steroids, most commonly dexamethasone, are a standard treatment for GBM and ASTRO G4 and are administered both before and after the surgical intervention and during chemotherapy/radiotherapy. The goal is to reduce the perilesional vasogenic edema as well as to prevent and even treat increased intracranial pressure. However, steroid administration is associated with a multitude of side effects, such as abnormalities in glucose metabolism, gastrointestinal complications, myopathies, insomnia, and anxiety. Although most complications are reversible after treatment discontinuation, 50% of patients have persistent disturbances in glucose metabolism after discontinuing the treatment [23,24,29,64–66].

The mean blood glucose levels were higher in the tumor groups compared to the control group, secondary to dexamethasone administration (treatment was administered for 1 to 3 days prior to glucose determination), with a statistically significant difference between the two groups (p-value = 0.0003, Table 2). These increased values show changes in the glucose metabolism, which in turn lead to an increase in the fuel needed for tumor development. On the other hand, the mean blood glucose level in ASTRO G4 patients was 8.9 mg/dL higher than in GBM patients. This slightly higher value can be explained by the administration of higher doses of glucocorticoids in patients with ASTRO G4 because the imaging aspects of astrocytoma grade 3/4 are characterized by peripheral low T1 signal and high T2 signal areas, sometimes without contrast enhancement on the T1C+ sequences, which can erroneously be interpreted as larger perilesional edematous areas (Figure 2d–f, red circle indicates tumor boundary). Zhou et al. analyzed 10 articles in a systematic review that included a total of 2230 patients diagnosed with GBM or ASTRO G4 and concluded that dexamethasone administration significantly decreases patient prognosis [67]. The results presented by us also raise questions about the doses and timing of dexamethasone usage throughout the course of the disease.

Another important marker calculated was GKI, designed to prove the effectiveness of various nutritional interventions which lead to lower blood sugar levels and increased KB levels. Artificial intelligence (AI) has the potential to play a significant role in evaluating markers like GKI and assessing their effectiveness in various nutritional interventions aimed at reducing blood sugar levels and increasing KB levels. Furthermore, AI can help in optimizing personalized dietary plans for individuals based on their unique metabolic responses. It can consider factors like genetics, lifestyle, and medical history to recommend tailored nutritional interventions that are more likely to achieve the desired GKI outcomes. In summary, AI can enhance our understanding of the impact of nutritional interventions on markers like GKI by efficiently analyzing complex data and providing evidence-based insights to guide dietary recommendations for individuals seeking to manage their blood sugar and ketone levels [68].

Due to the changes in blood glucose values secondary to steroid administration, GKI values were altered in the tumor groups, with a statistically significant difference between the three groups of patients (p-value = 0.008, CI 95%, Table 1). Although we do not expect significant changes between patients with GBM and those with ASTRO G4, the GKI value was 34.4 mm higher in the group of patients with ASTRO G4. These values emphasize the need to manage the two pathologies individually, highlighting the GBM heterogeneity.

While our study provides valuable information, there are several limitations to consider like the relatively small number of patients and the fact that the two tumoral groups of patients had to receive dexamethasone to decrease the perilesional edema which has led to elevations in the levels of blood glucose and GKI.

5. Conclusions

Highlighting new markers that are feasible to acquire (such as KB and GKI) which could also become additional therapeutic targets represent important steps toward treatment individualization and survival rate prolongation in patients with GBM and ASTRO G4.

Although this study was performed on a small group of patients, we have demonstrated statistically significant differences in the peripheral blood values of KBs and GKI between these two pathologies (GBM and ASTRO G4) and compared them to a control group; therefore, these two pathologies need to be viewed and managed as two distinct pathologies. We can also emphasize that KB values over 0.5 mM represent a negative prognostic factor in patients with GBM.

Establishing individualized adjuvant therapies based on reducing blood glucose levels and increasing KB levels in patients with ASTRO G4 could lead to survival rate improvements in this category of patients, considering that the KB values in these patients are like those of healthy subjects (below 0.2 mM). In contrast, nutritional changes may be ineffective in patients with GBM due to the heterogeneity and adaptive mechanisms of this pathology.

Our study also raises the need for larger clinical trials which are aimed to demonstrate the benefits of dexamethasone administration in patients with GBM and ASTRO G4.

Author Contributions: Conceptualization, C.T. and A.B.; methodology, F.T. and A.K.; software, G.S. and C.T.; validation, C.T., A.B. and C.B.; formal analysis, C.T. and A.K.; investigation, G.S.; resources, F.T.; data curation, F.T.; writing—original draft preparation, G.S.; writing—review and editing, A.B.; visualization, A.B.; supervision, C.B.; project administration, A.B.; funding acquisition, C.T., A.B. and C.B. All authors have read and agreed to the published version of the manuscript.

Funding: This research was funded by "George Emil Palade" University of Medicine, Pharmacy, Science and Technology of Targu Mures, research grant number 10126/2/17.12.2020.

Institutional Review Board Statement: The study was conducted in accordance with the Declaration of Helsinki and approved by the Ethics Committee of the Emergency Clinical County Hospital of Targu Mures, Romania (No. 30291/08.12.2020).

Informed Consent Statement: Informed consent was obtained from all subjects involved in the study.

Data Availability Statement: MDPI Research Data Policies" at https://www.mdpi.com/ethics.

Conflicts of Interest: The authors declare no conflict of interest.

References

1. Taphoorn, M.J.B.; Sizoo, E.M.; Bottomley, A. Review on Quality of Life Issues in Patients with Primary Brain Tumors. *Oncologist* **2010**, *15*, 618–626. [CrossRef]
2. Luo, C.; Song, K.; Wu, S.; Hameed, N.U.F.; Kudulaiti, N.; Xu, H.; Wu, J.S.; Qin, Z.Y. The prognosis of glioblastoma: A large, multifactorial study. *Br. J. Neurosurg.* **2021**, *35*, 555–561. [CrossRef]
3. Ohgaki, H.; Kleihues, P. The definition of primary and secondary glioblastoma. *Clin. Cancer Res.* **2013**, *19*, 764–772. [CrossRef] [PubMed]
4. Bouwens van der Vlis, T.A.M.; Kros, J.M.; Mustafa, D.A.M.; van Wijck, R.T.A.; Ackermans, L.; van Hagen, P.M.; van der Spek, P.J. The complement system in glioblastoma multiforme. *Acta Neuropathol. Commun.* **2018**, *6*, 91. [CrossRef]
5. Maroon, J.; Seyfried, T.; Donohue, J.; Bost, J. The role of metabolic therapy in treating glioblastoma multiforme. *Surg. Neurol. Int.* **2015**, *6*, 61. [CrossRef]
6. Seyfried, T.N.; Flores, R.; Poff, A.M.; D'Agostino, D.P.; Mukherjee, P. Metabolic therapy: A new paradigm for managing malignant brain cancer. *Cancer Lett.* **2015**, *356*, 289–300. [CrossRef]
7. Ostrom, Q.T.; Gittleman, H.; Farah, P.; Ondracek, A.; Chen, Y.; Wolinsky, Y.; Stroup, N.E.; Kruchko, C.; Jill, S.B.S. CBTRUS statistical report: Primary brain and central nervous system tumors diagnosed in the United States in 2006–2010. *Neuro-oncology* **2013**, *15*, ii1–ii56. [CrossRef] [PubMed]
8. Philips, A.; Henshaw, D.L.; Lamburn, G.; O'Carroll, M.J. Brain tumours: Rise in glioblastoma multiforme incidence in England 1995–2015 Suggests an Adverse Environmental or Lifestyle Factor. *J. Environ. Public Health* **2018**, *2018*, 7910754. [CrossRef] [PubMed]
9. Brodbelt, A.; Greenberg, D.; Winters, T.; Williams, M.; Vernon, S.; Collins, V.P. Glioblastoma in England: 2007–2011. *Eur. J. Cancer* **2015**, *51*, 533–542. [CrossRef]
10. Elsakka, A.M.A.; Bary, M.A.; Abdelzaher, E.; Elnaggar, M.; Kalamian, M.; Mukherjee, P.; Seyfried, T.N. Management of Glioblastoma Multiforme in a Patient Treated With Ketogenic Metabolic Therapy and Modified Standard of Care: A 24-Month Follow-Up. *Front. Nutr.* **2018**, *5*, 20. [CrossRef]
11. Mittal, S.; Pradhan, S.; Srivastava, T. Recent advances in targeted therapy for glioblastoma. *Expert Rev. Neurother.* **2015**, *15*, 935–946. [CrossRef] [PubMed]
12. Louis, D.N.; Perry, A.; Reifenberger, G.; von Deimling, A.; Figarella-Branger, D.; Cavenee, W.K.; Hiroko, O.; Otmar, D.W.; Paul, K.; David, W.E. The 2016 World Health Organization Classification of Tumors of the Central Nervous System: A summary. *Acta Neuropathol.* **2016**, *131*, 803–820. [CrossRef] [PubMed]
13. Louis, D.N.; Perry, A.; Wesseling, P.; Brat, D.J.; Cree, I.A.; Figarella-Branger, D.; Cynthia, H.; Ng, H.K.; Stefan, M.P.; Guido, R.; et al. The 2021 WHO classification of tumors of the central nervous system: A summary. *Neuro-oncology* **2021**, *23*, 1231–1251. [CrossRef] [PubMed]
14. de Gooijer, M.C.; Guillén Navarro, M.; Bernards, R.; Wurdinger, T.; van Tellingen, O. An Experimenter's Guide to Glioblastoma Invasion Pathways. *Trends Mol. Med.* **2018**, *24*, 763–780. [CrossRef] [PubMed]
15. Pencheva, N.; de Gooijer, M.C.; Vis, D.J.; Wessels, L.F.A.; Würdinger, T.; van Tellingen, O.; Rene, B. Identification of a Druggable Pathway Controlling Glioblastoma Invasiveness. *Cell Rep.* **2017**, *20*, 48–60. [CrossRef]
16. Bensalma, S.; Turpault, S.; Balandre, A.C.; De Boisvilliers, M.; Gaillard, A.; Chadéneau, C.; Jean, M.M. PKA at a Cross-Road of Signaling Pathways Involved in the Regulation of Glioblastoma Migration and Invasion by the Neuropeptides VIP and PACAP. *Cancers* **2019**, *11*, 123. [CrossRef]
17. Strickland, M.; Stoll, E.A. Metabolic Reprogramming in Glioma. *Front. Cell Dev. Biol.* **2017**, *26*, 5–43. [CrossRef]
18. Agnihotri, S.; Zadeh, G. Metabolic reprogramming in glioblastoma: The influence of cancer metabolism on epigenetics and unanswered questions. *Neuro-oncology* **2016**, *18*, 160–172. [CrossRef]
19. Masui, K.; Onizuka, H.; Cavenee, W.K.; Mischel, P.S.; Shibata, N. Metabolic reprogramming in the pathogenesis of glioma: Update. *Neuropathology* **2019**, *39*, 3–13. [CrossRef]
20. Tran, Q.; Lee, H.; Kim, C.; Kong, G.; Gong, N.; Kwon, S.H.; Park, J. Revisiting the Warburg Effect: Diet-Based Strategies for Cancer Prevention. *Biomed Res. Int.* **2020**, *4*, 8105735. [CrossRef]
21. Woolf, E.C.; Syed, N.; Scheck, A.C. Tumor metabolism, the ketogenic diet and β-hydroxybutyrate: Novel approaches to adjuvant brain tumor therapy. *Front. Mol. Neurosci.* **2016**, *9*, 122. [CrossRef] [PubMed]

22. Zhang, S.; Xie, C. The role of OXCT1 in the pathogenesis of cancer as a rate-limiting enzyme of ketone body metabolism. *Life Sci.* **2017**, *183*, 110–115. [CrossRef] [PubMed]
23. Duma, M.N.; Oszfolk, N.I.; Boeckh-Behrens, T.; Oechsner, M.; Zimmer, C.; Meyer, B.; Paul, T.P.; Stephanie, E.C. Positive correlation between blood glucose and radiotherapy doses to the central gustatory system in Glioblastoma Multiforme patients. *Radiat. Oncol.* **2019**, *14*, 97. [CrossRef]
24. Seliger, C.; Ricci, C.; Meier, C.R.; Bodmer, M.; Jick, S.S.; Bogdahn, U.; Peter, U.; Michael, F.L. Diabetes, use of antidiabetic drugs, and the risk of glioma. *Neuro-oncology* **2016**, *18*, 340–349. [CrossRef] [PubMed]
25. Caniglia, J.L.; Jalasutram, A.; Asuthkar, S.; Sahagun, J.; Park, S.; Ravindra, A.; Andrew, J.T.; Guda, M.R.; Kiran, K.V. Beyond glucose: Alternative sources of energy in glioblastoma. *Theranostics* **2021**, *11*, 2048–2057. [CrossRef]
26. Libby, C.J.; Tran, A.N.; Scott, S.E.; Griguer, C.; Hjelmeland, A.B. The pro-tumorigenic effects of metabolic alterations in glioblastoma including brain tumor initiating cells. *Biochim. Biophys. Acta-Rev. Cancer* **2018**, *1869*, 175–188. [CrossRef]
27. Chang, H.T.; Olson, L.K.; Schwartz, K.A. Ketolytic and glycolytic enzymatic expression profiles in malignant gliomas: Implication for ketogenic diet therapy. *Nutr. Metab.* **2013**, *10*, 47. [CrossRef]
28. Lin, H.; Patel, S.; Affleck, V.S.; Wilson, I.; Turnbull, D.M.; Joshi, A.R.; Ross, M.; Elizabeth, A.S. Fatty acid oxidation is required for the respiration and proliferation of malignant glioma cells. *Neuro-oncology* **2017**, *19*, 43–54. [CrossRef]
29. Sperry, J.; Condro, M.C.; Guo, L.; Braas, D.; Vanderveer-Harris, N.; Kim, K.K.O.; Whitney, B.P.; Ajit, D.; Albert, L.; Heather, C.; et al. Glioblastoma Utilizes Fatty Acids and Ketone Bodies for Growth Allowing Progression during Ketogenic Diet Therapy. *iScience* **2020**, *23*, 101453. [CrossRef]
30. Vallejo, F.A.; Shah, S.S.; de Cordoba, N.; Walters, W.M.; Prince, J.; Khatib, Z.; Ricardo, J.K.; Steven, V.; Regina, M.G. The contribution of ketone bodies to glycolytic inhibition for the treatment of adult and pediatric glioblastoma. *J. Neurooncol.* **2020**, *147*, 317–326. [CrossRef]
31. Azzalin, A.; Brambilla, F.; Arbustini, E.; Basello, K.; Speciani, A.; Mauri, P.; Paola, B.; Lorenzo, M. A New Pathway Promotes Adaptation of Human Glioblastoma Cells to Glucose Starvation. *Cells* **2020**, *9*, 1249. [CrossRef] [PubMed]
32. Seyfried, T.N.; Shivane, A.G.; Kalamian, M.; Maroon, J.C.; Mukherjee, P.; Zuccoli, G. Ketogenic Metabolic Therapy, Without Chemo or Radiation, for the Long-Term Management of IDH1-Mutant Glioblastoma: An 80-Month Follow-Up Case Report. *Front. Nutr.* **2021**, *8*, 682243. [CrossRef] [PubMed]
33. Abdelwahab, M.G.; Fenton, K.E.; Preul, M.C.; Rho, J.M.; Lynch, A.; Stafford, P.; Adrienne, C.S. The ketogenic diet is an effective adjuvant to radiation therapy for the treatment of malignant glioma. *PLoS ONE* **2012**, *7*, e36197. [CrossRef] [PubMed]
34. Schönfeld, P.; Reiser, G. Why does brain metabolism not favor burning of fatty acids to provide energy? Reflections on disadvantages of the use of free fatty acids as fuel for brain. *J. Cereb. Blood Flow Metab.* **2013**, *33*, 1493–1499. [CrossRef] [PubMed]
35. Friendlander, A.H.; Ettinger, R.L. Karnofsky performance status scale. *Spec. Care Dent.* **2009**, *4*, 147–180. [CrossRef] [PubMed]
36. Meidenbauer, J.J.; Mukherjee, P.; Seyfried, T.N. The glucose ketone index calculator: A simple tool to monitor therapeutic efficacy for metabolic management of brain cancer. *Nutr. Metab.* **2015**, *12*, 12. [CrossRef]
37. Loewen, S.C.; Anderson, B.A. Reliability of the Modified Motor Assessment Scale and the Barthel Index. *Phys. Ther.* **1988**, *68*, 1077–1081. [CrossRef]
38. Bodien, Y.G.; Barra, A.; Temkin, N.R.; Barber, J.; Foreman, B.; Vassar, M.; Claudia, R.; Sabrina, R.T.; Amy, J.M.; Geoffrey, T.M.; et al. Diagnosing Level of Consciousness: The Limits of the Glasgow Coma Scale Total Score. *J. Neurotrauma* **2021**, *38*, 3295–3305. [CrossRef]
39. Kothari, R.U.; Brott, T.; Broderick, J.P.; Barsan, W.G.; Sauerbeck, L.R.; Zuccarello, M.; Khoury, J. The ABCs of measuring intracerebral hemorrhage volumes. *Stroke* **1996**, *27*, 1304–1350. [CrossRef]
40. Stupp, R.; Mason, W.P.; van den Bent, M.J.; Weller, M.; Fisher, B.; Taphoorn, M.J.B.; Karl, B.; Alba, A.B.; Christine, M.; Ulrich, B.; et al. Radiotherapy plus concomitant and adjuvant temozolomide for glioblastoma. *N. Engl. J. Med.* **2005**, *352*, 987–996. [CrossRef]
41. Spetzler, R.F.; Sanai, N. The quiet revolution: Retractorless surgery for complex vascular and skull base lesions. *J. Neurosurg.* **2012**, *116*, 291–300. [CrossRef] [PubMed]
42. Lai, A.; Kharbanda, S.; Pope, W.B.; Tran, A.; Solis, O.E.; Peale, F.; William, F.F.; Kanan, P.; Jose, A.C.; Ajay, P.; et al. Evidence for sequenced molecular evolution of IDH1 mutant glioblastoma from a distinct cell of origin. *J. Clin. Oncol.* **2011**, *29*, 4482–4490. [CrossRef] [PubMed]
43. Guo, J.; Xue, Q.; Liu, K.; Ge, W.; Liu, W.; Wang, J.; Wang, J.; Zhang, M.; Li, Q.-Y.; Cai, D.; et al. Dimethylaminomicheliolide (DMAMCL) Suppresses the Proliferation of Glioblastoma Cells via Targeting Pyruvate Kinase 2 (PKM2) and Rewiring Aerobic Glycolysis. *Front. Oncol.* **2019**, *9*, 993. [CrossRef] [PubMed]
44. Rieger, J.; Bähr, O.; Maurer, G.D.; Hattingen, E.; Franz, K.; Brucker, D.; Stefan, W.; Ulrike, K.; Johannes, F.C.; Michael, W.; et al. ERGO: A pilot study of ketogenic diet in recurrent glioblastoma. *Int. J. Oncol.* **2014**, *45*, 1843–1852. [CrossRef] [PubMed]
45. Sanzey, M.; Abdul Rahim, S.A.; Oudin, A.; Dirkse, A.; Kaoma, T.; Vallar, L.; Christel, H.M.; Rolf, B.; Anna, G.; Simone, P.N. Comprehensive analysis of glycolytic enzymes as therapeutic targets in the treatment of glioblastoma. *PLoS ONE* **2015**, *10*, e0123544. [CrossRef] [PubMed]
46. Stanke, K.M.; Wilson, C.; Kidambi, S. High Expression of Glycolytic Genes in Clinical Glioblastoma Patients Correlates With Lower Survival. *Front. Mol. Biosci.* **2021**, *8*, 752404. [CrossRef] [PubMed]

47. Zahra, K.; Dey, T.; Ashish, S.; Mishra, P.; Pandey, U. Pyruvate Kinase M2 and Cancer: The Role of PKM2 in Promoting Tumorigenesis. *Front. Oncol.* **2020**, *10*, 159. [CrossRef]
48. Laffel, L. Ketone bodies: A review of physiology, pathophysiology and application of monitoring to diabetes. *Diabetes Metab. Res. Rev.* **1999**, *15*, 412–426. [CrossRef]
49. Wenger, K.J.; Wagner, M.; Harter, P.N.; Franz, K.; Bojunga, J.; Fokas, E.; Detlef, I.; Claus, R.; Johannes, R.; Elke, H.; et al. Maintenance of energy homeostasis during calorically restricted ketogenic diet and fasting-MR-spectroscopic insights from the ergo2 trial. *Cancers* **2020**, *12*, 3549. [CrossRef]
50. Lakomy, R.; Kazda, T.; Selingerova, I.; Poprach, A.; Pospisil, P.; Belanova, R.; Pavel, F.; Vaclav, V.; Martin, S.; Radim, J.; et al. Real-World Evidence in Glioblastoma: Stupp's Regimen After a Decade. *Front. Oncol.* **2020**, *10*, 840. [CrossRef]
51. Minniti, G.; De Sanctis, V.; Muni, R.; Filippone, F.; Bozzao, A.; Valeriani, M.; Osti, M.F.; Paula, U.D.; Lanzetta, G.; Tombolini, V.; et al. Radiotherapy plus concomitant and adjuvant temozolomide for glioblastoma in elderly patients. *J. Neurooncol.* **2008**, *88*, 97–103. [CrossRef] [PubMed]
52. Stupp, R.; Taillibert, S.; Kanner, A.; Read, W.; Steinberg, D.M.; Lhermitte, B.; Steven, T.; Ahmed, I.; Manmeet, S.A.; Karen, F.; et al. Effect of tumor-treating fields plus maintenance temozolomide vs maintenance temozolomide alone on survival in patients with glioblastoma a randomized clinical trial. *JAMA* **2017**, *318*, 2306–2316. [CrossRef] [PubMed]
53. Mofatteh, M.; Mashayekhi, M.S.; Arfaie, S.; Chen, Y.; Malhotra, A.K.; Alvi, M.A.; Sader, N.; Antonick, V.; Fatehi Hassanabad, M.; Mansouri, A.; et al. Suicidal ideation and attempts in brain tumor patients and survivors: A systematic review. *Neuro-Oncol. Adv.* **2023**, *12*, 5. [CrossRef] [PubMed]
54. Hagihara, K.; Kajimoto, K.; Osaga, S.; Nagai, N.; Eku, S.; Hideyuki, N.; Hitomi, S.; Mai, N.; Mariko, T.; Hideaki, K.; et al. Promising Effect of a New Ketogenic Diet Regimen in Patients with Adanced Cancer. *Nutrients* **2020**, *12*, 1473. [CrossRef]
55. Panhans, C.M.; Gresham, G.; Amaral, J.L.; Hu, J. Exploring the Feasibility and Effects of a Ketogenic Diet in Patients With CNS Malignancies: A Retrospective Case Series. *Front. Neurosci.* **2020**, *14*, 390. [CrossRef]
56. Allen, B.G.; Bhatia, S.K.; Anderson, C.M.; Eichenberger-Gilmore, J.M.; Sibenaller, Z.A.; Mapuskar, K.A.; Joshua, D.S.; John, M.B.; Douglas, R.S.; Melissa, A.F. Ketogenic diets as an adjuvant cancer therapy: History and potential mechanism. *Redox Biol.* **2014**, *2*, 963–970. [CrossRef]
57. Carneiro, L.; Leloup, C. Mens Sana in corpore Sano: Does the glycemic index have a role to play? *Nutrients* **2020**, *12*, 2989. [CrossRef]
58. Garcia, J.H.; Jain, S.; Aghi, M.K. Metabolic Drivers of Invasion in Glioblastoma. *Front. Cell Dev. Biol.* **2021**, *9*, 683276. [CrossRef]
59. Cruz Da Silva, E.; Mercier, M.C.; Etienne-Selloum, N.; Dontenwill, M.; Choulier, L. A Systematic Review of Glioblastoma-Targeted Therapies in Phases II, III, IV Clinical Trials. *Cancers* **2021**, *13*, 1795. [CrossRef]
60. De Feyter, H.M.; Behar, K.L.; Rao, J.U.; Madden-Hennessey, K.; Ip, K.L.; Hyder, F.; Lester, R.D.; Jean-Francois, G.; Robin, A.G.; Douglas, R. A ketogenic diet increases transport and oxidation of ketone bodies in RG2 and 9L gliomas without affecting tumor growth. *Neuro-oncology* **2016**, *18*, 1079–1087. [CrossRef]
61. Grieco, M.; Giorgi, A.; Gentile, M.C.; d'Erme, M.; Morano, S.; Maras, B.; Tiziana, F. Glucagon-Like Peptide-1: A Focus on Neurodegenerative Diseases. *Front. Neurosci.* **2019**, *13*, 1112. [CrossRef]
62. Zhang, C.; Wang, M.; Ji, F.; Peng, Y.; Wang, B.; Zhao, J.; Wu, J.; Zhao, H. A Novel Glucose Metabolism-Related Gene Signature for Overall Survival Prediction in Patients with Glioblastoma. *Biomed Res. Int.* **2021**, *22*, 8872977. [CrossRef]
63. Sargaço, B.; Oliveira, P.A.; Antunes, M.L.; Moreira, A.C. Effects of the Ketogenic Diet in the Treatment of Gliomas: A Systematic Review. *Nutrients* **2022**, *14*, 1007. [CrossRef] [PubMed]
64. Schwartzbaum, J.; Edlinger, M.; Zigmont, V.; Stattin, P.; Rempala, G.A.; Nagel, G.; Nikas, H.; Hanno, U.; Bernhard, F.; Goran, W.; et al. Associations between prediagnostic blood glucose levels, diabetes, and glioma. *Sci. Rep.* **2017**, *7*, 1436. [CrossRef] [PubMed]
65. Tieu, M.T.; Lovblom, L.E.; McNamara, M.G.; Mason, W.; Laperriere, N.; Millar, B.A.; Cunthia, M.; Tim, R.K.; Bruce, A.P.; Caroline, C. Impact of glycemia on survival of glioblastoma patients treated with radiation and temozolomide. *J. Neurooncol.* **2015**, *124*, 119–126. [CrossRef] [PubMed]
66. Seliger, C.; Genbrugge, E.; Gorlia, T.; Chinot, O.; Stupp, R.; Nabors, B.; Michael, W.; Peter, H. Use of metformin and outcome of patients with newly diagnosed glioblastoma: Pooled analysis. *Int. J. Cancer* **2020**, *146*, 803–809. [CrossRef]
67. Zhou, L.; Shen, Y.; Huang, T.; Sun, Y.; Alolga, R.N.; Zhang, G.; Ge, Y. The Prognostic Effect of Dexamethasone on Patients With Glioblastoma: A Systematic Review and Meta-Analysis. *Front. Pharmacol.* **2021**, *12*, 727707. [CrossRef]
68. Mohammad, M. Neurosurgery and artificial intelligence. *AIMS Neurosci.* **2021**, *8*, 477–495. [CrossRef]

Disclaimer/Publisher's Note: The statements, opinions and data contained in all publications are solely those of the individual author(s) and contributor(s) and not of MDPI and/or the editor(s). MDPI and/or the editor(s) disclaim responsibility for any injury to people or property resulting from any ideas, methods, instructions or products referred to in the content.

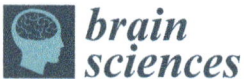

Article

Melatonin in Combination with Albendazole or Albendazole Sulfoxide Produces a Synergistic Cytotoxicity against Malignant Glioma Cells through Autophagy and Apoptosis

Miguel Hernández-Cerón [1,†], Víctor Chavarria [2,†], Camilo Ríos [1,3], Benjamin Pineda [2], Francisca Palomares-Alonso [4], Irma Susana Rojas-Tomé [4] and Helgi Jung-Cook [5,*]

1. Doctorate in Biological and Health Sciences, Universidad Autónoma Metropolitana, Mexico City 04960, Mexico; miguelqfbuamx@gmail.com (M.H.-C.); crios@correo.xoc.uam.mx (C.R.)
2. Neuroimmunology and Neuro-Oncology Unit, Instituto Nacional de Neurología y Neurocirugía (INNN), Mexico City 14269, Mexico; vchavarria@innn.edu.mx (V.C.); benjamin.pineda@innn.edu.mx (B.P.)
3. Laboratorio de Neurofarmacología Molecular, Departamento de Sistemas Biológicos, Universidad Autónoma Metropolitana, Unidad Xochimilco, Mexico City 04960, Mexico
4. Neuropsycopharmacology Lab, Instituto Nacional de Neurología y Neurocirugía, Mexico City 14269, Mexico; francisca.palomares@innn.edu.mx (F.P.-A.); isrtome@hotmail.com (I.S.R.-T.)
5. Pharmacy Department, Universidad Nacional Autónoma de México, Mexico City 04510, Mexico
* Correspondence: helgi@unam.mx
† These authors contributed equally to this work.

Abstract: Glioblastoma is the most aggressive and lethal brain tumor in adults, presenting diffuse brain infiltration, necrosis, and drug resistance. Although new drugs have been approved for recurrent patients, the median survival rate is two years; therefore, new alternatives to treat these patients are required. Previous studies have reported the anticancer activity of albendazole, its active metabolite albendazole sulfoxide, and melatonin; therefore, the present study was performed to evaluate if the combination of melatonin with albendazole or with albendazole sulfoxide induces an additive or synergistic cytotoxic effect on C6 and RG2 rat glioma cells, as well as on U87 human glioblastoma cells. Drug interaction was determined by the Chou–Talalay method. We evaluated the mechanism of cell death by flow cytometry, immunofluorescence, and crystal violet staining. The cytotoxicity of the combinations was mainly synergistic. The combined treatments induced significantly more apoptotic and autophagic cell death on the glioma cell lines. Additionally, albendazole and albendazole sulfoxide inhibited proliferation independently of melatonin. Our data justify continuing with the evaluation of this proposal since the combinations could be a potential strategy to aid in the treatment of glioblastoma.

Keywords: glioblastoma; melatonin; albendazole; albendazole sulfoxide; synergism

Citation: Hernández-Cerón, M.; Chavarria, V.; Ríos, C.; Pineda, B.; Palomares-Alonso, F.; Rojas-Tomé, I.S.; Jung-Cook, H. Melatonin in Combination with Albendazole or Albendazole Sulfoxide Produces a Synergistic Cytotoxicity against Malignant Glioma Cells through Autophagy and Apoptosis. *Brain Sci.* 2023, 13, 869. https://doi.org/10.3390/brainsci13060869

Academic Editors: Luis Exequiel Ibarra, Laura Natalia Milla Sanabria and Nuria Arias-Ramos

Received: 10 May 2023
Revised: 23 May 2023
Accepted: 25 May 2023
Published: 27 May 2023

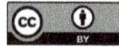

Copyright: © 2023 by the authors. Licensee MDPI, Basel, Switzerland. This article is an open access article distributed under the terms and conditions of the Creative Commons Attribution (CC BY) license (https://creativecommons.org/licenses/by/4.0/).

1. Introduction

Glioblastoma (GB) is the most frequent malignant tumor of the central nervous system (CNS) in adults, and it has a poor prognosis. Currently, the standard treatment involves maximal surgical resection, followed by radiotherapy and chemotherapy; however, the median overall survival is between 12 and 15 months [1]. In 2017, bevacizumab, an angiogenesis inhibitor, received Food and Drug Administration approval for the treatment of adults with recurrent GB that has progressed following prior therapy; however, the median overall survival did not exceed 24 months [2]. The poor prognosis of GB treatment is related to the low specificity of chemotherapeutic agents, the difficulty of most antitumor agents to access the CNS due to the blood–brain barrier (BBB), as well as the limitation to intracellular accumulation of drugs in tumor cells mediated by efflux transporters [3–5]. Therefore, these challenges point to the need to develop new therapies for this disease.

Drug repositioning has been a successful strategy to investigate existing drugs for additional clinical indications, with evidence supporting the anticancer effects of benzimidazole carbamates [6,7]. In this category, albendazole (ALB) has been addressed in different cancer models, including GB [8–10], with a well-tolerated high dose as anticancer treatment in clinical trials [11].

After oral administration, ALB is rapidly transformed into the chiral active metabolite albendazole sulfoxide [(+)-ALBSO; (−)-ALBSO)], which possesses anthelmintic activity, and into the non-chiral metabolite albendazole sulfone, which lacks pharmacologic activity. Studies from microsomal investigations in several species suggests that CYP3A4 and flavin-containing monooxygenase (FMO) are major enzymes responsible for the formation of sulfoxide metabolites from ALB [12]. Lee et al. reported that the ALBSO formation from ALB is also mediated by the CYP2J2 isoform, and significantly higher than those by the CYP3A4 isoform [13]. ALBSO readily crosses the BBB due to its high lipid solubility, presenting high availability in CNS, with almost half the concentration in cerebrospinal fluid than in plasma [14,15]. ALB and ALBSO are classically known for their affinity for tubulin and alteration of the microtubule assembly [16]. In addition, ALB has been reported is pleiotropic drugs with multiple effects on cells, including the inhibition of phosphorylation signaling pathways [17] and induction of oxidative stress promoting DNA fragmentation [18].

Melatonin (MLT), an endogenous indolamine synthesized primarily by the pineal gland, regulates numerous processes in humans, such as the sleep–wake cycle, immunomodulation, and endocrine function. MLT is primarily metabolized to 6-hydroxymelatonin, but MLT can also be deacetylated to 5-methoxytryptamine and N^1-acetyl-5-methoxykynuramine in the CNS, with antioxidant properties to capture reactive oxygen species and reactive nitrogen species [19–21]. MLT is a highly lipophilic molecule that can diffuse through the cell membrane to interact with intracellular targets [22]. Several studies have shown the potential use of MLT in the treatment of cancer [23], including GB, with synergistic activity when combined with other drugs, attributed to the inhibition of multiple pro-survival pathways, the inhibition of efflux pumps, and the regulation of autophagy [24–27].

The present study was performed to evaluate if the combination of MLT with ALB or with ALBSO induces an additive or synergistic cytotoxic effect in glioma cells. Likewise, the cell death mechanisms involved were investigated. The assays were conducted on three of the most widely used cell lines (C6, RG2, and U87).

2. Materials and Methods

2.1. Reagents, Drugs, and Antibodies

Dulbecco's Modified Eagle Medium (DMEM), antibiotic-antimycotic solution (10,000 units of penicillin, 10 mg of streptomycin, and 25 µg of amphotericin B per mL), 10× trypsin solution, albendazole (ALB), albendazole sulfoxide (ALBSO), melatonin (MLT), propidium iodide (PI), crystal violet, and 3-(4,5-dimethylthiazol-2-yl)-2,5-diphenyltetrazolium bromide (MTT) were obtained from Sigma-Aldrich (St. Louis, MO, USA). Fetal bovine serum (FBS) was obtained from Biowest (Nuaillé, Pays de la Loire, France). MACS bovine serum albumin was obtained from Miltenyi Biotec (Bergisch Gladbach, Germany). APC-Annexin V Apoptosis Detection Kit with 7-AAD was obtained from BioLegend (San Diego, CA, USA). Dimethyl sulfoxide (DMSO) and ethanol (Merck, Readington Township, NJ, Germany) were of analytical reagent grade. Acridine orange (AO) was obtained from Polysciences (Warrington, PA, USA). The goat polyclonal antibody anti-MAP LC3 was obtained from Santa Cruz Biotechnology (Dallas, TX, USA), and the anti-goat IgG-FITC antibody was obtained from Abcam (Cambridge, UK).

2.2. Glioma Cells and Cell Culture

C6 and RG2 rat malignant glioma cell lines and U87 human glioblastoma cell line were acquired from the American Type Culture Collection (ATCC, Manassas, VA, USA). Cells were maintained in DMEM with 10% FBS and 1% antibiotic-antimycotic solution in a 37 °C incubator with 5% CO_2 atmosphere and 98% relative humidity. Cells were maintained in culture flasks until they reached 80–90% confluence. Confluent cells were washed with phosphate-buffered saline (PBS) and detached by incubation in $1\times$ trypsin solution, for collection and seeding.

2.3. Concentration-Effect and Combination Study

For concentration-effect study, the stock solutions of ALB 2000 µM and ALBSO 20,000 µM were prepared in DMSO. Additionally, a stock solution of MLT 200 mM was prepared in ethanol. The stock solutions were serially diluted in DMEM to prepare working solutions of each drug to obtain final concentrations 0.16, 0.24, 0.36, 0.55, 0.83, and 1.25 µM for ALB; 2, 4, 8, 16, 32, and 64 µM for ALBSO; and 0.18, 0.37, 0.75, 1.5, 3, and 6 mM for MLT. DMSO and ethanol concentrations in DMEM did not exceed 0.5% and 3%, respectively. Solutions of DMSO and ethanol were used as vehicle control. To evaluate the cytotoxic effect of the treatments, 3×10^3 cells were seeded into 96-well tissue culture plates. Then, 24 h later, the cells were incubated with 100 µL of working solutions of ALB, ALBSO, MLT, and vehicle. After 72 h of treatment, the medium was removed, and cells were washed with PBS, and then 100 µL of MTT solution at a concentration of 5 mg/mL in DMEM was added to each well and incubated for 3 h at 37 °C. Afterward, the medium was aspirated, and blue formazan crystals were solubilized with 100 µL of DMSO. Absorbance was determined using a microplate reader (Synergy LX, BioTek, Winooski, VT, USA) at 570 nm. Six replicates were evaluated for each treatment, and the experiments were repeated at least four times. The cell viability percentage was calculated by the formula:

$$(\text{Absorbance of treated group}/\text{Absorbance of vehicle}) \times 100$$

The median dose effect (Dm) equivalent to mean inhibitory concentration (IC_{50}) of the concentration–response curves was calculated using the Chou–Talalay method [28,29] and CompuSyn.exe® software (Version 1.0), developed from the physical–chemical principle of the mass-action law analysis via mathematical induction and deduction.

Once the Dm values of each drug were calculated, they were used to design the combination study. The experimental procedures for preparing the solutions and assessing the cell viability were the same as described in the concentration-effect study. DMEM with maximum 0.5% of DMSO and 3% of ethanol was prepared as vehicle control. Each experiment was performed in triplicate over six repetitions. The combination index (CI) was calculated from the Chou–Talalay method using CompuSyn.exe® software (Version 1.0), which represents a quantitative measure of the extent of drug interaction with the following ranges: CI = 0.1–0.90 (synergism), 0.90–1.10 (nearly additive), and 1.10 to >10 (antagonism) [28,29].

2.4. Determination of Cell Death Mechanisms

The combinations selected for the study were those that presented the greatest cytotoxic effect. In the C6 cell line, the concentrations were ALB 0.6 µM-MLT 0.6 mM and ALBSO 20 µM-MLT 1 mM, while for the RG2 cell line, the concentrations were ALB 0.6 µM-MLT 0.6 mM and ALBSO 26 µM-MLT 0.9 mM. For the U87 cell line, the concentrations used were ALB 0.45 µM-MLT 0.45 mM and ALBSO 18 µM-MLT 0.45 mM. In addition, the effect of individual drugs at the same concentrations was evaluated. For the experiments, 2×10^4 cells were seeded into 24-well tissue culture plates. Then, 24 h later, the cells were incubated with 1 mL of working solutions of the combinations and vehicle. After 48 h of treatment, the culture medium was transferred to flow cytometry tubes, and the cells were washed with PBS. Then, cells were detached by adding 1X trypsin solution and were harvested into the same centrifuge tubes. The samples were centrifuged at 2000 rpm for 5 min, and the supernatants were discarded, taking care not to throw the button of sedimented cells.

2.4.1. Apoptosis Detection with Annexin V and 7-AAD Double Stain

To detect annexin V bound to phosphatidylserine (PS) in the extracellular plasma membrane and 7-AAD bound to DNA, the Apoptosis detection with Annexin V and 7-AAD double stain assay was used [30]. To carry out these determinations, the treatments were prepared and processed as indicated in Section 2.4. After centrifuging and removing the supernatant, the pellet was resuspended with APC-labeled Annexin V and 7AAD in 100 µL of binding buffer. After 15 min of incubation at room temperature in the dark, 400 µL of binding buffer was added to analyze the cells by flow cytometry within 1 h after treatment. A total of 10,000 events were acquired in a FACS Calibur flow cytometer (BD Biosciences, Franklin Lakes, NJ, USA). Analysis was performed using CellQuest Pro and FlowJo v10 software. The dot plots were divided in quadrants to quantify the viable cells (Q4: Annexin V−/7AAD−), total apoptotic cells (Q3: early apoptosis, Annexin V+/7AAD− plus Q2: late apoptosis, Annexin V+/7AAD+) and necrotic cells (Q1: Annexin V−/7AAD+). The fluorescence distribution was shown as a colored dot plot analysis. Data were obtained from three independent experiments performed in triplicate.

2.4.2. Evaluation of Autophagy

Detection of Acidic Vesicular Organelles

Autophagy is characterized by the formation and promotion of acidic vesicular organelles (AVOs) [31]. We used the lysosomotropic agent acridine orange (AO), which moves freely across biological membranes when it is uncharged; its protonated form accumulates in acidic cell compartments, where it forms aggregates that fluoresce bright red, as we have previously reported [32]. Flow cytometry with AO staining was employed to detect and quantify the cells with AVOs. In AO-stained cells, the cytoplasm and nucleus fluoresce bright green and dim red, respectively, whereas acidic compartments fluoresce bright red. Therefore, we measured the change in the intensity of the red fluorescence to obtain the percentage of cells with AVOs. To carry out these determinations, the treatments were prepared and processed as indicated in Section 2.4. Briefly, after centrifuging and removing the supernatant, cells were resuspended and stained with 300 µL of a solution of 1 µg/mL AO in DMEM for 15 min at room temperature and analyzed on a CytoFlex SRT cell sorter (Beckman Coulter, Brea, CA, USA), measuring the green (FL-1, x-axis) vs. the red (FL-3, y-axis) fluorescence of AO in a linear scale. Dot plots are divided in quadrants, where the sum of the upper-left and the upper-right quadrants of the dot plot (red fluorescent events) was used to represent the percentage of autophagic cells. These assays were performed in triplicate.

LC3 immunofluorescence Staining

The microtubule-associated protein 1 light-chain 3 (LC3) is essential for amino-acid starvation-induced autophagy and is associated with the autophagosome membrane [33]. In this case, 1.5×10^4 glioma cells were seeded on chamber slide dishes (BD Biosciences, Franklin Lakes, NJ, USA), and treated with the drug concentrations and vehicle indicated in Section 2.4. After 48 h of treatment, cells were fixed with cold methanol for 30 min, washed twice with PBS and blocked with 2% bovine serum albumin for 10 min three times. After that, cells were incubated with the goat polyclonal antibody anti-MAP LC3 (1:400) for 30 min at room temperature. Then, cells were washed twice with PBS, blocked with 2% bovine serum albumin three times for 10 min, and incubated by additional 30 min in darkness with an anti-goat IgG-FITC antibody (1:400), washed again with PBS, and finally mounted with DAPI-mounting fluid. Images were obtained on a Leica DMLS microscope, with a 100× objective using the Leica Application Suite software (v. 4.0).

2.5. Proliferation Assay

For this test, the crystal violet dye was used, which binds to proteins and DNA molecules of attached cells, where cell proliferation can be calculated in relation to the amount of biomass present after treatment, since dead cells are shed, reducing the staining with crystal violet [34]. Briefly, 2×10^3 cells were seeded into 96-well plates and treated with the drug concentrations indicated in Section 2.4. Media were removed, and cells were fixed with a solution of cold ethanol (70%) for 30 min at room temperature after 1, 3, 5, and 7 days of treatment. Finally, cells were stained with a crystal violet solution (0.1%) for 30 min, and the supernatants were discarded. Crystals were dissolved with 100 µL of 10% glacial acetic acid solution, and absorbance was measured in a spectrophotometer Eon at 570 nm. The relative cell proliferation of each treatment group was calculated by the formula:

Absorbance of "X" group on each day (day 1, 3, 5, 7)/Absorbance of "X" group on day 1

where the "X" group represents a specific treatment group, dividing the absorbances obtained on days 1, 3, 5, and 7 by the absorbances of the same treatment group on day 1, individually, obtaining the relative cell proliferation. Analysis of the proliferation assay was performed by comparing the relative cell proliferation between the treatment groups on each day.

2.6. Statistical Analysis

Data were expressed as the mean ± standard deviation (SD). GraphPad Prism 6 software (v. 6.07) was used for statistical analysis, normality of the data was assessed with the Kolmogorov–Smirnov test, and statistical analysis was performed with the Kruskal–Wallis test followed by a Dunn's multiple comparison test.

3. Results

3.1. ALB, ALBSO, and MLT Induced a Cytotoxic Effect on C6, RG2, and U87 Cell Lines

We found that all three drugs induced a cytotoxic effect in a concentration-dependent manner (Figure 1). In addition, the Dm values for ALB were 0.6 µM, 0.6 µM, and 0.9 µM in the C6, RG2, and U87 cell lines, respectively. For the ALBSO, the Dm values were 20 µM, 26 µM and 36 µM in the C6, RG2, and U87 cells, respectively. In the case of MLT, the obtained Dm values were 1 mM, 0.9 mM, and 0.9 mM, for C6, RG2, and U87 cells, respectively.

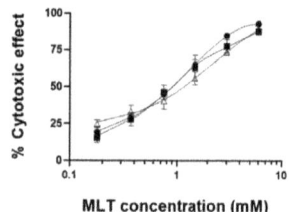
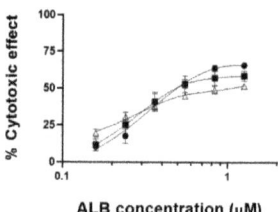
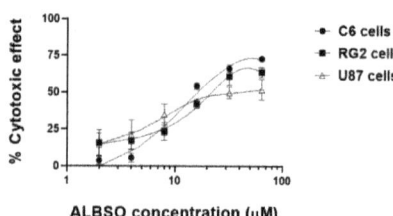

Figure 1. Concentration-effect curves of individual drugs. Cytotoxic effect after 72 h, in the three cell lines evaluated by the MTT reduction assay. Data obtained from four independent experiments, each with six replicates. Each dot represents mean ± SD.

3.2. The Combination of MLT with ALB or ALBSO Induced a Synergistic Cytotoxicity

Due to the ability of ALB, ALBSO, as well as MLT to induce cytotoxicity in the C6, RG2, and U87 cells, we tested whether the combination of ALB with MLT and ALBSO with MLT could induce an additive or synergistic cytotoxic effect. Based on the Dm of each drug, we combined ALB with MLT in a 1:1 ratio concentration for all cell lines. In the case of the combination of ALBSO with MLT, the ratio concentrations were 20:1 for C6 cells, 29:1 for RG2 cells and 40:1 for U87 cells. The results showed that most of the combinations caused a higher percentage of cytotoxicity than the single drugs. According to the Chou–Talalay method, most of the combinations of ALB-MLT caused a synergistic cytotoxic effect (CI < 1.00). In the case of ALBSO-MLT, most of the combinations caused a synergistic cytotoxic effect in the C6 and U87 lines, while in the RG2 line, this synergy was found only in the combinations with the highest concentrations (Figure 2).

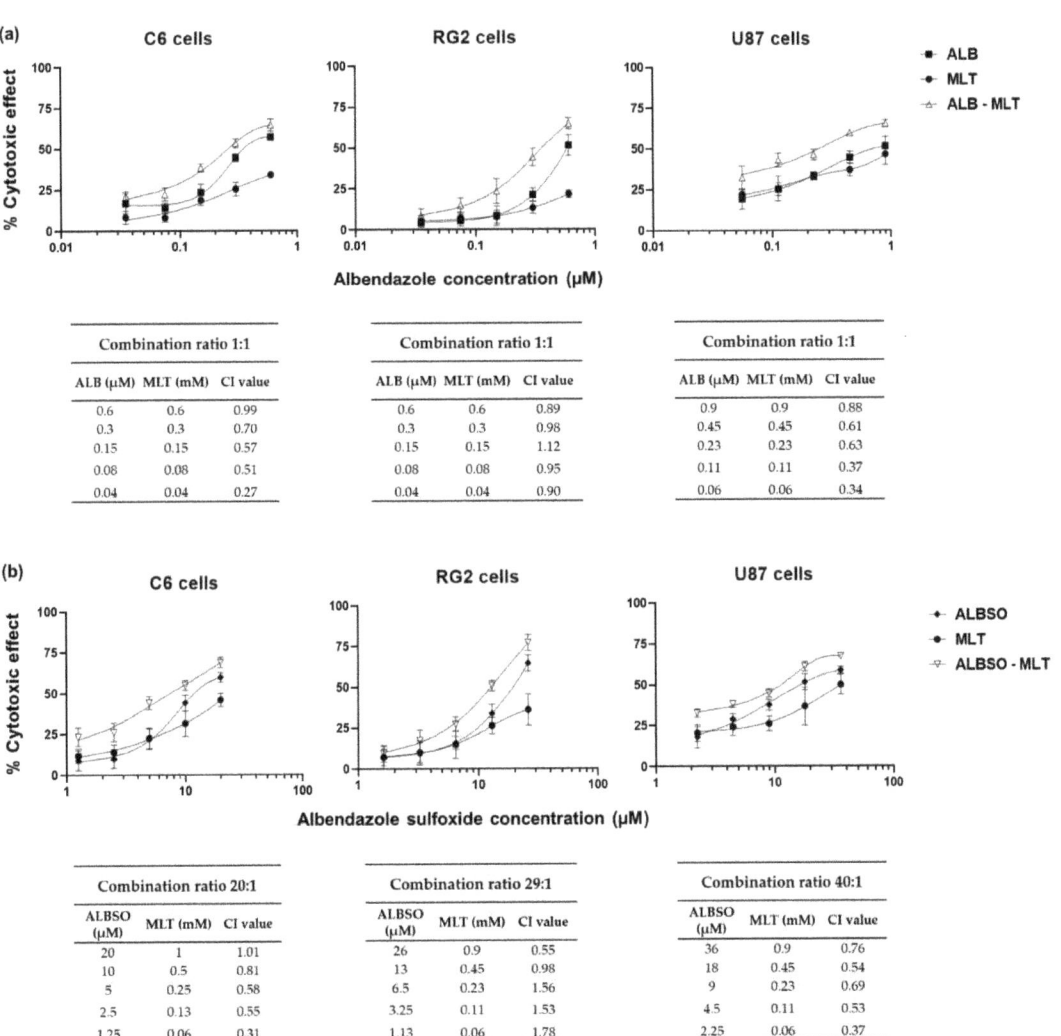

Figure 2. The combinations of MLT with ALB or ALBSO showed synergistic and/or additive effects. Graphic representation of the cytotoxic effect of the individual drugs and their combination, after 72 h of treatment, and the CI results in the three cell lines, for the combination of ALB with MLT (**a**) and ALBSO with MLT (**b**). Data obtained from three independent experiments in triplicate. Each dot represents mean ± SD.

3.3. Effect of the Combinations of MLT with ALB or ALBSO on the Cell Death Mechanisms
3.3.1. The Combinations of MLT with ALB or ALBSO Induced Apoptosis

Regarding the evaluation of the mechanisms involved in the decrease of tumor cell viability, our results showed that the combination of ALB 0.6 µM-MLT 0.6 mM induced apoptosis in 36% of C6 cells, statistically higher compared to 4.3% produced by the vehicle ($p < 0.01$), while MLT and ALB induced apoptosis only in 9.4 and 22.8% of cells, respectively

(Figure 3a,d). Similarly, the combination of ALBSO 20 µM-MLT 1 mM induced a statistical increase in apoptotic C6 cells, with a mean of 43.4% ($p < 0.01$).

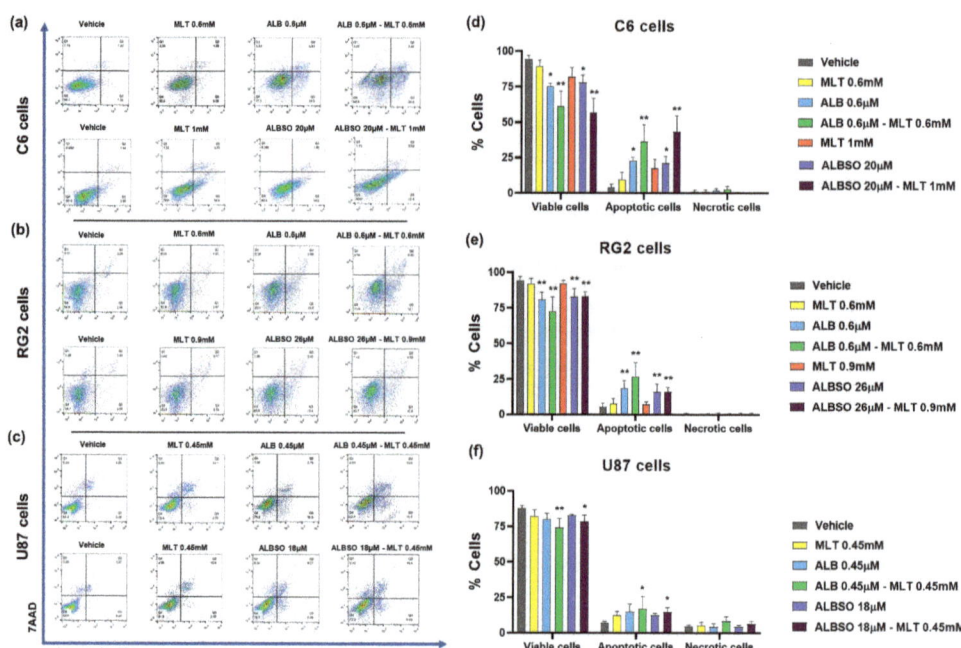

Figure 3. The combinations of MLT with ALB or ALBSO induced apoptosis. Representative dot plots and percentage of cells stained with Annexin V-APC/7AAD, quantified by flow cytometry after 48 h of treatment on C6 cells (**a,d**), RG2 cells (**b,e**), and U87 cells (**c,f**). The dot plots were divided in quadrants to quantify the viable cells (Q4: Annexin V-/7AAD-), total apoptotic cells (Q3: early apoptosis, Annexin V+/7AAD- plus Q2: late apoptosis, Annexin V+/7AAD+) and necrotic cells (Q1: Annexin V-/7AAD+). Data obtained from three independent experiments in triplicate (* $p < 0.05$, ** $p < 0.01$, compared to vehicle). Each bar represents mean ± SD.

In the RG2 cell line, the combination of ALB 0.6 µM-MLT 0.6 mM induced apoptosis in 26.7% of cells, statistically higher than the vehicle with 5.4% ($p < 0.01$), while MLT and ALB induced apoptosis in 7.8 and 18.7% of cells, respectively. While the treatment with ALBSO 26 µM-MLT 0.9 mM and ALBSO 26 µM alone induced similar percentages of apoptotic cells, with 16.2 and 16.1% ($p < 0.01$), respectively (Figure 3b,e).

In the U87 cells, the combination of ALB 0.45 µM-MLT 0.45 mM increased the apoptotic cells, with 17.1% ($p < 0.01$), while the vehicle produced 7.1%, MLT alone produced 12.4%, and ALB alone produced 15.1% of apoptotic cells. Likewise, the combination ALBSO 18 µM-MLT 0.45 mM showed similar percentages of apoptosis, with 15% of apoptotic cells ($p < 0.01$) (Figure 3e,f). Regarding the percentage of necrotic cells, there were no statistical differences between groups.

3.3.2. The Combinations of MLT with ALB or ALBSO Induced Autophagy

ALB has been reported to induce autophagy in human colon adenocarcinoma cells [35]; thus, we evaluated the contribution of autophagy to the cytotoxicity induced by the drug combinations. First, we verified the formation of LC3 puncta by immuno-fluorescence microscopy of glioblastoma cells. As seen in Figure 4a, the C6 cells show a higher expression of LC3 and the formation of the LC3 punctuate pattern after the treatment with ALB 0.6 µM, and in combination with MLT 0.6 mM, as well as when treated with ALBSO 20 µM, and in combination with MLT 1 mM. Similarly, the RG2 cells had a higher expression of LC3 and showed LC3 aggregation after the treatment with ALB 0.6 μM and in combination with MLT 0.6 mM, as well as when treated with ALBSO 26 μM and in combination with MLT 0.9 mM, as seen in Figure 4b. In addition, results in the U87 cells showed LC3 puncta formation after the treatment with ALB 0.45 μM and in combination with MLT 0.45 mM, as well as with ALBSO 18 μM treatment and in combination with MLT 0.45 mM, as seen in Figure 4c.

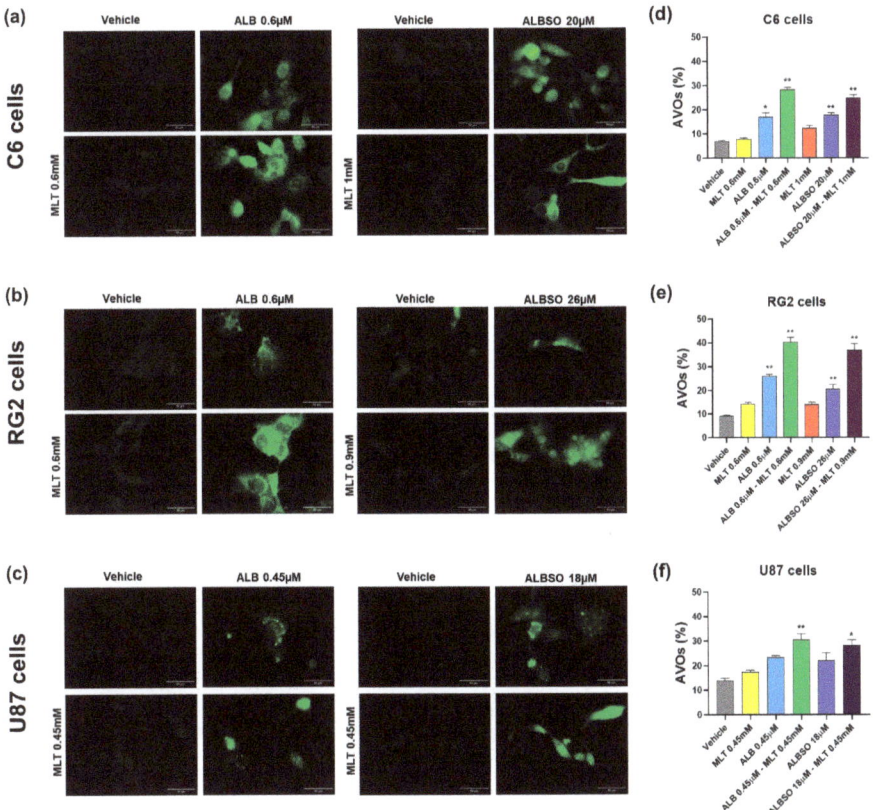

Figure 4. The combinations of MLT with ALB or ALBSO induced autophagy. Representative images of LC3-staining pattern by immunofluorescence and percentage of cells with AVOs quantified by flow cytometry after 48 h of treatment on C6 cells (**a,d**), RG2 cells (**b,e**), and U87 cells (**c,f**). Data obtained from three independent experiments in triplicate (* $p < 0.05$, ** $p < 0.01$, compared to vehicle). Scale bar equals 50 μm in microphotographs. Each bar represents mean ± SD in graphs.

Next, we quantified the generation of AVOs in the tumor cells with AO staining by flow cytometry, indicating the percentage of cells with AVOs. In the C6 cells, the combination of ALB 0.6 μM-MLT 0.6 mM induced AVOs in 28.3% cells, statistically higher than the vehicle with 6.9%, MLT alone (7.8%), and ALB alone (17.1%) ($p < 0.01$), as seen in Figure 4d. Similarly, the combination ALBSO 20 μM-MLT 1 mM increased the C6 cells with AVOs, with a mean of 24.8%, statistically higher than MLT alone (12.4%) and ALBSO alone (17.9%) ($p < 0.01$). In the RG2 cells, the combination of ALB 0.6 μM-MLT 0.6 mM induced the highest percent of cells with AVOs (40.4%), statistically higher than the vehicle (9%), the MLT alone (14.1%), and the ALB alone (26%) ($p < 0.01$). Similarly, the combination of ALBSO 26 μM-MLT 0.9 mM induced a higher percent of RG2 cells with AVOs (37%), when compared to MLT alone (14%) and ALBSO alone (20.6%) ($p < 0.01$), as seen in Figure 4e. In the case of U87 cells, the combinations ALB 0.45 µM-MLT 0.45 mM and ALBSO 18 µM-MLT 0.45 mM induced a significative increase in cells with AVOs, showing values of 30.5% ($p < 0.01$) and 28.3% ($p < 0.05$), respectively, when compared to vehicle (13.7%), as seen in Figure 4f.

3.4. The Treatment with ALB and ALBSO Inhibited Proliferation, Independently of MLT

Then, we evaluated the proliferation rate of tumor cells by crystal violet staining during 7 days of treatment on C6 cells (Figure 5a), RG2 cells (Figure 5b), and U87 cells (Figure 5c). In addition, for the C6 cells, we found a significant suppression of proliferation from day 3 until day 7 of treatment with ALB 0.6 µM or ALBSO 20 µM, independently of the combination with MLT ($p < 0.01$), as seen in Figure 5d. A similar result was obtained in the RG2 cells, where the treatment with ALB 0.6 µM or ALBSO 26 µM suppressed the cell proliferation, finding a significant difference after day 3 when comparing both combinations of ALB-MLT and ALBSO-MLT to the vehicle ($p < 0.05$), as seen in Figure 5e. Figure 5f shows the proliferation rate of U87 cells, finding a significant suppression of cell proliferation after 3 days of treatment ($p < 0.05$) with ALB 0.45 µM or ALBSO 18 µM, despite the presence of MLT, showing a higher difference on days 5 and 7 ($p < 0.001$).

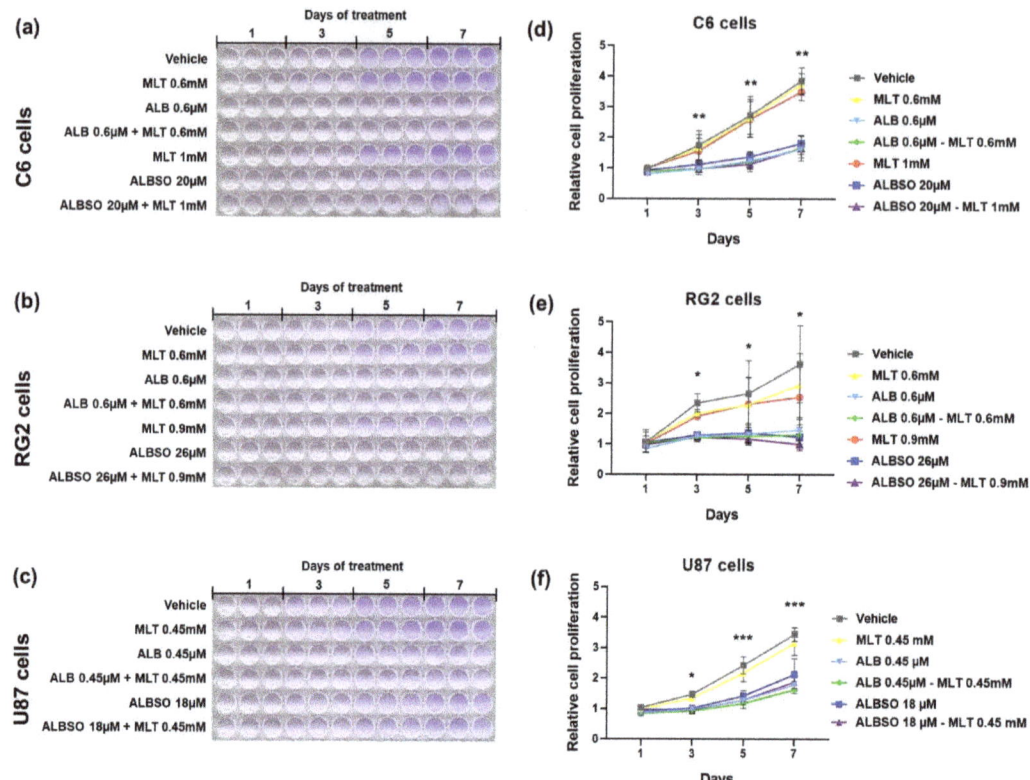

Figure 5. The treatment with ALB and ALBSO inhibited proliferation, independently of MLT. Representative images of crystal violet-stained cells in 96-well plates and graph with relative cell proliferation obtained after 1, 3, 5, and 7 days of treatment on C6 cells (**a,d**), RG2 cells (**b,e**), and U87 cells (**c,f**). Data obtained from three independent experiments in triplicate (* $p < 0.05$, ** $p < 0.01$, *** $p < 0.001$, compared to vehicle). Each dot represents mean ± SD.

4. Discussion

Glioblastoma remains to be the most aggressive brain tumor in adults. Although in recent decades advances in the treatment of GB have been achieved, recurrence is often inevitable, and the survival of patients remains low; therefore, new treatment strategies are under evaluation, such as monoclonal antibodies, viral therapies, vaccines, drug repositioning, and drug combinations [36,37]. In recent years, the combination of drugs with different mechanisms of action is gaining more relevance in the treatment of GB, with the aim to increase the efficacy, lower drug doses, and counteract mechanisms of drug-resistance, among others [38].

In the present study, we evaluated the combination of ALB with MLT, since both drugs have demonstrated antitumor activity through different mechanisms of action [25,39]; therefore, we investigated if the combination could potentially synergize their antitumor effect. Likewise, we evaluated the combination of MLT with ALBSO, considering that ALBSO, the main metabolite of ALB, has shown the highest levels in plasma and cerebrospinal fluid after the oral administration of ALB [40]. The assays were conducted on three of the most widely used cell lines in the GB research, namely, the U87 human glioblastoma cell line and the C6 and RG2 rat malignant glioma cell lines, that have proven to be highly homologous to the GB [41].

Our results corroborate the cytotoxic effect that the ALB and MLT have on the C6 and U87 glioma cell lines [42–45]. In addition, the cytotoxic effect of these drugs on the RG2 line is reported for the first time. In all cell lines, MLT was the most effective and ALB the most potent. To date, there are few studies that have determined the IC_{50} values for ALB or MLT in glioma cells. Marslin et al. evaluated the cytotoxic effect of ALB in the U87 cell line and reported a value of 50.1 µM for ALB [10], which is higher than those found in the present study (0.9 µM). The difference could be related to the exposure time, since in our study the incubation time was 72 h, and in the previous study, it was performed at 24 h.

This is the first study demonstrating the antitumor activity of ALBSO against glioma cells. The only prior report of the antitumor activity of ALBSO shows the induction of apoptosis of breast cancer cells in vitro [46]. The antitumor activity of ALBSO is relevant given that it is highly available in the brain, so it could reach therapeutic concentrations in brain tumors such as GB. The results showed that this metabolite was as effective as ALB in inducing cytotoxicity against the glioma cells.

When the combination study was performed, we found that both ALB-MLT and ALBSO-MLT combinations produced an additive or synergistic cytotoxic effect on most combination ratios in all three glioma cell lines. It is worth noting that apoptosis was the main cell death mechanism associated with the treatments using the drugs alone and in combination, finding necrosis in a minimal percentage on the three glioma cell lines. Ehteda et al. found that the combination of ALB with 2-methoxyestradiol synergizes the induction of apoptosis of colon cancer cells and improves the survival of HCT-116 tumor-bearing nude mice [47]. The synergy was based on the sum effect of microtubule-binding activity of both drugs, which differs from our approach, which is based on the possible sum of the different mechanisms of action attributed to ALB and MLT, as mentioned above [17,18,24,27]. On the other hand, MLT also has shown a chemosensitizing effect, since MLT downregulates the expression of ABC transporter ABCG2, inducing the synergistic cytotoxicity when combined with TMZ against GB cells and GB-stem cells [26].

The formation of a punctuate pattern of LC3 is associated with the initiation of autophagy, via the aggregation of LC3 and the formation of the autophagosome, and directly correlated to the increase in AVOs in glioma cells, as an indication of the fusion of the autophagosome and lysosome [48]. Previous reports indicate that benzimidazoles, as mebendazole and ALB, can induce autophagy on GB cells [49] and colon adenocarcinoma cells [35], respectively, while the blockade of autophagy in cholangiocarcinoma cells, after its induction with ALB, has been associated with increased apoptosis of tumor cells [50]. Meanwhile, MLT has shown the ability to suppress autophagy in ovarian granulosa cells [51], as well as in rat brain neurons, through the reduction of reactive oxygen species [52]; however, the oxidative capacity of MLT metabolites has also been reported [53]. The autophagy in GB cells has been associated with the induction of cell death as a response to sustained cell damage, related to the accumulation of AVOs and the loss of the protective effect of autophagy [54]. In this regard, the interplay between the induction of apoptosis and autophagy is proposed to potentiate cell death in cancer cells and promote the effectiveness of anti-tumor molecules [55].

Previous reports show that the anti-proliferative effect of MLT is attributed to the suppression of miR-155 on U87 cells; however, these effects were found with very low concentrations of MLT (1 μM), compared to the concentrations used in this study [44]. MLT has shown a synergistic anti-proliferative effect when combined with sorafenib, by dual suppression of the STAT3 pathway in pancreatic cancer cells in vitro and in vivo [56]. In the case of ALB, its antiproliferative activity on C6 cells has been previously attributed to the inhibition of enzymes involved in the glycolytic pathway and lower ATP concentration in vitro and in vivo, showing an enhanced effect when ALB is loaded on silver nanoparticles [45]. In a similar way, thiabendazole, another antiparasitic benzimidazole, has proven to be effective at inhibiting proliferation of several GB cell lines by the downregulation of mini-chromosome maintenance protein 2 (MCM2) [57]. Shu et al. demonstrated that ALB plus Palbociclib, a cyclin kinase 4/6 (CDK4/6) inhibitor, synergistically suppresses melanoma cell proliferation in vitro and in vivo, by the dual arrest of cell cycle progression [58].

The gold-standard drug in the treatment of GB is temozolomide (TMZ); however, in vitro evaluations indicate the need for high concentrations, ranging from 100 μM to more than 1000 μM, to induce the desired effect on glioma cells [59]. There is evidence of the potentiation of the cytotoxic effect of TMZ in combination with other treatments against glioma cells, where apoptosis and autophagy can be synergized [60,61]; therefore, the evaluation of the combined effect of MLT-ALB/ALBSO to potentiate the antitumor effect of TMZ is proposed as a follow-up to this work.

New directions are needed for the combinations of ALB, ALBSO, and MLT. Recently, ALB has also been reported to promote immunotherapy response by facilitating ubiquitin-mediated PD-L1 degradation in melanoma models [62]; likewise, MLT has shown antitumor potential by impairing many of the characteristics that sustain cancer progression [63], highlighting the importance of discovering other potential mechanisms of action that could benefit the current treatment of patients with cancer.

Future perspectives include the evaluation in an in vivo model of orthotopic malignant glioma, which will allow us to evaluate the impact of the combined administration of these drugs on molecular markers, tumor eradication, and survival time, given that survival is a parameter of great importance to determine the therapeutic efficacy of a drug in the management of GB [64]. Potential in vivo studies could be based on the use of classical immunocompetent orthotopic malignant glioma models, as we have previously reported with C6 cells implanted in the brain parenchyma of Wistar rats [65], or as the model performed with GL621 mouse glioma cells in C57BL/6 mice [66].

5. Conclusions

The combined mechanisms of the pleiotropic drugs, ALB, ALBSO, and MLT, are relevant for the additivity and synergism found against the glioma cells. Considering the safety and inexpensive profiles of these drugs, and their high availability to the CNS, their combination could be a potential therapeutic strategy against GB. Other studies would be necessary to evaluate the antitumoral activity of these combinations in in vivo models.

Author Contributions: Conceptualization, M.H.-C. and H.J.-C.; methodology, M.H.-C., V.C., B.P., F.P.-A., I.S.R.-T. and H.J.-C.; formal analysis, M.H.-C. and V.C.; investigation, M.H.-C., V.C., B.P., F.P.-A. and H.J.-C.; resources, M.H.-C., C.R., B.P., F.P.-A., I.S.R.-T. and H.J.-C.; data curation, M.H.-C., V.C., C.R., B.P., F.P.-A., I.S.R.-T. and H.J.-C.; writing—original draft preparation, M.H.-C., F.P.-A. and H.J.-C.; writing—review and editing, M.H.-C., V.C., C.R., B.P., F.P.-A., I.S.R.-T. and H.J.-C.; visualization, M.H.-C., C.R., B.P., F.P.-A. and H.J.-C.; supervision, C.R., B.P. and H.J.-C.; project administration,

M.H.-C., B.P., F.P.-A. and H.J.-C.; funding acquisition, M.H.-C., F.P.-A. and H.J.-C. All authors have read and agreed to the published version of the manuscript.

Funding: This research was funded by Consejo Nacional de Ciencia y Tecnología (CONACyT Mexico), grant number A1-S-40569.

Institutional Review Board Statement: Not applicable.

Informed Consent Statement: Not applicable.

Data Availability Statement: The data presented in this study are available on request to the corresponding author.

Acknowledgments: A student grant (419514) was provided to Miguel Hernández by Consejo Nacional de Ciencia y Tecnología (CONACyT Mexico). We thank Luis Tristán (Laboratory of Neurochemistry, INNN, Mexico), Edith Gonzales (Laboratory of Molecular Neuropharmacology and Nanotechnology, INNN, Mexico), and Nancy Ixtlahuaca-Barrientos for the technical assistance.

Conflicts of Interest: The authors declare no conflict of interest.

References

1. Stupp, R.; Hegi, M.E.; Mason, W.P.; van den Bent, M.J.; Taphoorn, M.J.; Janzer, R.C.; Ludwin, S.K.; Allgeier, A.; Fisher, B.; Belanger, K.; et al. Effects of radiotherapy with concomitant and adjuvant temozolomide versus radiotherapy alone on survival in glioblastoma in a randomised phase III study: 5-year analysis of the EORTC-NCIC trial. *Lancet Oncol.* **2009**, *10*, 459–466. [CrossRef]
2. Wick, W.; Osswald, M.; Wick, A.; Winkler, F. Treatment of glioblastoma in adults. *Ther. Adv. Neurol. Disord.* **2018**, *11*, 1756286418790452. [CrossRef] [PubMed]
3. Cruz, J.V.R.; Batista, C.; Afonso, B.H.; Alexandre-Moreira, M.S.; Dubois, L.G.; Pontes, B.; Moura Neto, V.; Mendes, F.A. Obstacles to Glioblastoma Treatment Two Decades after Temozolomide. *Cancers* **2022**, *14*, 3203. [CrossRef]
4. Bhatia, P.; Bernier, M.; Sanghvi, M.; Moaddel, R.; Schwarting, R.; Ramamoorthy, A.; Wainer, I.W. Breast cancer resistance protein (BCRP/ABCG2) localises to the nucleus in glioblastoma multiforme cells. *Xenobiotica* **2012**, *42*, 748–755. [CrossRef]
5. Lin, F.; de Gooijer, M.C.; Roig, E.M.; Buil, L.C.; Christner, S.M.; Beumer, J.H.; Würdinger, T.; Beijnen, J.H.; van Tellingen, O. ABCB1, ABCG2, and PTEN determine the response of glioblastoma to temozolomide and ABT-888 therapy. *Clin. Cancer Res.* **2014**, *20*, 2703–2713. [CrossRef] [PubMed]
6. Panic, G.; Duthaler, U.; Speich, B.; Keiser, J. Repurposing drugs for the treatment and control of helminth infections. *Int. J. Parasitol. Drugs Drug. Resist.* **2014**, *4*, 185–200. [CrossRef] [PubMed]
7. Son, D.S.; Lee, E.S.; Adunyah, S.E. The Antitumor Potentials of Benzimidazole Anthelmintics as Repurposing Drugs. *Immune Netw.* **2020**, *20*, e29. [CrossRef]
8. Castro, L.S.; Kviecinski, M.R.; Ourique, F.; Parisotto, E.B.; Grinevicius, V.M.; Correia, J.F.; Wilhelm Filho, D.; Pedrosa, R.C. Albendazole as a promising molecule for tumor control. *Redox Biol.* **2016**, *10*, 90–99. [CrossRef]
9. Pourgholami, M.H.; Akhter, J.; Wang, L.; Lu, Y.; Morris, D.L. Antitumor activity of albendazole against the human colorectal cancer cell line HT-29: In vitro and in a xenograft model of peritoneal carcinomatosis. *Cancer Chemother. Pharm.* **2005**, *55*, 425–432. [CrossRef]
10. Marslin, G.; Siram, K.; Liu, X.; Khandelwal, V.K.M.; Xiaolei, S.; Xiang, W.; Franklin, G. Solid Lipid Nanoparticles of Albendazole for Enhancing Cellular Uptake and Cytotoxicity against U-87 MG Glioma Cell Lines. *Molecules* **2017**, *22*, 2040. [CrossRef]
11. Pourgholami, M.H.; Szwajcer, M.; Chin, M.; Liauw, W.; Seef, J.; Galettis, P.; Morris, D.L.; Links, M. Phase I clinical trial to determine maximum tolerated dose of oral albendazole in patients with advanced cancer. *Cancer Chemother. Pharm.* **2010**, *65*, 597–605. [CrossRef]
12. Rawden, H.C.; Kokwaro, G.O.; Ward, S.A.; Edwards, G. Relative contribution of cytochromes P-450 and flavin-containing monoxygenases to the metabolism of albendazole by human liver microsomes. *Br. J. Clin. Pharm.* **2000**, *49*, 313–322. [CrossRef] [PubMed]
13. Lee, C.A.; Neul, D.; Clouser-Roche, A.; Dalvie, D.; Wester, M.R.; Jiang, Y.; Jones, J.P.; Freiwald, S.; Zientek, M.; Totah, R.A. Identification of novel substrates for human cytochrome P450 2J2. *Drug. Metab. Dispos.* **2010**, *38*, 347–356. [CrossRef]
14. Jung, H.; Cárdenas, G.; Sciutto, E.; Fleury, A. Medical treatment for neurocysticercosis: Drugs, indications and perspectives. *Curr. Top. Med. Chem.* **2008**, *8*, 424–433. [CrossRef] [PubMed]
15. Sotelo, J.; Jung, H. Pharmacokinetic optimisation of the treatment of neurocysticercosis. *Clin. Pharm.* **1998**, *34*, 503–515. [CrossRef] [PubMed]
16. Aguayo-Ortiz, R.; Méndez-Lucio, O.; Medina-Franco, J.L.; Castillo, R.; Yépez-Mulia, L.; Hernández-Luis, F.; Hernández-Campos, A. Towards the identification of the binding site of benzimidazoles to β-tubulin of Trichinella spiralis: Insights from computational and experimental data. *J. Mol. Graph. Model.* **2013**, *41*, 12–19. [CrossRef]
17. Yang, M.H.; Ha, I.J.; Um, J.Y.; Ahn, K.S. Albendazole Exhibits Anti-Neoplastic Actions against Gastric Cancer Cells by Affecting STAT3 and STAT5 Activation by Pleiotropic Mechanism(s). *Biomedicines* **2021**, *9*, 362. [CrossRef]

18. Kim, U.; Shin, C.; Kim, C.Y.; Ryu, B.; Kim, J.; Bang, J.; Park, J.H. Albendazole exerts antiproliferative effects on prostate cancer cells by inducing reactive oxygen species generation. *Oncol. Lett.* **2021**, *21*, 395. [CrossRef] [PubMed]
19. Macchi, M.M.; Bruce, J.N. Human pineal physiology and functional significance of melatonin. *Front. Neuroendocr.* **2004**, *25*, 177–195. [CrossRef] [PubMed]
20. Reiter, R.J.; Korkmaz, A. Clinical aspects of melatonin. *Saudi Med. J.* **2008**, *29*, 1537–1547.
21. Hardeland, R. Melatonin metabolism in the central nervous system. *Curr. Neuropharmacol.* **2010**, *8*, 168–181. [CrossRef] [PubMed]
22. Yu, H.; Dickson, E.J.; Jung, S.R.; Koh, D.S.; Hille, B. High membrane permeability for melatonin. *J. Gen. Physiol.* **2016**, *147*, 63–76. [CrossRef] [PubMed]
23. Liu, J.; Clough, S.J.; Hutchinson, A.J.; Adamah-Biassi, E.B.; Popovska-Gorevski, M.; Dubocovich, M.L. MT1 and MT2 Melatonin Receptors: A Therapeutic Perspective. *Annu. Rev. Pharm. Toxicol.* **2016**, *56*, 361–383. [CrossRef] [PubMed]
24. Moretti, E.; Favero, G.; Rodella, L.F.; Rezzani, R. Melatonin's Antineoplastic Potential Against Glioblastoma. *Cells* **2020**, *9*, 599. [CrossRef] [PubMed]
25. Li, Y.; Li, S.; Zhou, Y.; Meng, X.; Zhang, J.J.; Xu, D.P.; Li, H.B. Melatonin for the prevention and treatment of cancer. *Oncotarget* **2017**, *8*, 39896–39921. [CrossRef] [PubMed]
26. Martín, V.; Sanchez-Sanchez, A.M.; Herrera, F.; Gomez-Manzano, C.; Fueyo, J.; Alvarez-Vega, M.A.; Antolín, I.; Rodriguez, C. Melatonin-induced methylation of the ABCG2/BCRP promoter as a novel mechanism to overcome multidrug resistance in brain tumour stem cells. *Br. J. Cancer* **2013**, *108*, 2005–2012. [CrossRef]
27. Hsiao, S.Y.; Tang, C.H.; Chen, P.C.; Lin, T.H.; Chao, C.C. Melatonin Inhibits EMT in Bladder Cancer by Targeting Autophagy. *Molecules* **2022**, *27*, 8649. [CrossRef]
28. Chou, T.C.; Talalay, P. Quantitative analysis of dose-effect relationships: The combined effects of multiple drugs or enzyme inhibitors. *Adv. Enzym. Regul.* **1984**, *22*, 27–55. [CrossRef]
29. Chou, T.C. Theoretical basis, experimental design, and computerized simulation of synergism and antagonism in drug combination studies. *Pharm. Rev.* **2006**, *58*, 621–681. [CrossRef] [PubMed]
30. Zembruski, N.C.; Stache, V.; Haefeli, W.E.; Weiss, J. 7-Aminoactinomycin D for apoptosis staining in flow cytometry. *Anal. Biochem.* **2012**, *429*, 79–81. [CrossRef]
31. Kanzawa, T.; Kondo, Y.; Ito, H.; Kondo, S.; Germano, I. Induction of autophagic cell death in malignant glioma cells by arsenic trioxide. *Cancer Res.* **2003**, *63*, 2103–2108. [PubMed]
32. Romano-Feinholz, S.; Salazar-Ramiro, A.; Munoz-Sandoval, E.; Magana-Maldonado, R.; Hernandez Pedro, N.; Rangel Lopez, E.; Gonzalez Aguilar, A.; Sanchez Garcia, A.; Sotelo, J.; Perez de la Cruz, V.; et al. Cytotoxicity induced by carbon nanotubes in experimental malignant glioma. *Int. J. Nanomed.* **2017**, *12*, 6005–6026. [CrossRef]
33. Runwal, G.; Stamatakou, E.; Siddiqi, F.H.; Puri, C.; Zhu, Y.; Rubinsztein, D.C. LC3-positive structures are prominent in autophagy-deficient cells. *Sci. Rep.* **2019**, *9*, 10147. [CrossRef] [PubMed]
34. Feoktistova, M.; Geserick, P.; Leverkus, M. Crystal Violet Assay for Determining Viability of Cultured Cells. *Cold Spring Harb. Protoc.* **2016**, *2016*, 087379. [CrossRef] [PubMed]
35. Jung, Y.Y.; Baek, S.H.; Ha, I.J.; Ahn, K.S. Regulation of apoptosis and autophagy by albendazole in human colon adenocarcinoma cells. *Biochimie* **2022**, *198*, 155–166. [CrossRef]
36. Liu, H.; Qiu, W.; Sun, T.; Wang, L.; Du, C.; Hu, Y.; Liu, W.; Feng, F.; Chen, Y.; Sun, H. Therapeutic strategies of glioblastoma (GBM): The current advances in the molecular targets and bioactive small molecule compounds. *Acta Pharm. Sin. B* **2022**, *12*, 1781–1804. [CrossRef]
37. Mudduluru, G.; Walther, W.; Kobelt, D.; Dahlmann, M.; Treese, C.; Assaraf, Y.G.; Stein, U. Repositioning of drugs for intervention in tumor progression and metastasis: Old drugs for new targets. *Drug. Resist. Updat.* **2016**, *26*, 10–27. [CrossRef] [PubMed]
38. Yool, A.J.; Ramesh, S. Molecular Targets for Combined Therapeutic Strategies to Limit Glioblastoma Cell Migration and Invasion. *Front. Pharm.* **2020**, *11*, 358. [CrossRef]
39. Li, Y.Q.; Zheng, Z.; Liu, Q.X.; Lu, X.; Zhou, D.; Zhang, J.; Zheng, H.; Dai, J.G. Repositioning of Antiparasitic Drugs for Tumor Treatment. *Front. Oncol.* **2021**, *11*, 670804. [CrossRef]
40. González-Hernández, I.; Ruiz-Olmedo, M.I.; Cárdenas, G.; Jung-Cook, H. A simple LC-MS/MS method to determine plasma and cerebrospinal fluid levels of albendazole metabolites (albendazole sulfoxide and albendazole sulfone) in patients with neurocysticercosis. *Biomed. Chromatogr.* **2012**, *26*, 267–272. [CrossRef]
41. Giakoumettis, D.; Kritis, A.; Foroglou, N. C6 cell line: The gold standard in glioma research. *Hippokratia* **2018**, *22*, 105–112. [PubMed]
42. Martín, V.; Herrera, F.; Carrera-Gonzalez, P.; García-Santos, G.; Antolín, I.; Rodriguez-Blanco, J.; Rodriguez, C. Intracellular signaling pathways involved in the cell growth inhibition of glioma cells by melatonin. *Cancer Res.* **2006**, *66*, 1081–1088. [CrossRef]
43. Ariey-Bonnet, J.; Carrasco, K.; Le Grand, M.; Hoffer, L.; Betzi, S.; Feracci, M.; Tsvetkov, P.; Devred, F.; Collette, Y.; Morelli, X.; et al. In silico molecular target prediction unveils mebendazole as a potent MAPK14 inhibitor. *Mol. Oncol.* **2020**, *14*, 3083–3099. [CrossRef]
44. Gu, J.; Lu, Z.; Ji, C.; Chen, Y.; Liu, Y.; Lei, Z.; Wang, L.; Zhang, H.T.; Li, X. Melatonin inhibits proliferation and invasion via repression of miRNA-155 in glioma cells. *Biomed. Pharm.* **2017**, *93*, 969–975. [CrossRef] [PubMed]
45. Liang, J.; Zhu, Y.; Gao, C.; Ling, C.; Qin, J.; Wang, Q.; Huang, Y.; Lu, W.; Wang, J. Menthol-modified BSA nanoparticles for glioma targeting therapy using an energy restriction strategy. *NPG Asia Mater.* **2019**, *11*, 1–18. [CrossRef]

46. Belaz, K.R.A.; Denadai, M.; Almeida, A.P.; Lima, R.T.; Vasconcelos, M.H.; Pinto, M.M.; Cass, Q.B.; Oliveira, R.V. Enantiomeric resolution of albendazole sulfoxide by semipreparative HPLC and in vitro study of growth inhibitory effects on human cancer cell lines. *J. Pharm. Biomed. Anal.* **2012**, *66*, 100–108. [CrossRef]
47. Ehteda, A.; Galettis, P.; Pillai, K.; Morris, D.L. Combination of albendazole and 2-methoxyestradiol significantly improves the survival of HCT-116 tumor-bearing nude mice. *BMC Cancer* **2013**, *13*, 86. [CrossRef]
48. Thomé, M.P.; Filippi-Chiela, E.C.; Villodre, E.S.; Migliavaca, C.B.; Onzi, G.R.; Felipe, K.B.; Lenz, G. Ratiometric analysis of Acridine Orange staining in the study of acidic organelles and autophagy. *J. Cell. Sci.* **2016**, *129*, 4622–4632. [CrossRef]
49. Jo, S.B.; Sung, S.J.; Choi, H.S.; Park, J.S.; Hong, Y.K.; Joe, Y.A. Modulation of Autophagy is a Potential Strategy for Enhancing the Anti-Tumor Effect of Mebendazole in Glioblastoma Cells. *Biomol. Ther.* **2022**, *30*, 616–624. [CrossRef]
50. He, Q.; Yin, Y.; Pan, X.; Wu, Y.; Li, X. Albendazole-induced autophagy blockade contributes to elevated apoptosis in cholangiocarcinoma cells through AMPK/mTOR activation. *Toxicol. Appl. Pharm.* **2022**, *454*, 116214. [CrossRef]
51. Wu, D.; Zhao, W.; Xu, C.; Zhou, X.; Leng, X.; Li, Y. Melatonin suppresses serum starvation-induced autophagy of ovarian granulosa cells in premature ovarian insufficiency. *BMC Womens Health* **2022**, *22*, 474. [CrossRef] [PubMed]
52. Shi, L.; Liang, F.; Zheng, J.; Zhou, K.; Chen, S.; Yu, J.; Zhang, J. Melatonin Regulates Apoptosis and Autophagy Via ROS-MST1 Pathway in Subarachnoid Hemorrhage. *Front. Mol. Neurosci.* **2018**, *11*, 93. [CrossRef] [PubMed]
53. Ximenes, V.F.; Pessoa, A.S.; Padovan, C.Z.; Abrantes, D.C.; Gomes, F.H.; Maticoli, M.A.; de Menezes, M.L. Oxidation of melatonin by AAPH-derived peroxyl radicals: Evidence of a pro-oxidant effect of melatonin. *Biochim. Biophys. Acta* **2009**, *1790*, 787–792. [CrossRef]
54. Yao, K.C.; Komata, T.; Kondo, Y.; Kanzawa, T.; Kondo, S.; Germano, I.M. Molecular response of human glioblastoma multiforme cells to ionizing radiation: Cell cycle arrest, modulation of the expression of cyclin-dependent kinase inhibitors, and autophagy. *J. Neurosurg.* **2003**, *98*, 378–384. [CrossRef]
55. Bata, N.; Cosford, N.D.P. Cell Survival and Cell Death at the Intersection of Autophagy and Apoptosis: Implications for Current and Future Cancer Therapeutics. *ACS Pharm. Transl. Sci.* **2021**, *4*, 1728–1746. [CrossRef]
56. Fang, Z.; Jung, K.H.; Yan, H.H.; Kim, S.J.; Rumman, M.; Park, J.H.; Han, B.; Lee, J.E.; Kang, Y.W.; Lim, J.H.; et al. Melatonin Synergizes with Sorafenib to Suppress Pancreatic Cancer via Melatonin Receptor and PDGFR-β/STAT3 Pathway. *Cell. Physiol. Biochem.* **2018**, *47*, 1751–1768. [CrossRef]
57. Hu, Y.; Zhou, W.; Xue, Z.; Liu, X.; Feng, Z.; Zhang, Y.; Li, W.; Zhang, Q.; Chen, A.; Huang, B.; et al. Thiabendazole Inhibits Glioblastoma Cell Proliferation and Invasion Targeting Mini-chromosome Maintenance Protein 2. *J. Pharm. Exp. Ther.* **2022**, *380*, 63–75. [CrossRef]
58. Zhu, L.; Yang, Q.; Hu, R.; Li, Y.; Peng, Y.; Liu, H.; Ye, M.; Zhang, B.; Zhang, P.; Liu-Smith, F.; et al. Novel therapeutic strategy for melanoma based on albendazole and the CDK4/6 inhibitor palbociclib. *Sci. Rep.* **2022**, *12*, 5706. [CrossRef]
59. Lee, S.Y. Temozolomide resistance in glioblastoma multiforme. *Genes. Dis.* **2016**, *3*, 198–210. [CrossRef] [PubMed]
60. Golden, E.B.; Cho, H.Y.; Jahanian, A.; Hofman, F.M.; Louie, S.G.; Schönthal, A.H.; Chen, T.C. Chloroquine enhances temozolomide cytotoxicity in malignant gliomas by blocking autophagy. *Neurosurg. Focus.* **2014**, *37*, E12. [CrossRef]
61. Magaña-Maldonado, R.; Manoutcharian, K.; Hernández-Pedro, N.Y.; Rangel-López, E.; Pérez-De la Cruz, V.; Rodríguez-Balderas, C.; Sotelo, J.; Pineda, B. Concomitant treatment with pertussis toxin plus temozolomide increases the survival of rats bearing intracerebral RG2 glioma. *J. Cancer Res. Clin. Oncol.* **2014**, *140*, 291–301. [CrossRef] [PubMed]
62. Zhu, L.; Kuang, X.; Zhang, G.; Liang, L.; Liu, D.; Hu, B.; Xie, Z.; Li, H.; Liu, H.; Ye, M.; et al. Albendazole induces immunotherapy response by facilitating ubiquitin-mediated PD-L1 degradation. *J. Immunother. Cancer* **2022**, *10*, e003819. [CrossRef] [PubMed]
63. Talib, W.H.; Alsayed, A.R.; Abuawad, A.; Daoud, S.; Mahmod, A.I. Melatonin in Cancer Treatment: Current Knowledge and Future Opportunities. *Molecules* **2021**, *26*, 2506. [CrossRef] [PubMed]
64. deSouza, R.M.; Shaweis, H.; Han, C.; Sivasubramaniam, V.; Brazil, L.; Beaney, R.; Sadler, G.; Al-Sarraj, S.; Hampton, T.; Logan, J.; et al. Has the survival of patients with glioblastoma changed over the years? *Br. J. Cancer* **2016**, *114*, 146–150. [CrossRef] [PubMed]
65. Chavarria, V.; Ortiz-Islas, E.; Salazar, A.; Pérez-de la Cruz, V.; Espinosa-Bonilla, A.; Figueroa, R.; Ortíz-Plata, A.; Sotelo, J.; Sánchez-García, F.J.; Pineda, B. Lactate-Loaded Nanoparticles Induce Glioma Cytotoxicity and Increase the Survival of Rats Bearing Malignant Glioma Brain Tumor. *Pharmaceutics* **2022**, *14*, 327. [CrossRef]
66. Wu, S.; Calero-Pérez, P.; Arús, C.; Candiota, A.P. Anti-PD-1 Immunotherapy in Preclinical GL261 Glioblastoma: Influence of Therapeutic Parameters and Non-Invasive Response Biomarker Assessment with MRSI-Based Approaches. *Int. J. Mol. Sci.* **2020**, *21*, 8775. [CrossRef] [PubMed]

Disclaimer/Publisher's Note: The statements, opinions and data contained in all publications are solely those of the individual author(s) and contributor(s) and not of MDPI and/or the editor(s). MDPI and/or the editor(s) disclaim responsibility for any injury to people or property resulting from any ideas, methods, instructions or products referred to in the content.

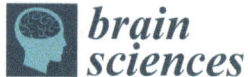

Article

Locomotion Outcome Improvement in Mice with Glioblastoma Multiforme after Treatment with Anastrozole

Irene Guadalupe Aguilar-García [1], Ismael Jiménez-Estrada [2], Rolando Castañeda-Arellano [3], Jonatan Alpirez [4], Gerardo Mendizabal-Ruiz [5], Judith Marcela Dueñas-Jiménez [6], Coral Estefania Gutiérrez-Almeida [4], Laura Paulina Osuna-Carrasco [5], Viviana Ramírez-Abundis [4] and Sergio Horacio Dueñas-Jiménez [4,*]

[1] Departamento de Biología Molecular y Genómica, Centro Universitario de Ciencias de la Salud, Universidad de Guadalajara, Guadalajara 44340, Mexico
[2] Departamento de Fisiología, Biofísica y Neurociencias, Centro de Investigación y Estudios Avanzados del Instituto Politécnico Nacional, Ciudad de Mexico 07000, Mexico
[3] Laboratorio de Farmacología, Centro de Investigación Multidisciplinario en Salud, Centro Universitario de Tonalá, Universidad de Guadalajara, Tonalá 45425, Mexico
[4] Departamento de Neurociencias, Centro Universitario de Ciencias de la Salud, Universidad de Guadalajara, Guadalajara 44340, Mexico
[5] Centro Universitario de Ciencias Exactas e Ingenierías, Universidad de Guadalajara, Guadalajara 44430, Mexico
[6] Departamento de Fisiología, Centro Universitario de Ciencias de la Salud, Universidad de Guadalajara, Guadalajara 44340, Mexico
* Correspondence: sergio.duenas@academicos.udg.mx; Tel.: +52-3310585313

Abstract: Glioblastoma Multiforme (GBM) is a tumor that infiltrates several brain structures. GBM is associated with abnormal motor activities resulting in impaired mobility, producing a loss of functional motor independence. We used a GBM xenograft implanted in the striatum to analyze the changes in Y (vertical) and X (horizontal) axis displacement of the metatarsus, ankle, and knee. We analyzed the steps dissimilarity factor between control and GBM mice with and without anastrozole. The body weight of the untreated animals decreased compared to treated mice. Anastrozole reduced the malignant cells and decreased GPR30 and ERα receptor expression. In addition, we observed a partial recovery in metatarsus and knee joint displacement (dissimilarity factor). The vertical axis displacement of the GBM+anastrozole group showed a difference in the right metatarsus, right knee, and left ankle compared to the GBM group. In the horizontal axis displacement of the right metatarsus, ankle, and knee, the GBM+anastrozole group exhibited a difference at the last third of the step cycle compared to the GBM group. Thus, anastrozole partially modified joint displacement. The dissimilarity factor and the vertical and horizontal displacements study will be of interest in GBM patients with locomotion alterations. Hindlimb displacement and gait locomotion analysis could be a valuable methodological tool in experimental and clinical studies to help diagnose locomotive deficits related to GBM.

Keywords: locomotion; glioblastoma; anastrozole

1. Introduction

Glioblastoma Multiforme (GBM) is the most aggressive type of glioma [1], with a median survival expectancy of 15–18 months after the diagnosis and a five-year survival rate of <10% [2]. GBM patients' standard treatment consists of surgical tumor resection, several radiotherapy cycles, and the chemotherapy drug temozolomide. Unfortunately, this combined intervention protocol is ineffective [3]. Therefore, it is essential to find a groundbreaking treatment for GBM [4]. Focal neurological deficits (i.e., motor weakness) typically occur in glioma patients and are associated with growth into motor areas. The striatal area has a significant role in controlling motor activities, and murine striatal glioblastoma models in this area allow the assessment of motor abilities [5]. Several studies involving this region show their participation in neurological disorders associated with abnormal motor activity [6,7]. Likewise, the degeneration in this structure impairs diverse motor and behavioral tasks [8]. However, more longitudinal studies of motor dysfunction in animal models are needed, as well as tools for early detection. The hindlimb displacement in mice walking over-ground has not been studied in murine striatal glioblastoma xenograft and could be an adequate model to test motor alterations.

Glioblastoma is a heterogeneous tumor with multiple redundant intracellular pathways, generating several subtypes [1,9]. Their expression is associated with the patient's survival outcome [10]. The estrogens directly bind classical or membrane estrogen receptors to initiate gene expression, suggesting diverse functions and tumoral properties. Third-generation aromatase inhibitors, such as anastrozole, have reduced estrogen levels by over 96%. This change is associated with decreased malignant cell viability and tumor growth [11]. This novel strategy should aim to target glioma growth and prevent the functional deterioration of spared brain networks. Based on these premises, we have set up a GBM mouse model by injecting C6 cells into the striatum to monitor locomotive behavioral dysfunction induced by tumor growth. The striatum in murine models is the topographic location showing the densest presence of gliomas. Moreover, the location of the xenograft in the striatum was due to the availability of sensitive behavioral tests that allowed the longitudinal assessment of motor abilities in the same animals. Additionally, this strategy allowed us to count the number of malignant cells and provided us with a new diagnosis tool to correlate tumor growth and hindlimb motor alterations.

2. Methods

2.1. Cells Culture

The rat C6 cell line (ATCC, CCL-107^{TM}) was cultured in DMEM-F12 high in glucose (Caisson DFL-14), supplemented with 10% fetal bovine serum (Gibco 26140, MO, USA) and 1% penicillin/streptomycin (Corning, 30-002-CL, AZ, USA). The cells underwent incubation at 37 °C in a humidified atmosphere containing 95% air and 5% CO_2. Afterward, cells were separated from the plate to implant them (1×10^6) in nude/nude mice into the right striatum.

2.2. Animals

We housed male Balb-C-nude/nude (Jackson lab: NU/J 002010), 6–7 weeks of age. The animals were kept under sterile conditions in boxes with sterile air exchange and light-dark cycles of 12×12 h, with controlled temperature between 23 and 25 °C, and free access to water and food until the day of surgery. All animal experiments were performed following the USA Guide for the Care and Use of Laboratory Animals, National Institutes of Health, The Mexican Regulation of Animal Care and Maintenance (NOM-062-ZOO-1999, 2001), and the institutional University of Guadalajara regulations.

2.3. Glioblastoma Xenograft and Mice Treatment

We formed two groups of mice; both groups received a C6 cells' xenograft; the first group was not treated (GBM group, $n = 5$), and the other one was treated with anastrozole (GBM+anastrozole, $n = 5$). We anesthetized mice with sevoflurane (3%). We made an incision in the brain midline of the scalp and a small hole in the skull following the stereotaxic coordinates (X = 1.34 mm, Y = 1.5 mm, and Z = 3.5 mm). We administered 1×10^6 cells in 2 µL of DMEM-F12 using a Hamilton syringe in mice's right striatum (See Supplementary Materials). Anastrozole (Sigma Aldrich A2736, MO, USA) was dissolved in DMSO 0.1 mM to obtain a final concentration of 500 µg/mL (stock solution) and stored at −20 °C. The drug (0.1 mg/kg) was administered through the tail vein with an insulin syringe (0.5 mL daily) for seven days.

2.4. Body Weight in Mice

The mice were randomly separated into 2 different groups: the GBM group and the GBM+anastrozole group. Then, they were fed with ad libitum access to food and water. The mice were kept with monitoring of food intake, water intake, and excretion, and were sacrificed at day 14. The body weight initially was 21 g ± 1 g in both groups.

2.5. Hematoxylin & Eosin Staining

The animals were anesthetized intraperitoneally with pentobarbital at 160 mg/kg of body weight and sacrificed by intracardiac perfusion using a saline solution (0.9%) and 4% paraformaldehyde. Brains were removed and placed in the same fixed solution at 4 °C. The brains were sectioned in the coronal plane at a thickness of thirty micrometers with a vibratome (Thermo Scientific, HM650V, MA, USA), and then processed for histology by Hematoxylin & Eosin staining. The slices were first submerged for two minutes in water and after three minutes in hematoxylin (Sigma H3136) and then three seconds in acid alcohol (1% HCl in 70% alcohol), washed with distilled water, and immersed in eosin (Sigma Aldrich 212954, MO USA) for a minute and a half before being washed with tap water for thirty seconds. For dehydration, the tissues were put in an increasing gradient of ethanol and xylol: 70% ethanol for 3 s, 90% ethanol for 3 s, and 96% alcohol for 3 min, twice in 100% ethanol for 5 min, and then twice in xylene for 5 min. We used entellan for mounting sections and observed them under a microscope (Carl-Zeiss Aalen, Germany) at 10× and 40×. We counted cells using a 40× objective, considering four fields of the ipsilateral hemisphere.

2.6. Immunofluorescence

We used immunofluorescence for GFAP, GRP30, and ERα. The brain sections were incubated at room temperature for 30 min in PBS 1x/Triton X-100 0.2%. Next, the tissue sections were incubated for 1 h in PBS 1X bovine albumin serum 1%. Then, the sections were incubated overnight with GFAP antibody (1:750, DAKO, Z0334, RRID: AB_10013382), anti-ERα mouse monoclonal (1:500, Abcam ab 66102 RRID: AB_310305), and anti-GPR30 mouse monoclonal (1:500, Abcam ab 39742 RRID: AB_1950438). Lastly, the secondary antibodies: FITC anti-rabbit IgG (1:500, Jackson AB_2337972) and Alexa fluor 594 polyclonal rabbit (1:1000, Abcam ab150080) were used for a 2 h incubation. We used a 40× oil immersion objective and the Olympus BX51WI microscope.

2.7. Tunnel Walk Recordings

We conducted a locomotion analysis studying the metatarsus, ankle, and knee joints' hindlimbs displacements. We used the dissimilarity factor (DF) and vertical/horizontal displacements of the mice's strides. We took the data registered before tumor implantation (control group) and after seven days (GBM group), as well as after fourteen days (GBM+anastrozole group) of xenograft implant. We took video recordings while the animals were walking on a transparent Plexiglas tunnel. The video was registered using two synchronized cameras recording left and right hindlimbs simultaneously. We set the cameras to record at 240 fps with a resolution of 1280 × 720 pixels. Post-processing was applied to the resulting videos to remove spherical distortion due to the lenses by estimating a homographic matrix using four points on the image [12]. A step cycle corresponds to when the metatarsus lifts off to when the metatarsus touches down. Using custom-made software, we marked knee, ankle, and metatarsus joints on each video frame for each step. We studied each joint's displacement curves and values through software developed in our laboratory. Each one of the animal's steps was captured on the video separately. During several steps, we generated displacement curves on the horizontal and vertical axes concerning time for each joint in the left and right hind limbs. All curves were normalized according to the stride using a value range from one to 100, employing a spline-based interpolation.

2.8. Dissimilarity Factor Analysis

We measured the dissimilarity factor (*DF*) to compare the control group steps versus glioblastoma and anastrozole-treated animals to determine the locomotion changes between animal groups. We compared their displacement curves and calculated the dissimilarity factor between them using the Euclidean distance between each of the points of the normalized curve on the horizontal (X) and vertical (Y) axes as

$$DF_{\langle a,b \rangle} = \frac{1}{200}\sqrt{\sum_{i=1}^{100}(x_a(i)-x_b(i))^2 + \sum_{i=1}^{100}(y_a(i)-y_b(i))^2} \quad (1)$$

where $DF<a,b>$ is the squared error between every point of the normalized curves, defined as difference factor (*DF*); "$x_a(i) - x_b(i)$" is the difference (*d*) between the coordinates in *x*, and "$y_a(i) - y_b(i)$" in *y* of every point in the graph, when comparing two steps (*a* and *b*); and "*i*" is the percent in the step cycle.

We compared the curves of every animal in the control and the experimental groups (GBM and GBM+anastrozole). We analyzed the curves of a control animal vs. all control animals and the steep curve of an experimental animal concerning all control animals [Leon-Moreno et al., 2020]. Then, we had these comparisons: control vs. control, GBM vs. control, and GBM+anastrozole vs. control. We estimated the *DF* values and analyzed statistical significances with an ANOVA test of unidirectional via and a post hoc Tukey.

2.9. Vertical/Horizontal Displacement Analysis

We analyzed the vertical and horizontal displacements separately. We took each joint's vertical/horizontal displacement data and averaged it per group. The measurement of the hindlimbs displacement of each group was six repetitions, per side, per mouse. Then, we compared the experimental groups (GBM and GBM+anastrozole) versus the control group. We evaluated significant differences at every two perceptual points of the step cycle between groups through a student's *t*-test (a = 0.05). A locally designed MATLAB script was used for the pattern comparison analysis.

3. Statistics

The dissimilarity factors were expressed as means ± SD. We analyzed the data using one-way ANOVA with Tukey post hoc. The data analysis for body weight, cell counting, and horizontal and vertical displacement was performed through an unpaired one-tailed student's *t*-test, and a *p*-value of * <0.05 was considered statistically significant. We conducted the statistical analysis using the Prism 9.0 software GraphPad and MATLAB R 2021b.

4. Results

4.1. Body Weight in GBM and GBM+Anastrozole Groups

We evaluated the mice's weight from the xenograft day until 14 days post-transplantation. During the first 11 days after transplantation, GBM+anastrozole mice maintained a weight between 20 and 22 g (Figure 1). On days 12 and 13, there was no weight loss in the GBM group, while the GBM+anastrozole animals remained unchanged. A significant difference in body weight between the GBM and GBM+anastrozole groups on days 12 and 13 ($p < 0.05$) was observed.

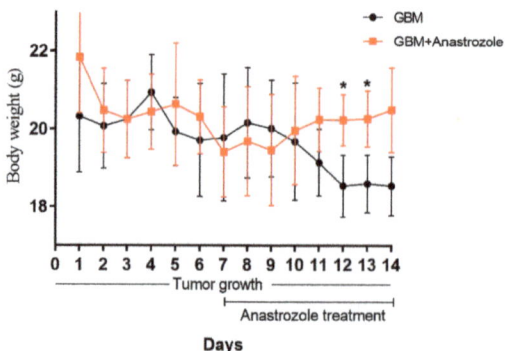

Figure 1. Body Weight in mice. Graph illustrating the body weight changes of mice monitored 14 days after xenograft. Data correspond to GBM and GBM+anastrozole. The GBM+anastrozole group showed a significant increase in body weight on the 12th and 13th days compared to the GBM group. The data show Mean ± SE values. The asterisks indicated statistical differences between groups (Mann–Whitney U test; $p < 0.05$).

4.2. Histopathological Changes in the Striatal Area of GBM and GBM+Anastrozole Mice

We analyzed the tumor volume of GBM vs. GBM+anastrozole (Figure 2A–C). The anastrozole-treated animals did not show statistical differences in tumor volume reduction at 14 days of treatment of 23.4 mm^3 ± 2.5, with respect to 27.5 mm^3 ± 3.2 of tumor volume of GBM (Figure 2F). However, the H&E staining showed that the glioma in mice treated with anastrozole exhibited better-defined tumor margins and fewer invasive cells to the GBM striatum compared with other brain regions.

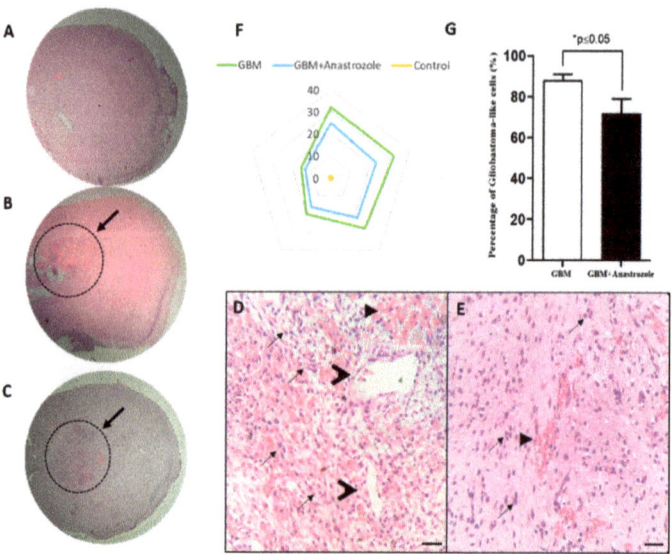

Figure 2. Histopathological changes in Striatum. (**A**) Photograph illustrating a transverse area in the right striatum of an untreated GBM mouse. (**B,C**) Administration of anastrozole does not reduce tumor growth in the mice glioma model. Glioblastoma tumor tissue shows morphological features that include a disordered arrangement of clear and large cells with condensed nuclei and darkly stained cytoplasm. Arrows point to necrotic centers indicating areas of necrosis. (**D,E**) Photograph of

an area in the striatum of a GBM+anastrozole mouse showing the arrangement of cells. Arrows head indicates vessels. Arrows without line shows necrotic area. Note that it contains fewer large cells and a reduced number of nuclei than the striatal GBM tissue. (**F**) The tumor volume was measured in mm^3. (**G**) Graph exhibiting data of the counted tumor cells in GBM and GBM+anastrozole groups. Bars represent mean ± SD (n = 5 animals). The asterisk indicates statistical differences between groups (*t*-student test; $p < 0.05$). Scale bar = 50 µm and 200 µm.

Gliomas present typical malignant cell characteristics of humans, such as nuclear atypia and multinucleation. They also exhibited areas of necrosis and palisade arrangement (Figure 2D). The contralateral striatal area showed a normal distribution of glial cells and no angiogenesis (Figure 2E). Compared with the GBM group, the GBM+anastrozole group exhibits fewer cells in the tumor tissue (Figure 2E). Some striatum slices in GBM+anastrozole mice did not show tumor cells. The treatment with anastrozole reduces (19%) the number of glioblastoma cells in the striatum as compared to the GBM group (Figure 2G).

4.3. Expression of ERα and GPR30 Receptors in the Study Groups

As shown in Figure 3, the striatal cells in the GBM group present intense ERα-GFAP staining at 14 days post-xenograft (Figure 3A). At the same time, cells in the GBM+anastrozole group exhibited a less intense expression of ERα (Figure 3B). Furthermore, GPR30 immunopositive cells are present in Glioblastoma multiforme. The GBM group shows a highly positive reaction to GPR30 cells, which co-localized mainly in the cell nucleus (Figure 3C). In contrast, anastrozole treatment strongly reduced the GPR30-positive cells in glioblastoma (Figure 3D).

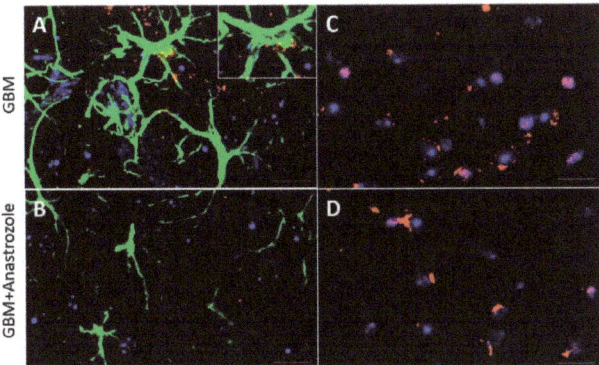

Figure 3. Expression of ERα and GPR30 immunopositive C6 cells. (**A**) Microphotograph showing the merge of GFAP immunopositive cells (green), ERα expression (red), and cell nuclei stained with DAPI (blue) in striatal tissue of GBM. (**B**) In GBM+anastrozole mice, striatal cells and striatal tissue exhibited a decrease in staining to ERα in GFAP and DAPI. The insert clearly shows GFAP-immunofluorescence with ERα co-expression in glioblastoma cells. (**C,D**) The microphotographs show GPR30 expression (red) and nuclei (blue) in striatal tissue slides of GBM and GBM+anastrozole animals, respectively. GBM tissue exhibits more nuclei and higher GPR30 expression than those observed in GBM+anastrozole tissue. Scale bar = 30 µm.

4.4. Changes in Mice Locomotion with Glioblastoma and Those Treated with Anastrozole

We analyzed the hindlimb displacement in all study groups and compared dissimilarity factors before and after xenograft in the same animal. We observed a significant effect on the DF of mice 14 days following the xenograft. The left metatarsus DF of the control group had a statistical difference (* $p = 0.029$, Figure 4A) compared to the GBM group.

The left metatarsus DF in the GBM vs. GBM+anastrozole mice groups' curves does not exhibit statistical differences (Figure 4A). In the left ankle, there was no difference between the study groups (Figure 4B). The left knee DF showed statistically significant changes between the GBM and the control group (* p = 0.0178). The differences were also present in GBM vs. GBM+anastrozole group (* p = 0.0137). There were no differences between the control and anastrozole-treated groups. (Figure 4C). So, there was a recovery in the DF of treated animals.

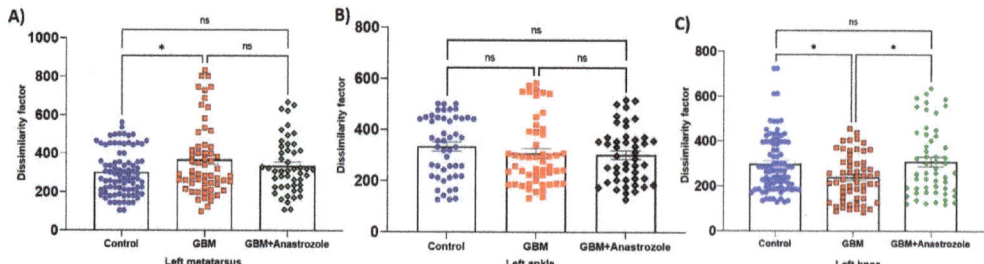

Figure 4. Dissimilarity factor changes in metatarsus, ankle, and knee of the left hindlimb in GBM-control and GBM+anastrozole groups. (**A**) The dissimilarity factor (DF) in the left hindlimb metatarsus has a statistical difference between the control and GBM groups (* p < 0.027). (**B**) The DF in the ankle did not show differences among the control, GBM, and GBM+anastrozole groups. (**C**) The DF exhibited a significant difference between control versus GBM (* p < 0.0178) and GBM versus GBM+anastrozole (* p < 0.0137). The data show Mean ± SD values. The asterisks indicated statistical differences between groups using an ANOVA test.

4.5. The Horizontal Displacement among Different Study Groups

The left metatarsus, ankle, and knee horizontal displacement did not show a statistical difference among the study groups. Note that control vs. GBM (*), control vs. GBM+anastrozole (+), and GBM vs. GBM+anastrozole (x) are similar (Figure 5A–C). In contrast, the right metatarsus horizontal displacement shows a statistical difference in GBM vs. GBM+anastrozole group from bins 86 to 100 with a 16% difference (* p < 0.05, Figure 5D). The right ankle horizontal displacement showed a statistical difference between GBM vs. GBM+anastrozole (x) groups from the bins 72 to 100 with a 28% difference, and GBM+anastrozole vs. control (+) shows the difference from the bin 68–70 with a 2% difference (Figure 5E). In the right knee, horizontal displacement shows statistical changes in GBM+anastrozole vs. control (+) from bins 70 to 100 with a 32% difference, and in GBM+anastrozole vs. GBM (x), from bins 82 to 100 with a 24% difference (Figure 5F).

4.6. Changes in Vertical Displacement

The left metatarsus did not differ among the studied groups (Figure 6A). In contrast, the right metatarsus exhibited changes in the control group vs. GBM+anastrozole (+) from bins 66 to 72 with an 8% difference, in GBM+anastrozole vs. GBM (x) from bins 56 to 58 with a 4% difference, and also in the GBM vs. control (*) group from bins 50 to 54 with a 6% difference (Figure 6D).

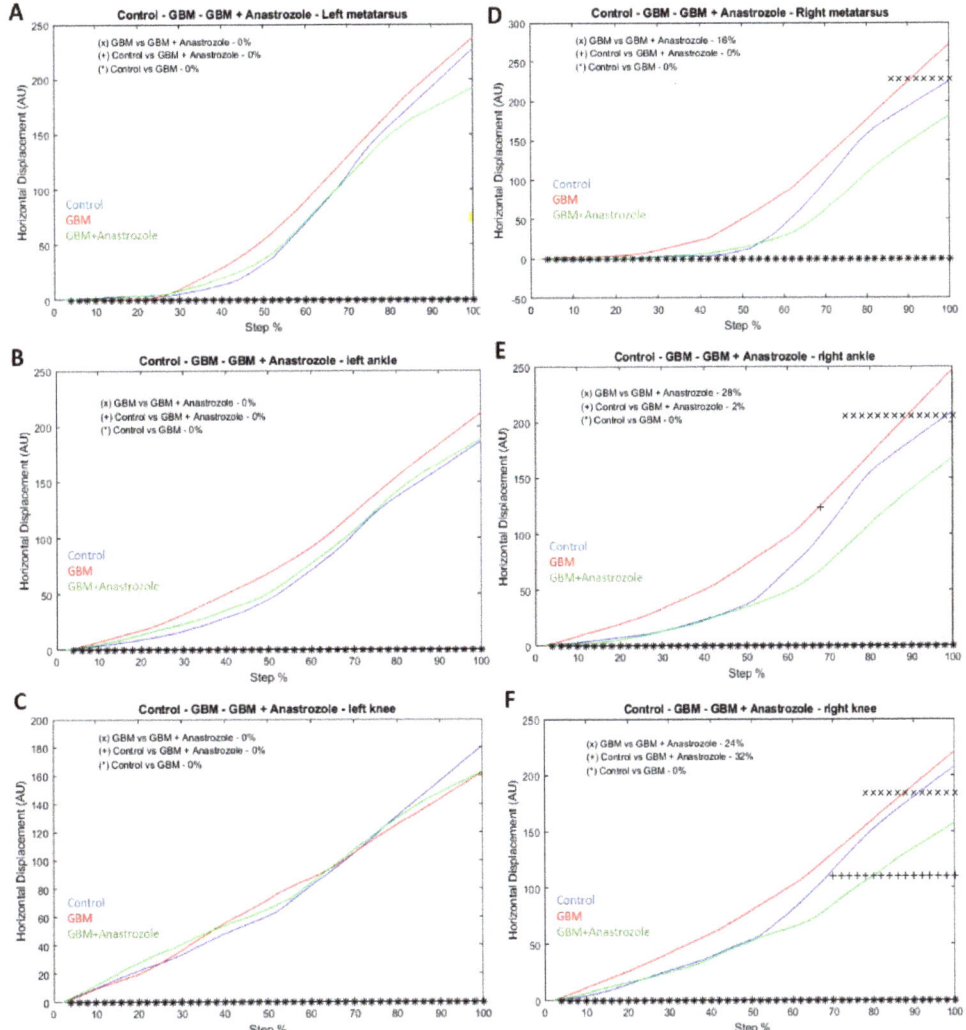

Figure 5. Left and right hindlimb metatarsus, ankle, and knee displacement in the horizontal axis. The left metatarsus, ankle, and knee horizontal displacement does not show a statistical difference among the control and GBM groups. (**A**–**C**). The right metatarsus horizontal displacement significantly changed in GBM vs. GBM+anastrozole groups (* $p < 0.05$, (**D**)). The right ankle horizontal displacement showed significant changes in the step cycle in the GBM vs. GBM+anastrozole groups (**E**). The right knee horizontal displacement showed significant changes among the GBM and GBM+anastrozole groups, and the GBM+anastrozole versus control groups (* $p < 0.05$, (**F**)). The symbols (*, +, x) over zero (0) indicate statistical differences between groups (student test; $p < 0.05$). Every symbol corresponds to two bins.

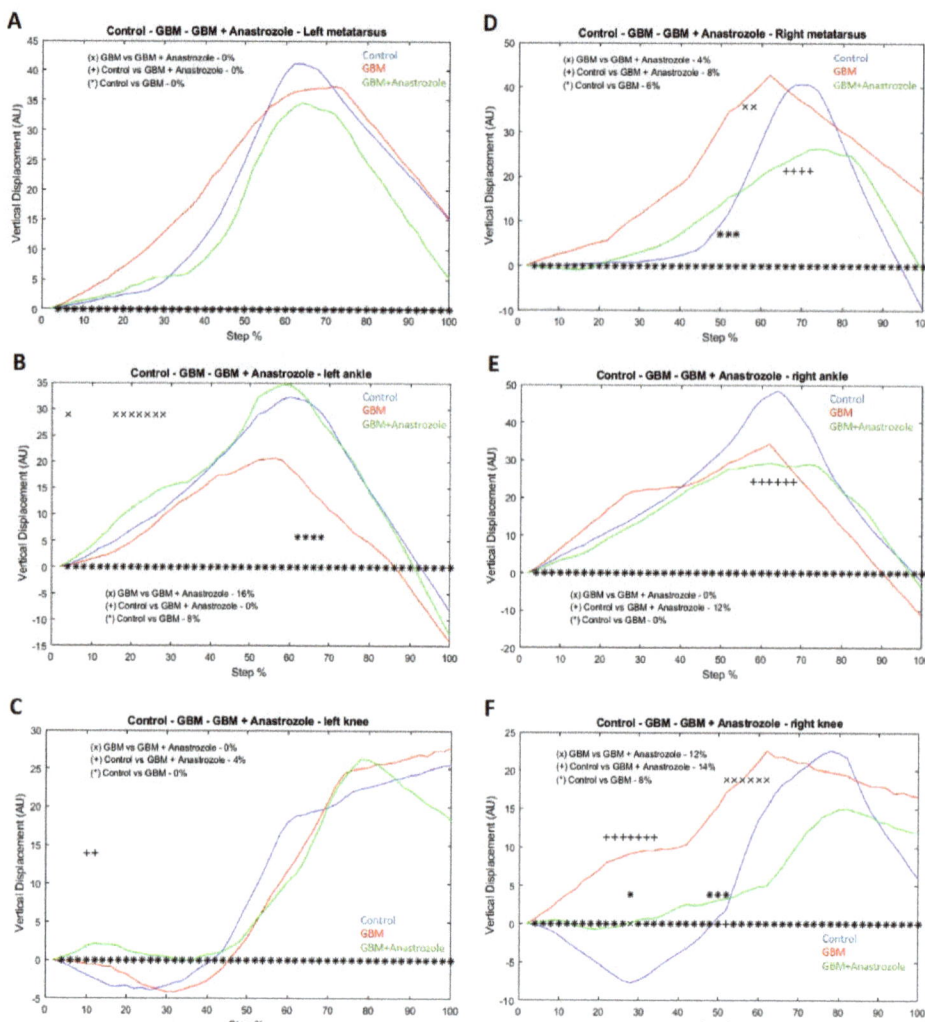

Figure 6. Left and right hindlimb metatarsus, ankle, and knee displacement in the vertical axis. The left metatarsus vertical displacement was not statistically significant among groups during the step cycle (**A**). The left ankle vertical displacement shows significant changes in some periods of the step cycle (**B**). It occurred between control versus GBM group and GBM+anastrozole versus GBM (* $p < 0.05$). The left knee vertical displacement changes significantly at the beginning of the step cycle. It appeared between control and GBM+anastrozole groups (**C**). The right metatarsus shows a statistically significant difference in various bins of the step cycle. The changes were observed in GBM versus GBM+anastrozole group, GBM+anastrozole versus control, and control versus GBM (* $p < 0.05$) (**D**). The right ankle vertical displacement showed a statistically significant change in the middle of the step cycle. It occurred between the control versus GBM+anastrozole groups (* $p < 0.05$) (**E**). The right knee vertical displacement shows a statistical difference in several parts of the step cycle. It occurred between the GBM and the GBM+anastrozole groups, control versus GBM+anastrozole, and control versus GBM groups (* $p < 0.05$) (**F**). The symbols (*, +, x) over zero (0) indicated statistical differences between groups (student test; $p < 0.05$). Every symbol above zero corresponds to two bins with a significant statistical difference.

The left ankle vertical displacement showed statistically significant changes between control vs. GBM (*) from bins 60 to 68 with an 8% difference, and GBM compared to GBM+anastrozole (x) from bins 18 to 34 with a 16% difference ($p < 0.05$ * Figure 6B). The right ankle showed a difference between control and GBM+anastrozole from bins 58 to 70 with a 12% difference (Figure 6E).

The left knee vertical displacement between control vs. GBM+anastrozole groups changed from bins 50 to 52 with a 4% difference (Figure 6C). The right knee vertical displacement between GBM+anastrozole vs. GBM groups changed from bins 52 to 62 with a 12% difference, GBM+anastrozole vs. control from bins 20 to 34 with a 14% difference, and GBM vs. control from bins 26 to 28 and 46 to 52 with an 8% difference (* $p < 0.05$, Figure 6F).

5. Discussion

The body weight loss in animals treated with anastrozole occurred in rats [13,14] and in the transgenic female 3xTgAD mice [15]. This work described changes in body weight, with mice maintaining their weight on days 12 and 13. Breast cancer patients commonly report weight gain after tamoxifen or aromatase inhibitor administration [16]. Thus, we suggest that anastrozole could contribute to maintaining weight through steroid regulation of body weight mass.

The histopathological characteristics of the GBM developed in the striatum are similar to those observed in patients with GBM. There is tissue necrosis, neovascularization, and an arrangement palisade pattern of the tumor cells [17]. Glioma cells are reduced on the 14th post-treatment day, indicating an anastrozole antiproliferative and apoptotic effect. Such results agree with work reported for lung and breast cancers [18,19].

We observed a qualitative decrease in the expression of estrogen receptors (ERα and GPR30) in tumor GBM+anastrozole xenografted tissue. An increase in estrogen and its receptors is associated with tumor growth in different cancer types [20]. The increase in ERα expression was related to reduced GBM patient survival [21]. Clinical trials have shown that anastrozole is better than selective estrogen modulators against breast cancer [22,23]. This effect is due to a systemic reduction of 17ß-estradiol and negative ERα expression regulation [24]. The recently discovered estrogen receptor GPR30 is present in several cancer cells [25]. The expression of this receptor plays an essential role in the tumor growth of gastric cancer [26], breast cancer [27], and endometrial cancer [28], among others. This study found that ERα and GPR30 decreased expression in the GBM anastrozole-treated group. The reduced number of tumor cells could be due to low estrogen alpha and GPER receptor expression and estrogen levels [10,29]. Further experiments are needed to quantify estrogen receptor expression in GBM-treated anastrozole mice.

Brain tumors are related to cognitive and motor deficits [30,31]. Brain tumors significantly affect motor networks due to alterations in cortical areas [32,33]. They also affect functional connectivity between cortical and subcortical motor areas [34]. A study reported important aspects concerning tumor growth evaluation and specific motor behavioral alterations, particularly gait instability, in a rat model [35]. In clinical studies of GBM, gait instability is a common motor symptom caused by tumor invasion [36,37]. GBM models in rats show regions of focal invasion into brain tissue, similar to the diffuse infiltrating pattern seen in GBM patients [38]. Glioblastoma growth into motor areas is associated with an alteration in gait locomotion. A critical area related to locomotion is the striatum, and modifications in this area may produce complications in the rhythmic alternation of limbs [39]. The striatum modulates treadmill locomotion in rats and humans during free walking [6,40]. The GBM can produce diverse motor alterations because it has no defined limits.

In our experiments, we observed a reduction in the dissimilarity factors and, consequently, an improvement in the left hindlimb metatarsus and knee displacement in GBM+anastrozole mice. Thus, anastrozole improved gait locomotion, probably due to a brain tumor reduction in the right motor area (Figure 4). Concerning the step cycle changes, the horizontal and vertical displacement of the right side showed differences between the study groups. GBM tumor growth in the striatum may lead to impaired hindlimb displacement and motor impairment in each step cycle [37]. Further studies are needed to establish the relationship between lesion location resulting in the effects of tumors, or the pathways producing changes in the spinal cord central pattern generators [41]. Following the motor deficit found in our experiments, treatment and rehabilitation will depend on previous treatments, tumor area swelling, and invasivity.

The locomotor system comprises centers in the brainstem controlling spinal circuitry. The motor deficits of several hindlimb joint displacements could be attributed to the dispersed commands to engage the joint generator circuits [42,43].

In mice walking over-ground, we found changes in the right metatarsus, ankle, and knee joints after anastrozole. It seems possible that GBM progression and regression occur differentially in the right and left brain stems. Further studies are necessary to evaluate the recovery of brain stem–spinal cord pathways and their relationship with tumor size reduction. It will be interesting to study why anastrozole reduces the horizontal displacement in the right hindlimb. Reducing the step cycle's variability could help stabilize locomotion and navigation. The hindlimbs' right gait compensation could stabilize the correct hindlimb gait.

Additionally, our study showed that the alterations in vertical displacement were more dispersed than horizontal displacement in both hindlimbs. The neural pathways that activate the displacement are not known, and neither are the tumor dimensions nor the precise infiltration. Anastrozole produces differential effects in the tumoral cells. We need to study the spatial tumor dimensions to propose an anastrozole effect to obtain a clear conclusion.

An important finding is that the vertical axis of the displacement of GBM+anastrozole is similar to the control group, which implies that anastrozole regulates the changes due to GBM in the ankle joint displacement.

The pyramidal pathways project to motor neurons and the CPG (Central Pattern Generator). They adapt the basic locomotor pattern to environmental constraints [44,45]. They could participate in adapting the motor system to the brain stem alterations produced by the tumor.

In this study, the variations found in horizontal and vertical displacements in the different joints suggest independent burst pattern generators for each joint of both hindlimbs on several projections coming from the brain stem.

6. Conclusions

We addressed the functional relevance of the antineoplastic effect of anastrozole treatment by regulating the ERα and GPR30 expression in GBM xenograft. Thus, anastrozole partially recovered joint displacement by modifications in vertical and horizontal displacements in different phases of the step cycle. It will be interesting to study whether similar results occur in some patients with GBM exhibiting locomotion alterations. Hindlimb displacement and gait locomotion analysis could be a valuable methodological tool in experimental and clinical studies to develop new therapeutic approaches against locomotive deficits produced by GBM.

Supplementary Materials: The following supporting information can be downloaded at https://www.mdpi.com/article/10.3390/brainsci13030496/s1, Figure S1: Schematic diagram shows the experimental approach.

Author Contributions: I.G.A.-G.: writing—original draft preparation, investigation; R.C.-A.: conceptualization, validation, data curation; J.A.: software design for intrastep analysis; G.M.-R.: statistical analysis, data curation; C.E.G.-A.: revision and editing of the final manuscript; J.M.D.-J., V.R.-A. and L.P.O.-C.: methodology; I.J.-E. and S.H.D.-J.: funding acquisition, project conceptualization, and administration. All authors have read and agreed to the published version of the manuscript.

Funding: Acknowledgments: This work was partially supported by the Conacyt grant (2019-000006-01NACV-00352) and fellowships granted to Irene Aguilar García CONACyT (scholarship number 000235) and Ismael Jimenez Estrada by Sistema Nacional de Investigadores, México.

Institutional Review Board Statement: The animal study protocol was approved by Ethics Committee of Centro Universitario de Ciencias de la Salud (protocol code CONBIOETICA-14-CEI-002-20191003).

Informed Consent Statement: Not applicable.

Data Availability Statement: Not applicable.

Acknowledgments: Sandra Orozco Suarez generously provided the C6 cell line (C.M.N. Siglo XXI, Instituto Mexicano del Seguro Social).

Conflicts of Interest: The authors declare no conflict of interest.

References

1. Ghosh, D.; Nandi, S.; Bhattacharjee, S. Combination Therapy to Checkmate Glioblastoma: Clinical Challenges and Advances. *Clin. Transl. Med.* **2018**, *7*, 33. [CrossRef] [PubMed]
2. Stupp, R.; Mason, W.P.; van den Bent, M.J.; Weller, M.; Fisher, B.; Taphoorn, M.J.B.; Belanger, K.; Brandes, A.A.; Marosi, C.; Bogdahn, U.; et al. Radiotherapy plus Concomitant and Adjuvant Temozolomide for Glioblastoma. *N. Engl. J. Med.* **2005**, *352*, 987–996. [CrossRef] [PubMed]
3. Lonardi, S.; Tosoni, A.; Brandes, A.A. Adjuvant Chemotherapy in the Treatment of High Grade Gliomas. *Cancer Treat. Rev.* **2005**, *31*, 79–89. [CrossRef]
4. Birch, J.L.; Strathdee, K.; Gilmour, L.; Vallatos, A.; McDonald, L.; Kouzeli, A.; Vasan, R.; Qaisi, A.H.; Croft, D.R.; Crighton, D.; et al. A Novel Small-Molecule Inhibitor of MRCK Prevents Radiation-Driven Invasion in Glioblastoma. *Cancer Res.* **2018**, *78*, 6509–6522. [CrossRef] [PubMed]
5. Miyai, M.; Tomita, H.; Soeda, A.; Yano, H.; Iwama, T.; Hara, A. Current Trends in Mouse Models of Glioblastoma. *J. Neurooncol.* **2017**, *135*, 423–432. [CrossRef]
6. Shi, L.H.; Luo, F.; Woodward, D.J.; Chang, J.Y. Neural Responses in Multiple Basal Ganglia Regions during Spontaneous and Treadmill Locomotion Task in Rats. *Exp. Brain Res.* **2004**, *157*, 303–314. [CrossRef] [PubMed]
7. Gonzales, K.K.; Smith, Y. Cholinergic Interneurons in the Dorsal and Ventral Striatum: Anatomical and Functional Considerations in Normal and Diseased Conditions. *Ann. N. Y. Acad. Sci.* **2015**, *1349*, 1–45. [CrossRef] [PubMed]
8. Khan, S.; Yuldasheva, N.Y.; Batten, T.F.C.; Pickles, A.R.; Kellett, K.A.B.; Saha, S. Tau Pathology and Neurochemical Changes Associated with Memory Dysfunction in an Optimised Murine Model of Global Cerebral Ischaemia-A Potential Model for Vascular Dementia? *Neurochem. Int.* **2018**, *118*, 134–144. [CrossRef]
9. Yague, J.G.; Lavaque, E.; Carretero, J.; Azcoitia, I.; Garcia-Segura, L.M. Aromatase, the Enzyme Responsible for Estrogen Biosynthesis, Is Expressed by Human and Rat Glioblastomas. *Neurosci. Lett.* **2004**, *368*, 279–284. [CrossRef]
10. Dueñas Jiménez, J.M.; Candanedo Arellano, A.; Santerre, A.; Orozco Suárez, S.; Sandoval Sánchez, H.; Feria Romero, I.; López-Elizalde, R.; Alonso Venegas, M.; Netel, B.; de la Torre Valdovinos, B.; et al. Aromatase and Estrogen Receptor Alpha MRNA Expression as Prognostic Biomarkers in Patients with Astrocytomas. *J. Neurooncol.* **2014**, *119*, 275–284. [CrossRef]
11. Amir, E.; Seruga, B.; Niraula, S.; Carlsson, L.; Ocaña, A. Toxicity of Adjuvant Endocrine Therapy in Postmenopausal Breast Cancer Patients: A Systematic Review and Meta-Analysis. *J. Natl. Cancer Inst.* **2011**, *103*, 1299–1309. [CrossRef] [PubMed]
12. Ascencio-Piña, C.; Pérez-Cisneros, M.; Dueñaz-Jimenez, S.; Mendizabal-Ruiz, G. A System for High-Speed Synchronized Acquisition of Video Recording of Rodents during Locomotion. In *VIII Latin American Conference on Biomedical Engineering and XLII National Conference on Biomedical Engineering, Proceedings of CLAIB-CNIB 2019, Cancún, México, 2–5 October 2019*; Springer: Cham, Switzerland, 2020; pp. 309–314.
13. Kubatka, P.; Sadlonova, V.; Kajo, K.; Machalekova, K.; Ostatnikova, D.; Nosalova, G.; Fetisovova, Z. Neoplastic Effects of Exemestane in Premenopausal Breast Cancer Model. *Neoplasma* **2008**, *55*, 538–543.
14. Sadlonova, V.; Kubatka, P.; Kajo, K.; Ostatnikova, D.; Nosalova, G.; Adamicova, K.; Sadlonova, J. Side Effects of Anastrozole in the Experimental Pre-Menopausal Mammary Carcinogenesis. *Neoplasma* **2009**, *56*, 124–129. [CrossRef] [PubMed]
15. Overk, C.R.; Borgia, J.A.; Mufson, E.J. A Novel Approach for Long-Term Oral Drug Administration in Animal Research. *J. Neurosci. Methods* **2011**, *195*, 194–199. [CrossRef]
16. Sestak, I.; Cuzick, J. Preventive Therapy for Breast Cancer. *Curr. Oncol. Rep.* **2012**, *14*, 568–573. [CrossRef] [PubMed]
17. Broniscer, A.; Tatevossian, R.G.; Sabin, N.D.; Klimo, P.; Dalton, J.; Lee, R.; Gajjar, A.; Ellison, D.W. Clinical, Radiological, Histological and Molecular Characteristics of Paediatric Epithelioid Glioblastoma. *Neuropathol. Appl. Neurobiol.* **2014**, *40*, 327–336. [CrossRef]
18. Weinberg, O.K.; Marquez-Garban, D.C.; Fishbein, M.C.; Goodglick, L.; Garban, H.J.; Dubinett, S.M.; Pietras, R.J. Aromatase Inhibitors in Human Lung Cancer Therapy. *Cancer Res.* **2005**, *65*, 11287–11291. [CrossRef]

19. Forbes, J.F.; Sestak, I.; Howell, A.; Bonanni, B.; Bundred, N.; Levy, C.; Von Minckwitz, G.; Eiermann, W.; Neven, P.; Stierer, M.; et al. Anastrozole versus Tamoxifen for the Prevention of Locoregional and Contralateral Breast Cancer in Postmenopausal Women with Locally Excised Ductal Carcinoma in Situ (IBIS-II DCIS): A Double-Blind, Randomised Controlled Trial. *Lancet* **2016**, *387*, 866–873. [CrossRef]
20. Rothenberger, N.; Somasundaram, A.; Stabile, L. The Role of the Estrogen Pathway in the Tumor Microenvironment. *Int. J. Mol. Sci.* **2018**, *19*, 611. [CrossRef]
21. Hönikl, L.S.; Lämmer, F.; Gempt, J.; Meyer, B.; Schlegel, J.; Delbridge, C. High Expression of Estrogen Receptor Alpha and Aromatase in Glial Tumor Cells Is Associated with Gender-Independent Survival Benefits in Glioblastoma Patients. *J. Neurooncol.* **2020**, *147*, 567–575. [CrossRef]
22. Demark-Wahnefried, W.; Peterson, B.L.; Winer, E.P.; Marks, L.; Aziz, N.; Marcom, P.K.; Blackwell, K.; Rimer, B.K. Changes in Weight, Body Composition, and Factors Influencing Energy Balance Among Premenopausal Breast Cancer Patients Receiving Adjuvant Chemotherapy. *J. Clin. Oncol.* **2001**, *19*, 2381–2389. [CrossRef]
23. Winer, E.P.; Hudis, C.; Burstein, H.J.; Wolff, A.C.; Pritchard, K.I.; Ingle, J.N.; Chlebowski, R.T.; Gelber, R.; Edge, S.B.; Gralow, J.; et al. American Society of Clinical Oncology Technology Assessment on the Use of Aromatase Inhibitors As Adjuvant Therapy for Postmenopausal Women With Hormone Receptor–Positive Breast Cancer: Status Report 2004. *J. Clin. Oncol.* **2005**, *23*, 619–629. [CrossRef] [PubMed]
24. Smollich, M.; Götte, M.; Fischgräbe, J.; Radke, I.; Kiesel, L.; Wülfing, P. Differential Effects of Aromatase Inhibitors and Antiestrogens on Estrogen Receptor Expression in Breast Cancer Cells. *Anticancer Res.* **2009**, *29*, 2167–2171. [PubMed]
25. Vivacqua, A.; Lappano, R.; De Marco, P.; Sisci, D.; Aquila, S.; De Amicis, F.; Fuqua, S.A.W.; AndoÒ, S.; Maggiolini, M. G Protein-Coupled Receptor 30 Expression Is Up-Regulated by EGF and TGFα in Estrogen Receptor α-Positive Cancer Cells. *Mol. Endocrinol.* **2009**, *23*, 1815–1826. [CrossRef] [PubMed]
26. Tian, S.; Zhan, N.; Li, R.; Dong, W. Downregulation of G Protein-Coupled Estrogen Receptor (GPER) Is Associated with Reduced Prognosis in Patients with Gastric Cancer. *Med. Sci. Monit.* **2019**, *25*, 3115–3126. [CrossRef]
27. Tutzauer, J.; Sjöström, M.; Bendahl, P.O.; Rydén, L.; Fernö, M.; Fredrik Leeb-Lundberg, L.M.; Alkner, S. Plasma Membrane Expression of G Protein-Coupled Estrogen Receptor (GPER)/G Protein-Coupled Receptor 30 (GPR30) Is Associated with Worse Outcome in Metachronous Contralateral Breast Cancer. *PLoS ONE* **2020**, *15*, e0231786. [CrossRef]
28. Li, Y.; Jia, Y.; Bian, Y.; Tong, H.; Qu, J.; Wang, K.; Wan, X.-P. Autocrine Motility Factor Promotes Endometrial Cancer Progression by Targeting GPER-1. *Cell Commun. Signal.* **2019**, *17*, 22. [CrossRef]
29. Gutiérrez-Almeida, C.; Santerre, A.; León-Moreno, L.; Aguilar-García, I.; Castañeda-Arellano, R.; Dueñas-Jiménez, S.; Dueñas-jiménez, J. Proliferation and Apoptosis Regulation by G Protein-coupled Estrogen Receptor in Glioblastoma C6 Cells. *Oncol. Lett.* **2022**, *24*, 217. [CrossRef]
30. Lang, S.; Cadeaux, M.; Opoku-Darko, M.; Gaxiola-Valdez, I.; Partlo, L.A.; Goodyear, B.G.; Federico, P.; Kelly, J. Assessment of Cognitive, Emotional, and Motor Domains in Patients with Diffuse Gliomas Using the National Institutes of Health Toolbox Battery. *World Neurosurg.* **2017**, *99*, 448. [CrossRef]
31. IJzerman-Korevaar, M.; Snijders, T.J.; de Graeff, A.; Teunissen, S.C.C.M.; de Vos, F.Y.F. Prevalence of Symptoms in Glioma Patients throughout the Disease Trajectory: A Systematic Review. *J. Neurooncol.* **2018**, *140*, 485–496. [CrossRef]
32. Cochereau, J.; Herbet, G.; Duffau, H. Patients with Incidental WHO Grade II Glioma Frequently Suffer from Neuropsychological Disturbances. *Acta Neurochir.* **2016**, *158*, 305–312. [CrossRef]
33. Liouta, E.; Koutsarnakis, C.; Liakos, F.; Stranjalis, G. Effects of Intracranial Meningioma Location, Size, and Surgery on Neurocognitive Functions: A 3-Year Prospective Study. *J. Neurosurg.* **2016**, *124*, 1578–1584. [CrossRef]
34. Liouta, E.; Katsaros, V.K.; Stranjalis, G.; Leks, E.; Klose, U.; Bisdas, S. Motor and Language Deficits Correlate with Resting State Functional Magnetic Resonance Imaging Networks in Patients with Brain Tumors. *J. Neuroradiol.* **2019**, *46*, 199–206. [CrossRef]
35. Felix Souza, T.K.; Nucci, M.P.; Mamani, J.B.; Rodrigues da Silva, H.; Carvalho Fantacini, D.M.; Botelho de Souza, L.E.; Picanço-Castro, V.; Covas, D.T.; Vidoto, E.L.; Tannús, A.; et al. Image and Motor Behavior for Monitoring Tumor Growth in C6 Glioma Model. *PLoS ONE* **2018**, *13*, e0201453. [CrossRef]
36. Sciacero, P.; Girelli, G.F.; Cante, D.; Franco, P.; Borca, V.C.; Grosso, P.; Marra, A.; Bombaci, S.; Tofani, S.; La Porta, M.R.; et al. Cerebellar Glioblastoma Multiforme in an Adult Woman. *Tumori* **2014**, *100*, 74–78. [CrossRef]
37. Kushner, D.S.; Amidei, C. Rehabilitation of Motor Dysfunction in Primary Brain Tumor Patients. *Neuro-Oncol. Pract.* **2015**, *2*, 185–191. [CrossRef] [PubMed]
38. Jacobs, V.L.; Valdes, P.A.; Hickey, W.F.; de Leo, J.A. Current Review of in Vivo GBM Rodent Models: Emphasis on the CNS-1 Tumour Model. *ASN Neuro* **2011**, *3*, 171–181. [CrossRef]
39. Garcia-Rill, E. The Basal Ganglia and the Locomotor Regions. *Brain Res. Rev.* **1986**, *11*, 47–63. [CrossRef]
40. Wagner, J.; Stephan, T.; Kalla, R.; Brückmann, H.; Strupp, M.; Brandt, T.; Jahn, K. Mind the Bend: Cerebral Activations Associated with Mental Imagery of Walking along a Curved Path. *Exp. Brain Res.* **2008**, *191*, 247–255. [CrossRef] [PubMed]
41. Gosgnach, S. Synaptic Connectivity amongst Components of the Locomotor Central Pattern Generator. *Front. Neural Circuits* **2022**, *16*, 1–6. [CrossRef]
42. Grillner, S.; El Manira, A. Current Principles of Motor Control, with Special Reference to Vertebrate Locomotion. *Physiol. Rev.* **2020**, *100*, 271–320. [CrossRef]

43. Taccola, G.; Ichiyama, R.M.; Edgerton, V.R.; Gad, P. Stochastic Spinal Neuromodulation Tunes the Intrinsic Logic of Spinal Neural Networks. *Exp. Neurol.* **2022**, *355*, 114138. [CrossRef] [PubMed]
44. Rybak, I.A.; Dougherty, K.J.; Shevtsova, N.A. Organization of the Mammalian Locomotor CPG: Review of Computational Model and Circuit Architectures Based on Genetically Identified Spinal Interneurons. *Eneuro* **2015**, *2*, ENEURO.0069-15.2015. [CrossRef] [PubMed]
45. Song, J.; Pallucchi, I.; Ausborn, J.; Ampatzis, K.; Bertuzzi, M.; Fontanel, P.; Picton, L.D.; El Manira, A. Multiple Rhythm-Generating Circuits Act in Tandem with Pacemaker Properties to Control the Start and Speed of Locomotion. *Neuron* **2020**, *105*, 1048–1061.e4. [CrossRef] [PubMed]

Disclaimer/Publisher's Note: The statements, opinions and data contained in all publications are solely those of the individual author(s) and contributor(s) and not of MDPI and/or the editor(s). MDPI and/or the editor(s) disclaim responsibility for any injury to people or property resulting from any ideas, methods, instructions or products referred to in the content.

MDPI
St. Alban-Anlage 66
4052 Basel
Switzerland
www.mdpi.com

Brain Sciences Editorial Office
E-mail: brainsci@mdpi.com
www.mdpi.com/journal/brainsci

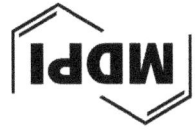

Disclaimer/Publisher's Note: The statements, opinions and data contained in all publications are solely those of the individual author(s) and contributor(s) and not of MDPI and/or the editor(s). MDPI and/or the editor(s) disclaim responsibility for any injury to people or property resulting from any ideas, methods, instructions or products referred to in the content.

www.ingramcontent.com/pod-product-compliance
Lightning Source LLC
LaVergne TN
LVHW070642100526
83820LV00013B/859